Nanocatalysis

Nanocatalysis

Synthesis of Bioactive Heterocycles

Edited by Keshav Lalit Ameta and Ravi Kant

CRC Press
Taylor & Francis Group
Boca Raton London New York

CRC Press is an imprint of the
Taylor & Francis Group, an **informa** business

First edition published 2022
by CRC Press
6000 Broken Sound Parkway NW, Suite 300, Boca Raton, FL 33487-2742

and by CRC Press
4 Park Square, Milton Park, Abingdon, Oxon, OX14 4RN

CRC Press is an imprint of Taylor & Francis Group, LLC

ISBN: 9780367693541 (hbk)
ISBN: 9780367693558 (pbk)
ISBN: 9781003141488 (ebk)

DOI: 10.1201/9781003141488

Typeset in Times
by Newgen Publishing UK

Contents

Figures

Tables

Preface

Catalysis is becoming a strategic field of research since it represents a new path to meet the challenges of energy and sustainability. These challenges are becoming main concerns for the global vision of societal challenges and the world economy. Catalysis research has become one of the most powerful tools in the pharmaceutical, petrochemical, and finechemical industries. One of the stimulating features of nanotechnology is its versatile use in almost any field. The discovery of nanoparticles with different sizes, shapes, and composition has stretched the limits of technology. Natural varieties of nanoparticles have emerged in daily life, which occur in every field from drugs and electronics to paints and cosmetics, and they are now emerging in the field of catalysis. The field of nanocatalysis (which involves a substance or material with catalytic properties that possesses at least one nanoscale dimension, either externally or in the internal structures) is undergoing rapid development. Nanocatalysis can help when designing catalysts that have excellent activity, greater selectivity, and high stability. Their properties can easily be adjubsted by tailoring the size, shape, and morphology of the nanomaterial.

Simple organic molecules are main basic building blocks that are found in nature and human beings. Heterocyclic compounds play a vital role in biological processes and are widespread as natural products. They are found widely in nature, in particular, in nucleic acids, plant alkaloids, anthocyanins, flavones, haem, and chlorophyll. Heterocycles have enormous potential as the most promising molecules as lead structures in heterocyclic chemistry, which is one of the most complex and intriguing branches of organic chemistry. Heterocyclic compounds are the largest and most varied family of organic compounds. Many broader aspects of heterocyclic chemistry have been recognized as disciplines of general significance that effect almost all aspects of modern organic chemistry, medicinal chemistry, and biochemistry. Heterocyclic compounds offer a high degree of structural diversity and have proved to be broadly and economically useful as therapeutic agents. Because heterocycles non-carbons are usually considered to replace carbon atoms, they are called heteroatoms, for example, they are different from carbon and hydrogen. Heteroatom atom pairs could be primarily responsible for the biological activity of the molecules.

Nanocatalysts exhibiting homogeneous and heterogeneous catalytic properties, which allow for rapid and selective chemical transformations that have the benefits of excellent product yield and ease of catalyst separation and recovery. This book will review the catalytic performance, synthesis, and characterization of nanocatalysts, which examines the current state-of-the-art and highlights new avenues for research, in particular, the synthesis of bioactive heterocycles. In addition, the authors will discuss new and emerging applications for nanocatalysts in the synthesis of biologically active heterocycles.

Therefore, this book will provide a summary of the nanocatalysed transformation of various bioactive heterocycles.

Contributors

Shikha Agarwal
Synthetic Organic Chemistry Laboratory, Department of Chemistry, MLSU, Udaipur, Rajasthan, India

Chetna Ameta
Department of Chemistry, University College of Science, M. L. Sukhadia University, Udaipur, Rajasthan, India

S. R. Bembalkar
Department of Chemistry, Deogiri College, Aurangabad, Maharashtra, India

R. M. Borade
Department of Chemistry, Government Institute of Forensic Science, Aurangabad, Maharashtra, India

Tushar M. Boralkar
Department of Medicinal Chemistry, National Institute of Pharmaceutical Education and Research-Raebareli (Transit Campus), Lucknow, India

R. Chandran
Department of Medicinal Chemistry, National Institute of Pharmaceutical Education and Research, Lucknow, Uttar Pradesh, India

Purnima Chaubisa
Department of Chemistry, University College of Science, M. L. Sukhadia University, Udaipur, Rajasthan, India

Sandeep Chaudhary
Department of Medicinal Chemistry, National Institute of Pharmaceutical Education and Research-Raebareli (Transit Campus), Lucknow, India

Laboratory of Organic and Medicinal Chemistry, Department of Chemistry, Malaviya National Institute of Technology, Jawaharlal Nehru Marg, Jaipur, India

Satish A. Dake
Department of Chemistry, Sunderrao Solanke Mahavidyalaya, Majalgaon, India

S. U. Deshmukh
Department of Chemistry, Deogiri College, Aurangabad, Maharashtra, India

Vedant V. Deshmukh
Department of Medicinal Chemistry, National Institute of Pharmaceutical Education and Research-Raebareli (Transit Campus), Lucknow, India

Surbhi Dhadda
Department of Chemistry (Centre of Advanced Study), University of Rajasthan, JLN Marg, Jaipur, Rajasthan, India

Dharmendra
Department of Chemistry, University College of Science, M. L. Sukhadia University, Udaipur, Rajasthan, India

Ajit K. Dhas
Department of Chemistry, Deogiri College, Aurangabad, Maharashtra, India

Anand B. Dhirbassi
Department of Chemistry, Deogiri College, Aurangabad, Maharashtra, India

Vidya D. Dofe
Department of Chemistry, Deogiri College, Aurangabad, Maharashtra, India

Divyani Gandhi
Synthetic Organic Chemistry Laboratory, Department of Chemistry, MLSU, Udaipur, Rajasthan, India

Rajita D. Ingle
Department of Chemistry, Deogiri College, Aurangabad, Maharashtra, India

Popat M. Jadhav
Department of Chemistry, Deogiri College,
  Aurangabad, Maharashtra, India

Mukesh Jain
Laboratory of Organic and Medicinal
  Chemistry, Department of Chemistry,
  Malaviya National Institute of Technology,
  Jawaharlal Nehru Marg, Jaipur, India

Nidhi Jangir
Department of Chemistry (Centre of Advanced
  Study), University of Rajasthan, JLN Marg,
  Jaipur, Rajasthan, India

S. B. Kale
Department of Applied Science, Government
  Polytechnic, Aurangabad, Maharashtra,
  India

A. B. Kanagare
Department of Chemistry, Deogiri
  College, Aurangabad, Maharashtra, India

Dinesh Kumar Jangid
Department of Chemistry (Centre of Advanced
  Study), University of Rajasthan, JLN Marg,
  Jaipur, Rajasthan, India

Arvnabh Mishra
Department of Industrial Chemistry, ISTAR,
  C. V. M. University, Vallabh Vidyanagar
  Anand, India

D. N. Pansare
Department of Chemistry, Deogiri College,
  Aurangabad, Maharashtra, India

C. S. Patil
Department of Chemistry, Deogiri College,
  Aurangabad, Maharashtra, India

R. P. Pawar
Department of Chemistry, Shiv Chattrapati
  College, Aurangabad, Maharashtra,
  India

Nusrat Sahiba
Synthetic Organic Chemistry Laboratory,
  Department of Chemistry, MLSU, Udaipur,
  Rajasthan, India

Jaiprakash N. Sangshetti
Department of Chemistry, Y. B. Chavan College
  of Pharmacy, Aurangabad, Maharashtra,
  India

Ayushi Sethiya
Synthetic Organic Chemistry Laboratory,
  Department of Chemistry, MLSU, Udaipur,
  Rajasthan, India

A. Sharma
Department of Medicinal Chemistry, National
  Institute of Pharmaceutical Education and
  Research, Lucknow, Uttar Pradesh, India

R. N. Shelke
Department of Chemistry, Sadguru Gadage
  Maharaj College Karad, Maharashtra, India

Atam B. Tekale
Department of Chemistry, Shri Shivaji College,
  Parbhani, Maharashtra, India

S. U. Tekale
Department of Chemistry, Deogiri College,
  Aurangabad, Maharashtra, India

S. B. Ubale
Department of Chemistry, Deogiri College,
  Aurangabad, Maharashtra, India

Yogeshwari Vyas
Department of Chemistry, University College
  of Science, M. L. Sukhadia University,
  Udaipur, Rajasthan, India

Ravi K. Yadav
Laboratory of Organic and Medicinal
  Chemistry, Department of Chemistry,
  Malaviya National Institute of Technology,
  Jawaharlal Nehru Marg, Jaipur, India

About the Editors

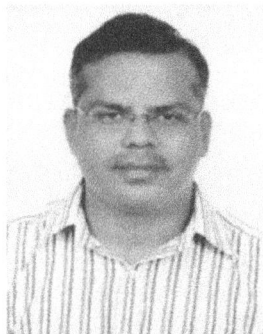

Keshav Lalit Ameta is Associate Professor at the Department of Chemistry, Sardar Patel University, Vallabh Vidyanagar, Gujarat, India. Prior to this, he was Professor of the Department of Chemistry, School of Liberal Arts and Sciences, Mody University of Science and Technology, Lakshmangarh, Rajasthan, India. His fields of research include green chemistry and nanotechnology in organic synthesis, heterocyclic, and medicinal chemistry. In addition, he has a keen interest in heterogeneous catalyzed organic synthesis and photocatalysis. Ameta has published over 80 research articles in the fields of synthetic organic chemistry, medicinal chemistry, and material science with publishers of international repute. Moreover, he was made an honored Fellow of the Linnean Society of Chemistry, United Kingdom in 2021 and a Fellow of the Indian Chemical Society in 2014. He has vast experience in teaching both graduate- and postgraduate-level students. He is actively associated with the American Chemical Society.

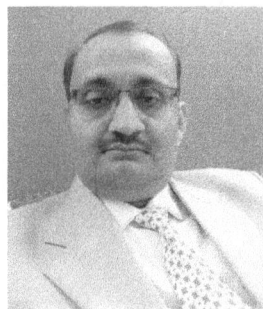

Ravi Kant is Professor of Chemistry, Faculty of Chemical Sciences with an additional responsibility as Director of Research and Consultancy, Shri Ramswaroop Memorial University Lucknow, Uttar Pradesh, India. For the last 21 years he has been involved in research into bioorganometallics, material science, and metalopharmaceutical chemistry. In addition, he teaches chemistry, applied chemistry, and pharmaceutical and medicinal chemistry to undergraduate and post-graduate students in engineering, science, and pharmaceutical sciences. He was the winner of Rashtriya Shiksha Gaurav Puraskar in 2015, the Young Scientist Award in 2018, and Best Faculty Award in 2017, along with more scientific recognition from the country. He is a Fellow of the Royal Society of Chemistry London, Linnean Society of London, Indian Science Congress Association, Uttar Pradesh Academy of Sciences, Indian Chemical Society, Chemical Research Society of India, and the Centre for Educational Growth and Research.

1 Nanocatalysed Synthesis of Lactams

R. Chandran and A. Sharma

Department of Medicinal Chemistry, National Institute of Pharmaceutical
Education and Research, Lucknow, Uttar Pradesh, India

1.1 INTRODUCTION

In various chemical reactions, catalysts play key roles in accelerating the transformation of reactants into products chemically. The careful selection of a catalyst enhances the reaction selectivity and eliminates chemical waste, which usually depends on the number of active sites and turnover frequency (TOF) or turnover number (TON) of the catalyst.[1,2] Tailoring and utilizing catalysts in ecological and economical approaches makes them a part of green chemistry as stated by Paul Anastas and John Warner in *12 Principles of Green Chemistry*.[3] Pharmaceutically, which is based on the catalytic material (e.g., solid or liquid) and the conditions employed during the catalytic reaction (e.g., liquid or gas phase), catalysis can be broadly classified as homogeneous or heterogeneous.[4] In a homogeneous catalyst, the catalyst and reactants are in the same phase and the reaction occurs in the gas or solid or mainly in the liquid phase. Therefore, a single-phase interaction between the reactant and accessible active catalytic sites is responsible for its higher activity and chemo, regio, enantioselectivity, or both. Complicated separation of the products from the catalyst remains a key issue because the catalysts and reactants exist in the same phase, which means that there are limited commercial applications.[4,5] Organometallics, a coordination complex, Bronsted and Lewis acids and organic molecules, or enzymes, or both are used as homogenous catalysts. Heterogeneous catalysts are usually in solid form and are similar to homogeneous catalysts in which the active catalytic moiety is entrapped or attached to the insoluble solid support (e.g., ion exchange resin, ceramic materials, and carbon (C) carriers) or soluble support (e.g., dendrimer, ionic liquid, soluble polymer, and supercritical fluid), which might be soluble in the reaction solvent but immiscible with the reaction product[6,7]. A heterogeneous catalysis reaction generally occurs in a two-phase (e.g., liquid–solid and gas–solid), or three-phase (i.e., liquid–solid–gas) system. These phases are responsible for the efficient separation, reusability, ease of handling, enhanced chemical and mechanical stability, and shelf-life, which makes them suitable for commercial applications.[7] Breaking the bond between the catalyst and insoluble solid support during chemical reactions leads to the leaching or dissolution of the catalyst in the reaction medium, and the catalytic activity for recycling and catalytic activity is lost due to the reduced interactions between the reactant and the active catalyst site because of the attached solid support, which are the main drawbacks faced in heterogeneous catalysis.[8] Metals, metal oxides, metal salts, and biocatalyst are commonly used heterogenous catalysts. This increases the need for advanced research into catalysts and catalytic activities to overcome the problems in classic catalysis. The emerging research topics of nanoscience and nanotechnology have improved the new catalytic system, which is known as nanocatalysts. This optimizes catalysis by increasing the number of catalytic active sites by decreasing the particle size in nanometers and they are anchored

DOI: 10.1201/9781003141488-1

or dispersed with nanosized support.[9] The recent rapid advances in nanotechnology and techniques have enabled nanocatalysts to be modified (e.g., size, shape, and morphology) specifically for the reaction of interest, to attain favorable and advantageous catalytic activity, selectivity, efficacy, stability, and sustainability.[10] Nanocatalyst are nanosized, with a large surface-to-volume ratio, which enhances the specific contact areas of the catalyst (e.g., edge, corner, or terrace) and results in better intrinsic catalytic performance and yield that is correlated with a homogeneous catalytic system. In addition, it helped catalyst separation, handling, and reuse, which was typically correlated with a heterogeneous catalytic system. Nanocatalysts offer the advantages of homogeneous and heterogeneous catalytic systems. Finally, nanocatalysts could be a candidate for green chemistry in chemical transformations.

The nucleation and uncontrolled growth of nanocatalyst into macroscopic structures (i.e., agglomeration) reduce catalytic activity and precipitate in the reaction mixture. This could be stabilized by adding stabilizers or protecting agents, or both, such as polymers, surfactants, dendrimers, ligands, and ionic liquids.[11,12] Nanosizing the catalytic noble and transition metals mean that they transition from metallic to atomic level and results in exceptional physical and chemical properties. Metal nanocatalysts are traditionally prepared by the deposition of metallic nanoparticles (NPs) in micro to nanosized inert supporting material (e.g., stable silicon oxide (SiO_2), aluminum oxide (Al_2O_3), titanium oxide (TiO_2), zirconium oxide (ZrO_2), valence-variable cerium oxide (CeO_2), iron oxides (Fe_2O_3 and Fe_3O_4), cobalt oxide (CoO), Co_3O_4, and ternary and quaternary metal oxides)[13]. Later, the capping of nanometallic catalysts in dendrimers, polymers, molecular monolayer, nanoshells, and nanocages were employed.[14,15]

Nanosized noble metals include silver (Ag), gold (Au), palladium (Pd), platinum (Pt), rhenium (Re), ruthenium (Ru), rhodium (Ru), osmium (Os), iridium (Ir), and transition metals include Fe, Co, nickel (Ni), copper (Cu), and Zinc (Zn), alloys include AuPt and noble metals (e.g., Pt, Pd), other transition metals alloys (e.g., Ni, Cu, and Co), core–shell (Rh–Pd), concentric core–shell nanostructures of metal– oxide (e.g., Ag, Au, Ni, Pt, and Co nanocores laminated with SiO_2, TiO_2, ZrO_2, CeO_2, Cr_2O_3, manganese oxide (MnO), Fe_3O_4, CoO, NiO, Cu_2O, or ZnO nanoshells), metal oxides (e.g., TiO_2, CeO_2, niobium pentoxide (Nb_2O_5), Fe_2O_3, and Co_3O_4) have been employed as a catalyst in C–C coupling reactions, C–heteroatom bond-forming reactions, oxidation and hydrogenation reactions, amination, hydrogenolysis, and rearrangement of organic compounds.

Strong interactions between metals show their crucial role in catalytic reactions. The synthesis of encapsulated metal NPs from metal NPs that used an organic capping agent provides the most effective approach to manage the shape, size, metal NP composition, and surface properties. Capping agents include polymers, ligands, surfactants, dendrimers, polycarboxylic acids, and polyhydroxy compounds[15].

Lactams are structurally cyclic amides that are nitrogen heterocycles. Most biologically active scaffolds in medicinal chemistry and drug discovery depend on the size of the ring. β-lactams are four-membered cyclic amides, which are known as 2-azetidinones, five-membered lactams are 2-pyrrolidinones, six-membered lactams are piperidinones, and seven-membered lactams are 2-azepanones in (Figure 1.1).

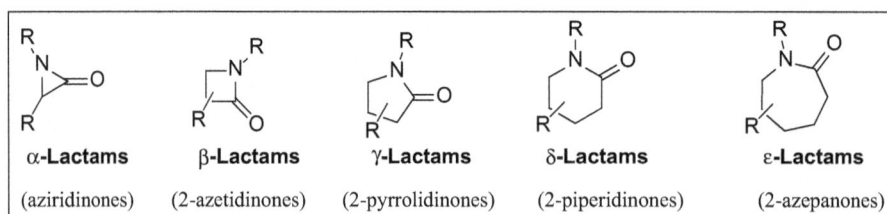

α-Lactams	β-Lactams	γ-Lactams	δ-Lactams	ε-Lactams
(aziridinones)	(2-azetidinones)	(2-pyrrolidinones)	(2-piperidinones)	(2-azepanones)

FIGURE 1.1   Class of lactams

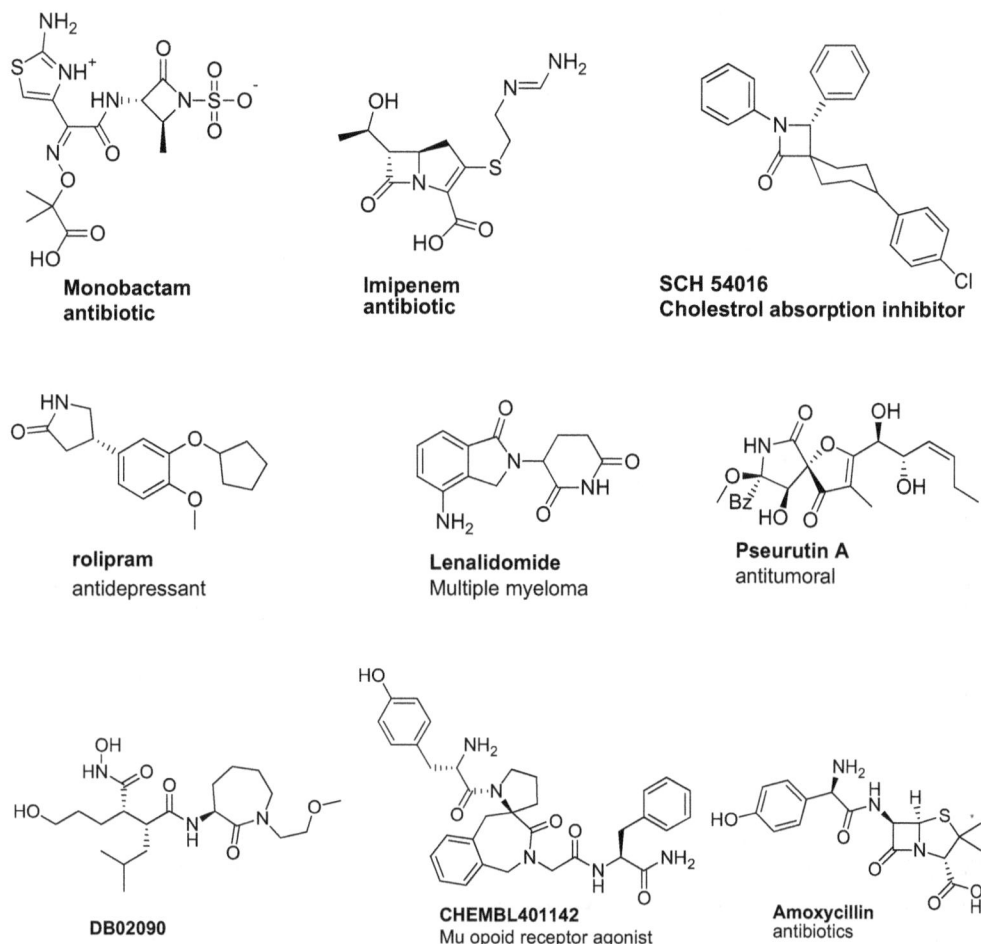

FIGURE 1.2 Biologically active lactam containing drugs

Lactams have diverse potential therapeutic values to treat various diseases. Their derivatives have potential medicinal values (Figure 1.2) as antibiotics, antidepressant, anticancer, and cholesterol-lowering agents.[16]

Lactams are synthesized from the amino acids, the Beckmann rearrangement of oximes, Schmidt ligation of hydrazoic acid, and cyclic ketones. Re(II) complexes mediated the coupling of amino alcohols to lactams, which leads to the byproduct hydrogen gas (H_2).

1.2 GOLD NANOPARTICLES

The exploration of Au NPs dates back to the fourth-century Romanian Lycurgus Cup, which gives off different colors depending upon the position of the light.[16] Scientifically, Francisci Antonii was the first philosopher and doctor who published a book on the preparation and medical use of colloidal Au in 1618. During the initial stages of exploration of transition, or noble metals, or both as catalysts, the catalytic activity of Au was relatively lower, chemically inert, and Au metal in bulk form cannot chemisorb reactant to accelerate chemical transformations.[17] In 1857, Micheal Faraday reported the preparation of a deep red colored colloidal Au by the reduction of a chloroauric aqueous solution with phosphorus (P) in carbon disulfide (CS_2).[18] Conventionally, a prepared Au catalyst is

TABLE 1.1
Supported Gold Catalyst and Its Application in Functional Group Conversion

Gold	Size	Reaction
Gold on titania[25]	30 nm	Hydrogenation
Gold on alumina[26]	3.8 nm	Hydrogenation
Au/Zno[27]	10–20 nm	Hydrogenation
Gold nanoparticles on an amorphous silica[28]	2–30 nm	Hydrogenation
Silica supported gold catalysts[24]	2–10 nm	Hydrogenation
Au/SiO$_2$[29]	6.6 nm	Oxidation
Au/BaCO$_3$[30]	3.5nm	Oxidation

supported on TiO$_2$, CeO$_2$, Fe$_2$O$_3$, ZrO$_2$, Al$_2$O$_3$, SiO$_2$, and a C solid supporting material to disperse, stabilize, and provide active sites for the reactants.[19] Improved catalytic activity of nanosized Au has been proved, where deposition–precipitation and coprecipitation techniques[20,21] were utilized to prepare Au NPs on a supporting material for carbon monoxide (CO) oxidation at –70°C. At nanosize, the catalytic activity of Au was improved as a result of changes in the chemical property, metallic state, increased active surface, and most importantly depends upon the type of supporting material used.[22] Various models, such as perimeter sites, two atomic layers, quantum size, extra or lacking electron, and the low coordination sites models have been proposed to understand the activity of nano Au catalysts[23]

An Au catalyst has been used as a catalyst of choice for oxidation, epoxidation, C–C bond formation, and hydrochlorination.[23] Hydrogenation was usually catalyzed by Ni, Pd, Ru, and Pt, and compared with a traditional catalyst nanosized Au catalyst showed active results (Table 1.1). An alternative for the preparation of an Au NPs catalyst by a common Au precursor was mainly auric chloride (e.g., AuCl$_3$ or Au$_2$Cl$_6$) or chloroauric acid, a complex salt of ethylenediamine complex [[Au(en)$_2$]Cl$_3$], and potassium aurocyanide (KAu(Cn)2).

Oxidation is one of the crucial reactions in the organic synthesis of chemical compounds. One of the important reactions is the oxidation of amines at the α-position to give the corresponding amides, which is for the synthesis of lactam from cyclic amines. For most of these reactions, chromium (Cr) and Mn catalysts are preferred but the use transition metal catalysts, such as Re complex, Cu or Pd catalysts are now used. It is important to have oxygen (O$_2$) as a terminal oxidant for the reaction to proceed. Although heterogeneous catalysts have several advantages, it is critical to devise methods that will lower the utilization and generation of hazardous chemicals or mediums during synthesis.[31,32]

Of note, an interesting change was observed for Au as a catalyst in green oxidation chemistry.[33–35] Au has been used as a catalyst for many reactions that include the oxidation of alcohols[36] and aldehydes,[37] the epoxidation of olefins,[38] and C–H bond activation in alkanes[39]. Lactams as a moiety are present in many synthetic and natural products and they act as a starting unit for many polymers, for example, ε-caprolactam is used to manufacture nylon 6,6. Lactams can be synthesized from oximes,[40] amino acids,[41] or cyclic ketones and hydrazoic acids[42]. In 1991,[43] a method was reported for lactam synthesis, which involved the direct coupling of amino alcohols that used a Re II complex. Recently, Au NPs have been explored for the synthesis of lactams under aerobic conditions. The following sections will present the use of Au NPs for the synthesis of lactams.

1.2.1 Polymer Confined Carbon Black–Gold and Gold and Cobalt Nanoparticles

The selective formation of lactams from amino alcohols using polymer confined carbon black –Au (PICB–Au) and PICB–Au or Co NPs as catalysts were reported.[44] PICB–Au and PICB–Au or Co NPs catalyst were prepared from the previously reported method in this study. In addition, the study

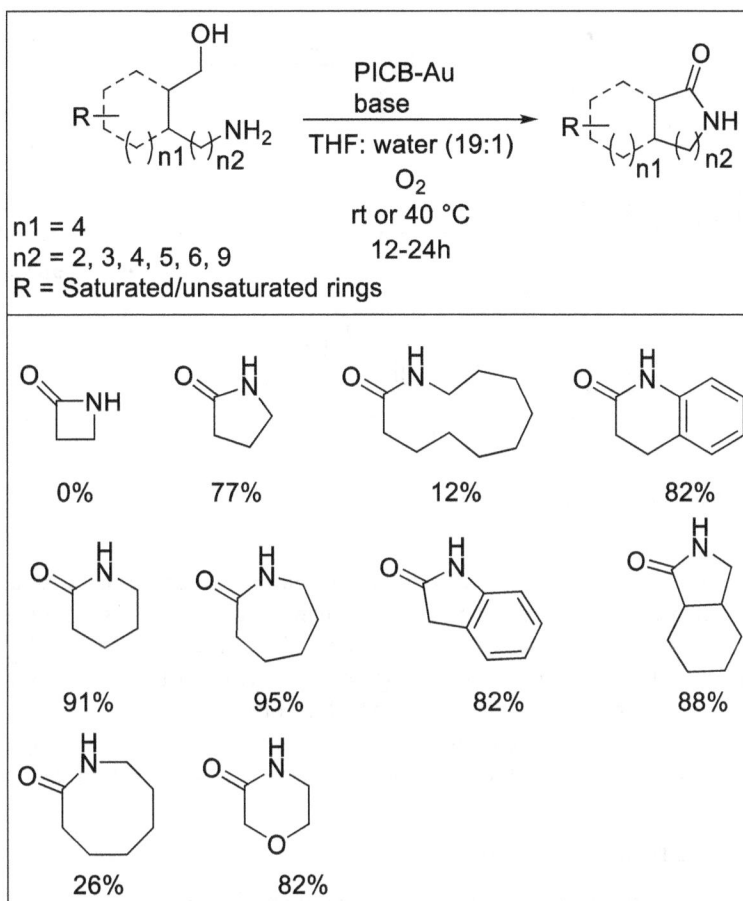

SCHEME 1.1   Synthesis of lactams from amino alcohols

was extended to synthesize lactams, such as PICB–Au and PICB–Au or Co catalysts. The effect of temperature, dilution, and catalyst was examined using 6-aminohexanol as a model substrate. Of interest, there was the reaction at room temperature (RT), and the reaction proceeded when the temperature was >40°C for the formation of lactam. However, lactam formation was not observed with a further increase in temperature. In addition, the high dilution of amino alcohols increased the selectivity toward lactam formation and increased the catalyst load for the reaction. The optimized reaction condition was 5 mol% of PICB–Au catalyst, one equivalent of a sodium hydroxide (NaOH) base at 40°C for 24 h. The obtained lactam product was >95 % pure after filtration, extraction, and acidic workup. However, the β lactam was not obtained in this reaction due to ring strain and polymerization. Finally, in the presence of benzyl alcohol presence, 5 mol% of PICB–Au or Co at RT, the amino alcohols converted into the desired lactam, such as 3,4-dihydroisoquinolin-1(2H)-one and isoindolin-1-one with >80 % yield.[44]

Five ring lactam synthesis were favored by this method; however, a ring size >8 exhibited poor yields due to the formation of oligomers. In addition, bicyclic lactam systems were synthesized by this method in sufficient yields (Scheme 1.1).

1.2.2   GOLD–TITANIA CATALYST FOR THE SYNTHESIS OF CAPROLACTAM

The use of Au-TiO$_2$ as a catalyst was discussed for the oxidation of 1,6-hexadiamine with O$_2$.[45] The deposition–precipitation method was used for the preparation of Au nanocatalyst. HAuCl$_4$.3H$_2$O was

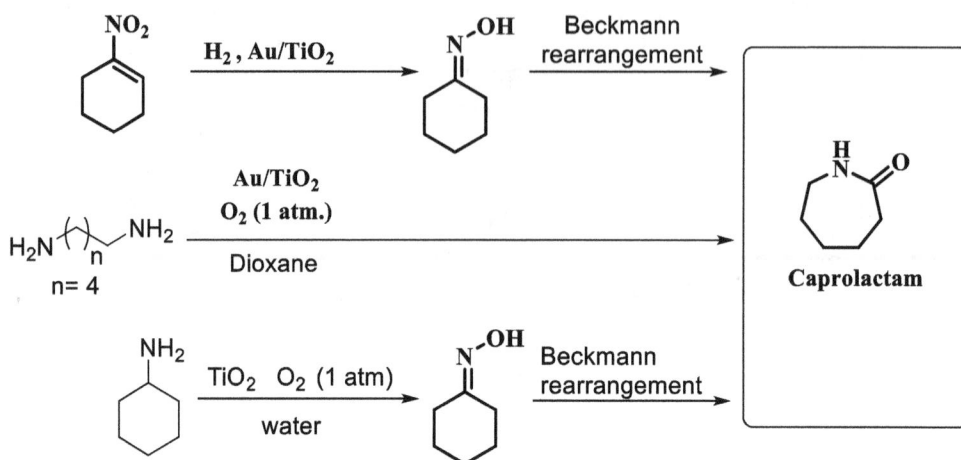

SCHEME 1.2 Methods for synthesis of caprolactam

the Au source (commercially available). In addition, they investigated the role of Au and TiO_2 in the reaction. Caprolactam was not formed when the reaction mixture was heated to $\geq 90°C$ for 18 h due to the formation of polymerized products. This same observation was evident when TiO_2 was used as a catalyst. Therefore, for the reaction, an Au–TiO_2 as a catalyst system was essential. A novel approach for the synthesis of caprolactam was mentioned, which involved the use of cyclohexylamine as the substrate. The catalyst Au–TiO_2 aided in the chemoselective hydrogenation of the substrate to yield cyclohexanone oxime, which was further converted into caprolactam (Scheme 1.2).[45]

1.2.3 GOLD-PALLADIUM NANOCATALYST

Levulinic acid (LA) and ethyl levulinate (EL) are the products that are obtained by the hydrolysis of biomass. They are important precursors that are used in the pharmaceutical industry, especially for the preparation of pyrrolidones. The traditional methods that are used for the conversion of LA/EL involved the use of metal catalysts (Pt- or Ru-based) and hazardous solvents like dimethyl sulfoxide (DMSO) used as reaction solvent under harsh conditions (e.g., $90°C$–$180°C$ and 5–55 atm. H_2). Poor yields were obtained due to the generation of undesirable byproducts. The use of AuPd as a catalyst was reported for the reductive amination of EL and LA to pyrrolidones under mild conditions (e.g., $85°C$, 1 atm. H_2, and no solvent),[46] as shown in Scheme 1.3.

The catalyst was prepared by the coreduction of Pd acetylacetonate and Au tetra-chloroaurate with borane morpholine in oleylamine. After the synthesis of the alloy, the nanocatalyst was supported on C and oleylamine was removed by acid treatment and washed to form a stable alloy C-$Au_{66}Pd_{34}$. High yields were isolated when a primary amine was used as the substrate with high TOF. In addition, the Pd present in the alloy functioned as LA and improved the rate of catalysis. The nanocatalyst could be reused and recycled 10 times without affecting its catalytic properties and composition. The approach was considered a greener process since there was no involvement of harmful solvents or harsh conditions, and the catalyst alloy of C-$Au_{66}Pd_{34}$ could be reused (Scheme 1.3).

1.2.4 POLY (N-VINYL-2-PYRROLIDONE)-STABILIZED NANO GOLD

The synthesis of different types of lactams that were obtained from the selective oxidation of cyclic amine with nanoclusters of Au stabilized with polyN-vinyl-2-pyrrolidone (PVP) as the catalyst have been reported.[47] The catalyst promoted the formation of intermediate imines followed by the generation of lactams in an aqueous medium under milder conditions. The effect of the solvent system,

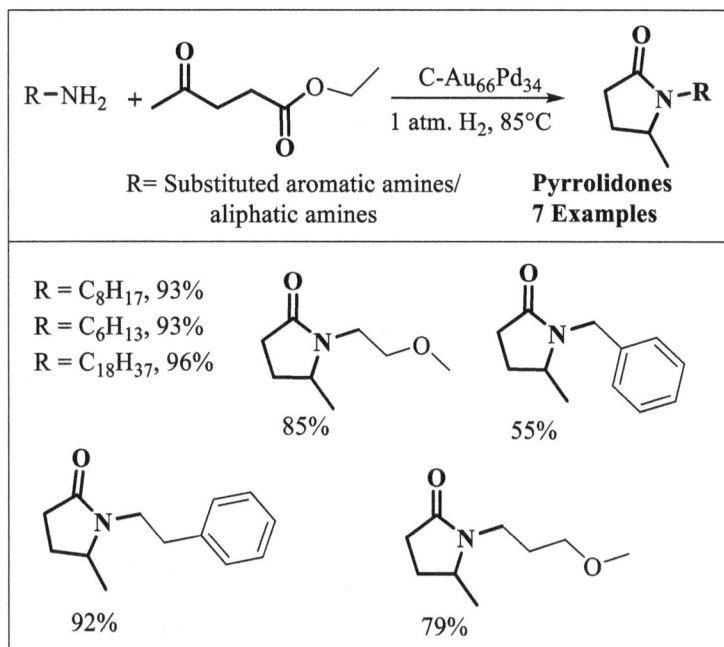

SCHEME 1.3 Synthesis of pyrrolidones

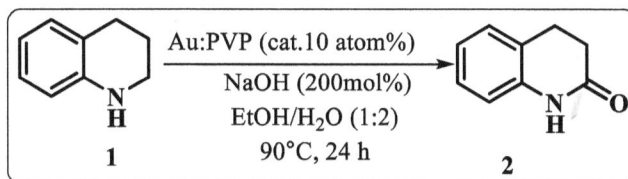

SCHEME 1.4 Synthesis of 3,4-dihydroquinolin-2(1*H*)-one

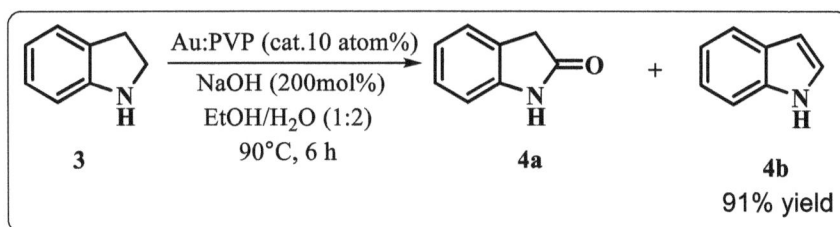

SCHEME 1.5 Synthesis of indole

base, temperature, and aromatization were investigated. The size of the nano Au catalyst played an important role.[47] Larger sizes (i.e., >20nm) reduced the catalytic activity of the nano Au particles. The reaction could not proceed if Au:PVP (i.e., 20 nm) was used under an argon atmosphere. The results indicated that oxygenation was promoted when O_2 was adsorbed onto the Au:PVP catalyst. A hydroalcoholic solvent system was preferred for synthesis and changing the system to water decreased the reaction rate and poor yields were obtained. The yield with water as the solvent was improved when the temperature was increased to 50°C. When the amount of Au:PVP was reduced to 1 atom%, the reaction was completed within 38 h at 50°C, with an 84% yield.

In Scheme 1.4, Au:PVP was used to catalyze the oxidation of benzo-fused cyclic amines to the corresponding lactam with an excellent yield. However, no reaction was observed with

1,2,3,4,5,6- hexahydrobenzo[*b*]azocine even at higher temperatures. The reaction of indoline (3), favored the synthesis of indole 99% (4b) rather than the desired lactam (4a), as shown in Scheme 1.5.

1.3   CATALYTIC APPLICATIONS OF COPPER NANOPARTICLES

NPs (i.e., mainly AU) have been used in China and Egypt for aesthetics, and the decoration of ceramics and glass. At the start of the seventeenth century, colloidal nanoparticles were developed. In 1987, catalytic activity in Au NPs <5 nm was developed for the oxidation of carbon monoxide (CO) to carbon dioxide (CO_2) by O_2.[48]

Cu and Cu-based NPs are some of the most abundant and inexpensive metals, which are exploited as a catalyst in organic reactions to combine with rare and expensive metals.[48] Various Cu conjugates, such as metallic Cu, Cur oxides, and hybrid nanostructures and Cu supported materials (i.e., SiO_2) are applied in catalysis. Cu is used as a catalyst in gas phase catalysis, electrocatalysis, and photocatalysis. Cu is abundant, low cost, and it is easy to make Cu-based nanomaterial, which means that this metal requires more research.[49,50] The application of Cu-based nanoparticles as a catalyst in chemical reactions,[51] is shown in Figure 1.3.

Available methods for the synthesis of 2-azetidinones include the Kinugasa reaction between Cu acetylides and nitrones,[52–54] the Staudinger reaction ([2+2] cycloaddition of ketene-imine cycloaddition),[54–58] and metallo–ester enolate–imine cyclocondensation.[59] In 1972,[60] the synthesis of β-lactams, which were catalyzed by Cu(I) via a one-pot method from terminal alkynes and nitrones, that used pyridine as a base was developed,[60] and led to optimal atom economy with readily accessible starting precursors.[61] $CuSO_4 \cdot 5H_2O$ or $Cu(Ac)_2.H_2O$ mediated synthesis of 2-azetidinones used sodium ascorbate as a reducing agent[62]. Then, a Kinugasa reaction was developed without a reducing agent that only used $Cu(ClO_4)_2.6H_2O$ as the catalyst.[63] Other research groups used other metals of Cu, such as $CuBr_2$ and $Cu(OTf)_2$.[64]

Recently, $CuFe_2O_4$ nanoparticles mediated Kinugasa reaction was developed for the synthesis of 2-azetidinones. The main characteristics of the $CuFe_2O_4$ nanoparticle are economic, inexpensive, stable in the air, and magnetically separable. Other research is being carried out into various organic reactions and transformations, such as the cross-coupling of phenol with aryl halides by C–O bonds, the synthesis of aryl azides, 1,4 diaryl-1,2,3- triazoles, click reactions by alkynes–azides by C–N cross-coupling, A3 coupling, and multicomponent reaction (i.e., Biginelli condensation).[65–68]

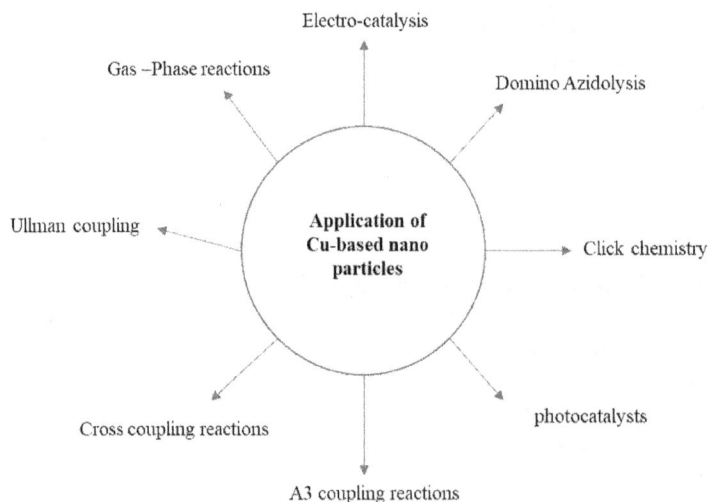

FIGURE 1.3   Application of Cu-based nano particles

1.3.1 COPPER FERRITE NANOPARTICLES

Highly efficient heterogeneous catalyst $CuFe_2O_4$ nanoparticles (15–20 nm)[69] were developed for the synthesis of 2-azetidinones, as shown in Scheme 1.6.

Here, terminal alkynes and nitrones were reacted in the presence of K_2CO_3 as the base and $CuFe_2O_4$ NPs as a heterogenous catalyst in N, N-dimethyl formamide (DMF), which led to the target product (only 43%). This was further evaluated with various solvents, such as DMF, tetrahydrofuran (THF),

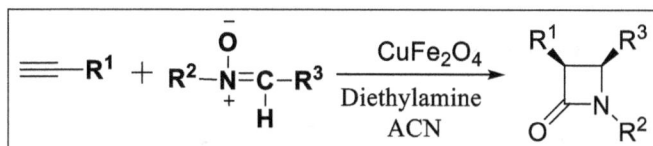

SCHEME 1.6 Synthesis of 2-azetidinones

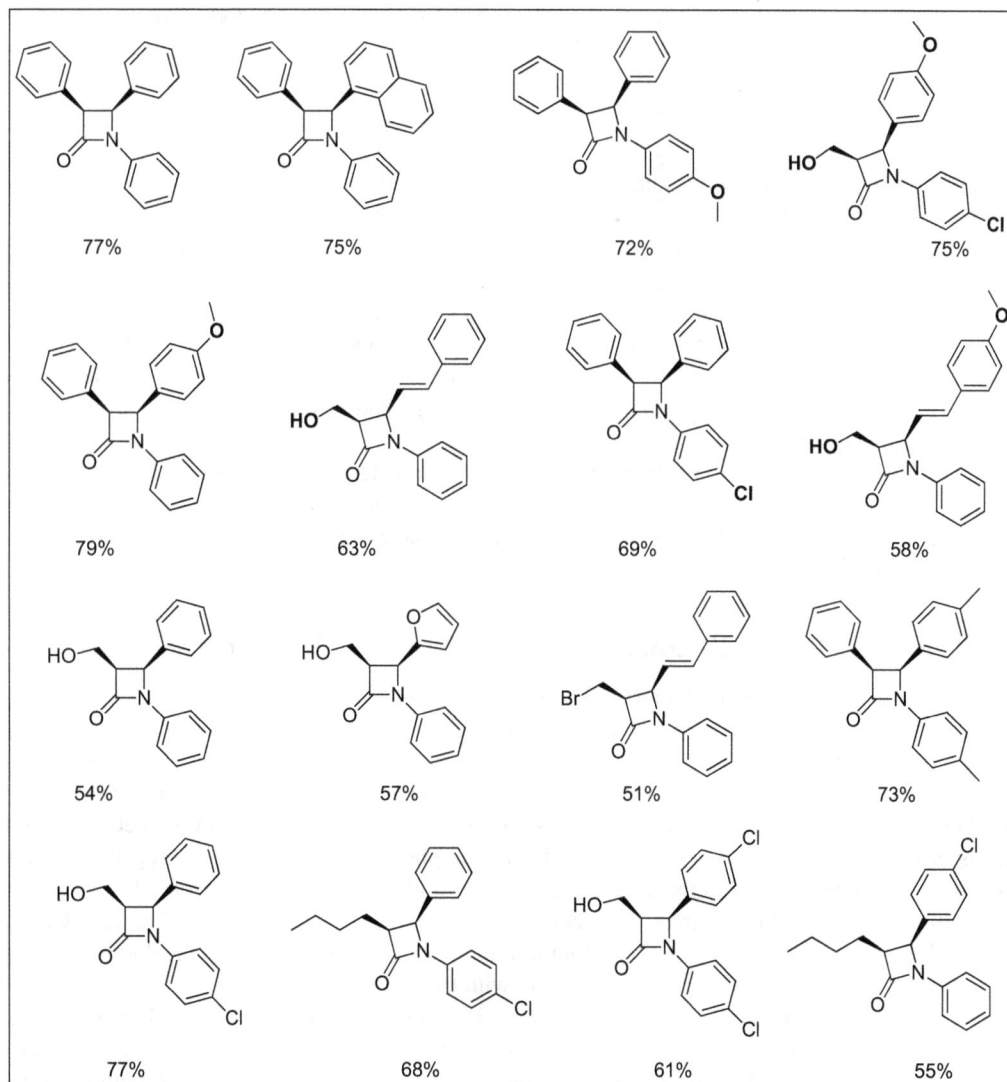

FIGURE 1.4 Substrate scope

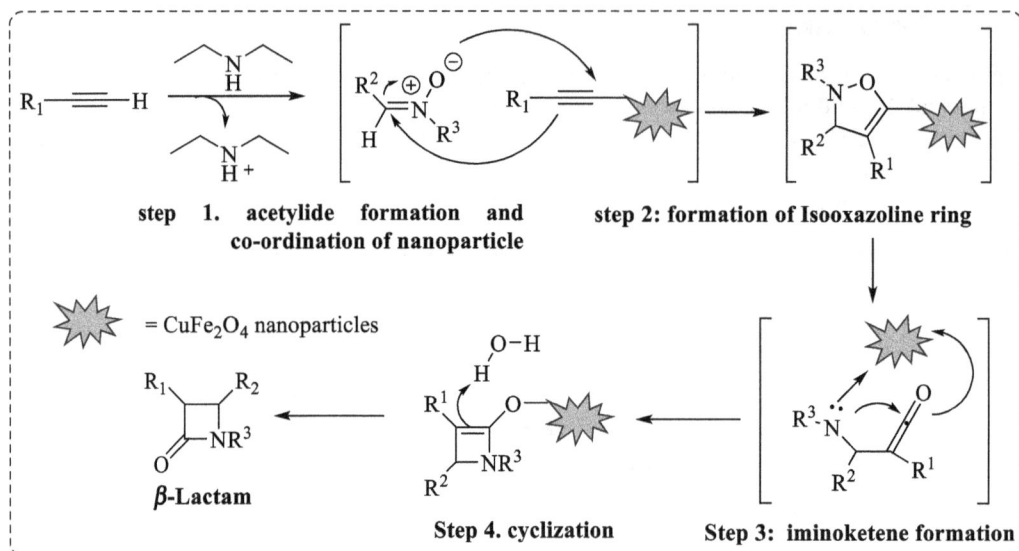

FIGURE 1.5 Plausible mechanism

acetonitrile (ACN), dimethyl sulfoxide (DMSO), and toluene for the yield of the product. ACN was the best solvent and $CuFe_2O_4$ NPs were readily separated by a magnetic field. Next, optimized bases (i.e., diethylamine (Et_2NH) were compared with other bases, such as K_2CO_3, triethylamine (TEA), and pyridine. Among the bases, organic bases gave maximum yield. Overall, 15% catalytic loading gave better results when the reaction was performed at RT compared with 0°C, and 50°C gave good to excellent yields of stereoselective cis 2-azetidinones. Purification was carried out by recrystallization with ethylacetate.[70] The substrate scope of the reaction is shown in Figure 1.4 Moderate to good yields of electron-donating and electron-withdrawing group substituents on the aromatic and aliphatic chain were obtained.

The mechanism involved the formation of acetylide (first step) followed by the coordination of $CuFe_2O_4$ NPs, the second step was the formation of an isooxazoline ring followed by an iminoketene intermediate. In the third step, $CuFe_2O_4$ assisted by iminoketene underwent cyclization to give the β-lactam ring shown in Figure 1.5.

1.3.2 BIOGENIC COPPER (II) OXIDE NANOPARTICLES FOR C–N CROSS-COUPLING

In the literature, recyclable CuNPs and CuO NPs (CuONPs) have been applied in C–N cross-coupling reactions.[48,71–73] The available methods have expensive, labor-intensive, use thermal conditions, and strong reducing agents.[74–76] Plant materials are widely available, which are cost-effective and easy to use and handle. Only a few plant extracts are known to convert metal ions into metal NPs.[77–81] Plant metabolites contain various phytochemicals that are used to make NPS or convert metal ions into metals or metal oxide NPs, the phytochemicals include phenolic acids, alkaloids, sugars, proteins, polyphenols, terpenoids, flavonols, flavones, chalcones, anthocyanin, and isoflavonoids.[82–85]

Recently, a highly efficient green protocol was developed for the synthesis of biogenic Cu (II) nanoparticles by the addition of a Cu (II) solution that used an *Ocimum sanctum* leaf extract at RT. *O. santum* leaves were boiled at 100°C for 10 min with triple distilled water. The extract was filtered and the filtered extract was mixed with 20 mL of 10µM solution of $CuSO_4$ in a 100 mL conical flask. Then, the mixture was maintained in a dark room until it changed color from brown to blackish brown. These color changes indicated the formation of Cu NPs. This is an effective method for the

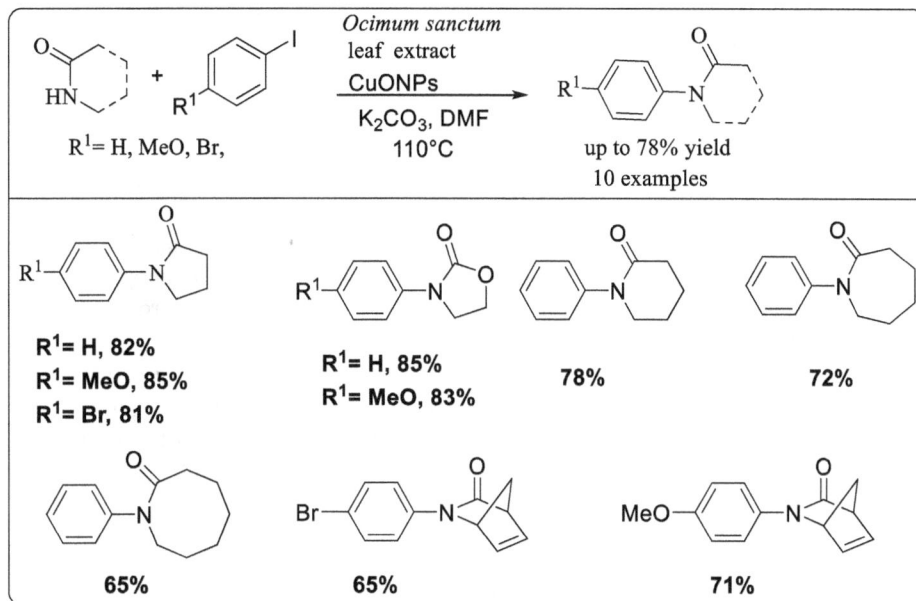

SCHEME 1.7   Synthesis of cyclic lactams

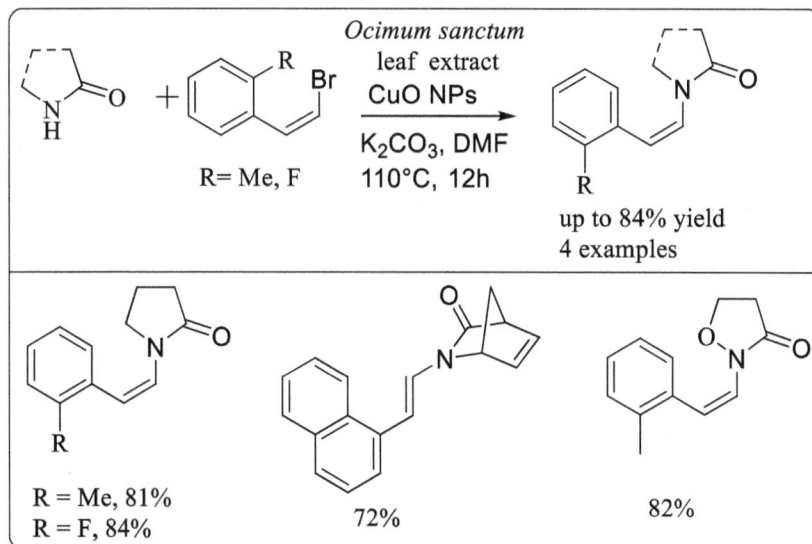

SCHEME 1.8   CuO catalyzed N-vinylation of cyclic amides

N-arylation of cyclic and acyclic amides with aryl and styryl halides as shown in Schemes 1.7 and 1.8. The advantages include that they are compatible with a wide range of substrates, have functional group tolerance, and have an acceptable yield. This protocol was extended to another heterocyclic synthesis for imidazole, pyrrole, indole, and carbazole.

The general protocol for the cyclic amide N-arylation was as follows: the 1 mmoL solution of amide and iodobenzene were stirred, 1.2 mmoL of K_2CO_3 and 3 mol% of CuO NPs in DMF was added and stirred at 110°C and the reaction was monitored by thin layer chromatography. The reaction mixture was allowed to cool and was extracted with ethyl acetate. Purification was carried out by column chromatography. After the reaction was complete, the catalyst was recycled by simple centrifugation and dried at 80°C.[86]

1.3.3 COPPER (II) OXIDE NANOPARTICLES TO COUPLE AMINES TO PYRROLIDINONE

The CuO NP mediated oxidative coupling of amines to pyrrolidinone was exploited (Scheme 1.9). Other various protocols that employed structurally diverse γ-lactams include Co catalyzed reductive coupling of nitrile with acrylamides[87] and intramolecular vinylation of iodonamides catalyzed by Cu iodide.[88] The synthesis of δ-substituted valero lactam by the reaction of aminophenyl ethyl ester with piperidinones involved 20% of CuO NP and 4 equivalent of tert-butyl hydroperoxide (TBHP), as shown in Scheme 1.10.

The following steps were involved in the reaction: (1) generation of tert-butoxyl radical; (2) abstraction of H at γ-C of 2-pyrrolidinone to form C-centered radical[89–92] (Figure 1.6); (3) formation of an iminium type intermediate by single electron transfer reaction (SET) of C-centered radical γ-carbon of 2-pyrrolidinone with CuO NP; and (4) the nucleophilic reaction of aniline to

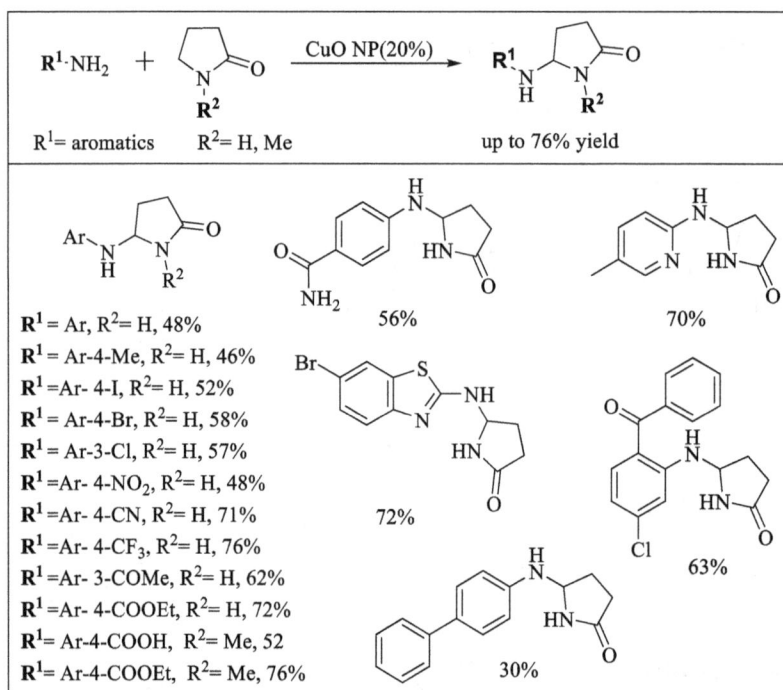

SCHEME 1.9 Coupling of amines to pyrrolidinone

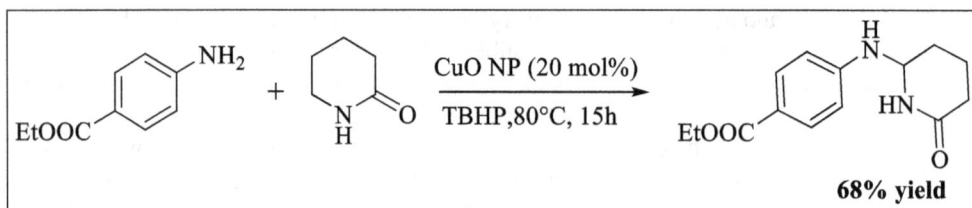

SCHEME 1.10 Preparation of δ-substituted valero lactam

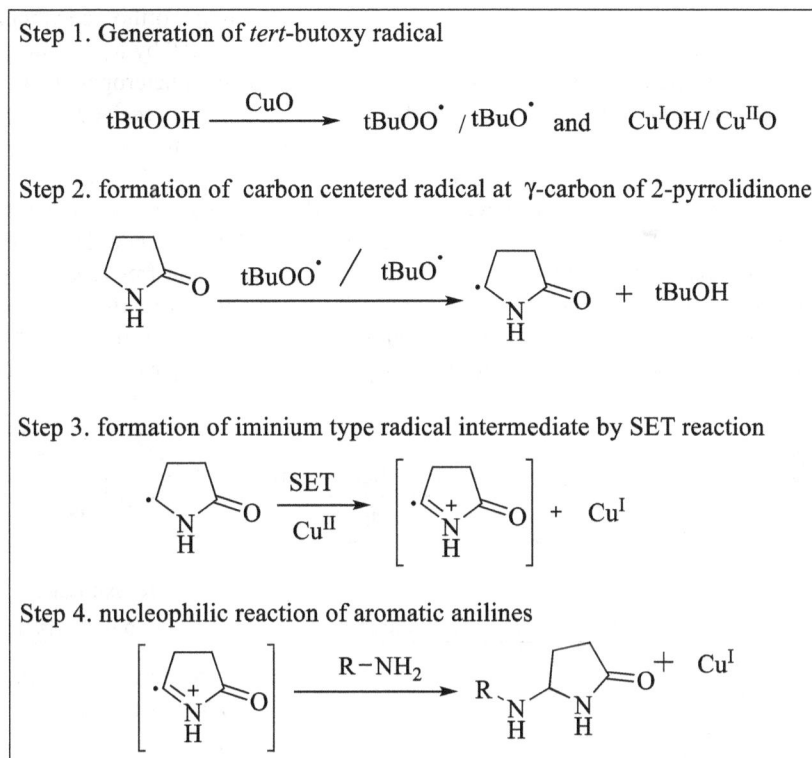

Step 1. Generation of *tert*-butoxy radical

$$tBuOOH \xrightarrow{\text{CuO}} tBuOO^{\bullet} / tBuO^{\bullet} \text{ and } Cu^IOH/Cu^{II}O$$

Step 2. formation of carbon centered radical at γ-carbon of 2-pyrrolidinone

$$\xrightarrow{tBuOO^{\bullet} / tBuO^{\bullet}} + tBuOH$$

Step 3. formation of iminium type radical intermediate by SET reaction

$$\xrightarrow[\text{Cu}^{II}]{\text{SET}} + Cu^I$$

Step 4. nucleophilic reaction of aromatic anilines

$$\xrightarrow{R-NH_2} + Cu^I$$

FIGURE 1.6   Plausible mechanism of reaction

give N-aryl-γ-amino-γ-lactam.[93–97] The mechanism involved SET, which depended on the nature of the Cu used as the precursor.

1.4   PLATINUM NANOPARTICLES FOR THE SYNTHESIS OF LACTAM

Pt was first used as a catalyst by C. F. Kuhlmann for ammonia oxidation, who filed a patent application for this invention in 1838.[98] PtNPs revolutionized nanotechnology, and played a crucial role in the chemical industry, biomedical applications, and the automotive sector. PtNPs display unique catalytic properties. Its stability at high temperatures and the large surface area is responsible for its unique nature.[99] They are used for various chemical reactions, such as oxidation, reductive amination, dehydrogenation, cyclization of keto acids, hydrogenation for the synthesis of biofuel, vitamins, and fats.[100]

1.4.1   PLATINUM AND PHOSPHOROS–TITANIUM DIOXIDE NANOCATALYSTS FOR THE SYNTHESIS OF PYRROLIDONES FROM LEVULINIC ACID

In general, organosilanes or formic acid are used as the H for reductive amination when converting LA to pyrrolidones.[101,102] However, limitations, such as corrosiveness, high cost, and harsh conditions hampered the large-scale application. Then, H_2 was used as the H source along with metal catalysts, such as Pt,[103,104] Pd,[105] Rh, Ru,[106] Co, and Ni.[107] However, this conversion is challenging. N-alkyl-5-methyl-2-pyrrolidone synthesis from LA was reported using Pt/P-TiO$_2$ at RT and pressure.[108] Pt/P-TiO$_2$ nanosheets showed excellent performance in the transformation of LA into substituted pyrrolidones. In addition, Pt/P-TiO$_2$ nanosheets were highly efficient in the reductive amination of levulinic esters, para-acetylbutyric acid, ortho-carboxybenzaldehyde, ortho-acetylbenzoic acid. The synthesis of N-substituted γ-lactams was reported for the first time[109] by a one-pot reaction by reductive amination of EL with nitro derivatives <10 bars of H_2 using a heterogenous Pt as a catalyst. However, this method required more equivalents of EL. Manzer[110] received a patent for his invention, the one-pot synthesis of N-substituted γ-lactams by reductive amination between LA and aryl cyano compounds that utilized metal catalysts, such as Pd, Rh, Ru, or Pt loaded onto Al_2O_3 or C under H_2. Then, another method was developed for the direct synthesis of N-substituted γ- and δ-lactams from keto acids with nitriles by reductive amination/cyclization under H_2 in the presence of a Pt-molybdenum oxide (Pt-MoO$_x$/TiO$_2$) catalyst.[111] This was a solvent-free reaction under mild conditions that included 7 bar H_2 and 110°C. Recently, Pt nanocatalysts were discovered on porous TiO$_2$ nanosheets for the reductive amination of levulinic acid or ester to pyrrolidones.[108] The efficient catalytic reactivity was observed due to the strong acidity of P–TiO$_2$ and Pt site lower electron

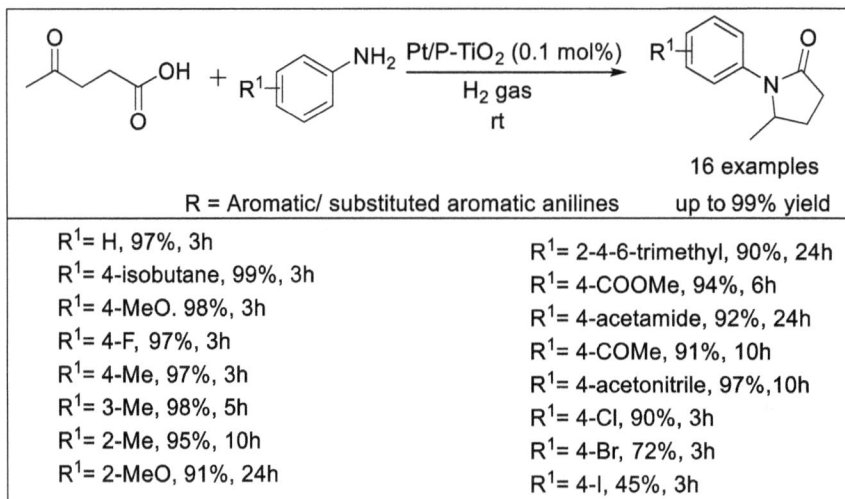

SCHEME 1.11   Substrate scope of aromatic derivative of pyrrolidones

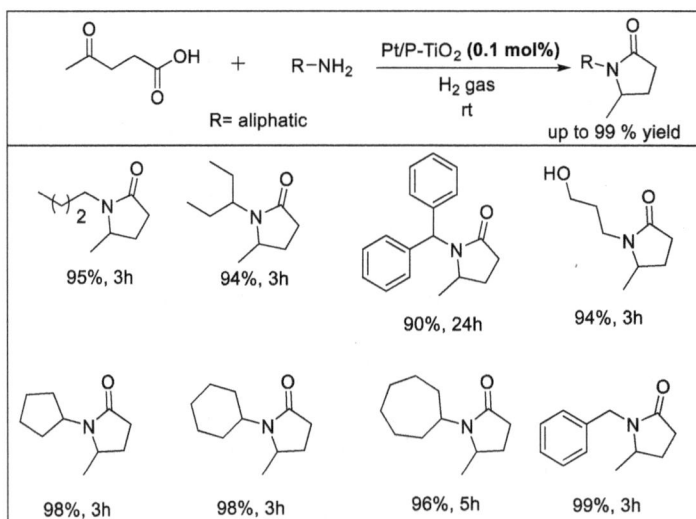

SCHEME 1.12   Substrate scope of aliphatic derivative of pyrrolidones

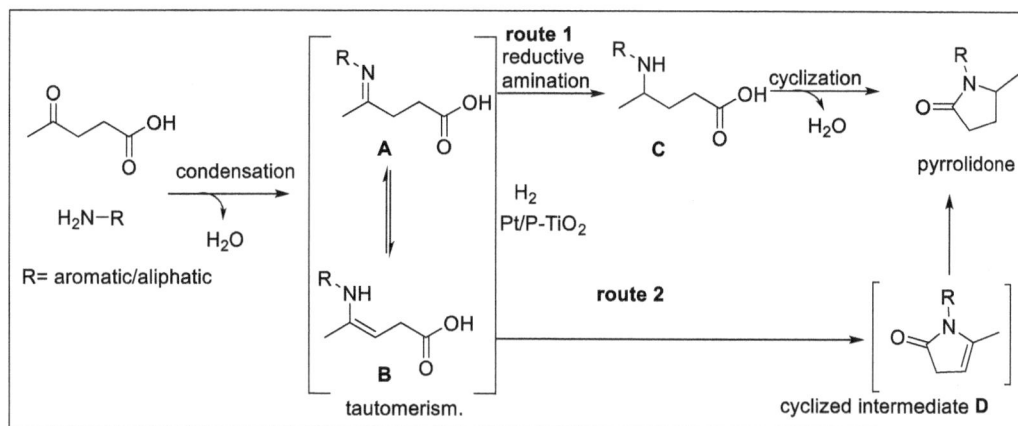

FIGURE 1.7 Plausible mechanism of reaction

density with the porous structure of the catalyst. The examples of various aromatic amines is shown in Scheme 1.11. Further methodology extended to aliphatic amines with a good to excellent yield of products as shown in Scheme 1.12.

The synthesis of pyrrolidinones from the reductive amination of LA involved LA and its ester undergoing condensation with an amine to form imine A and enamine B tautomerism. Two reaction pathways proceeded for the Pt/PTiO$_2$ catalyst. The first route indicated the formation of direct products by reductive amination. Due to the acidic site of Pt, N-substituted pyrrolidone formation was controlled by intramolecular cyclization. Then, form a cyclic intermediate D was formed and eventually hydrogenated through the Pt sites, which led to the final production of pyrrolidones[108] (Figure 1.7).

1.4.2 Heterogeneous Platinum Catalysts for Synthesis of γ-lactams from Nitrile

The reductive amination and cyclization of ketoacids (LA) with nitriles was reported (7 bar H$_2$, 110 °C under solvent-free condition) for the synthesis of N-substituted δand γ-lactams, where in Pt and MoOx coloaded TiO$_2$ (Pt-MoOx/TiO$_2$) catalyst was used,[111] as shown in Schemes 1.13 and 1.14. The basic reaction mechanism involved nitrile, which was hydrogenated to form imine A and primary amine B and led to two pathways. Pathway one (fast) begins from the thermal condensation of primary amine B and keto acid to form imine intermediate C. This undergoes hydrogenation to give intermediate D, which leads to cyclic amidation to form γ-lactam. Pathway two (slow) involves the formation of side product and starts from the reaction of imine A and primary amine B to form secondary imine E. This was hydrogenated to give secondary amine F. Then, it formed tertiary amine 5 after reacting with amine as shown in Figure 1.8.

1.5 IRON (III) OXIDE NANOPARTICLES FOR THE SYNTHESIS OF β-LACTAM THAT CONTAINS AN ARYL AMINO GROUP

Amines are valuable synthetic intermediates in organic synthesis. In general, amines are prepared by the reduction and hydrogenation of nitroarenes.[112–114] Most of the methods have disadvantages, such as they are hazardous reagents, the formation of byproducts, and harsh reaction conditions. Fe$_3$O$_4$ NPs were developed for the reduction of an aryl nitro group that was attached to the β-lactam.[115] The desired product (i.e., 98% yield) was synthesized in the presence of 10 mol% Fe$_3$O$_4$ NPs and hydrazine hydrate and the various examples are shown in Scheme 1.15. Fe$_3$O$_4$ NPs can be separated by magnetic separation. In addition, the effect of other solvents was investigated, such as DMSO, DMF, chloroform (CHCl$_3$), and CH$_3$CN, which led to failed reactions.[115]

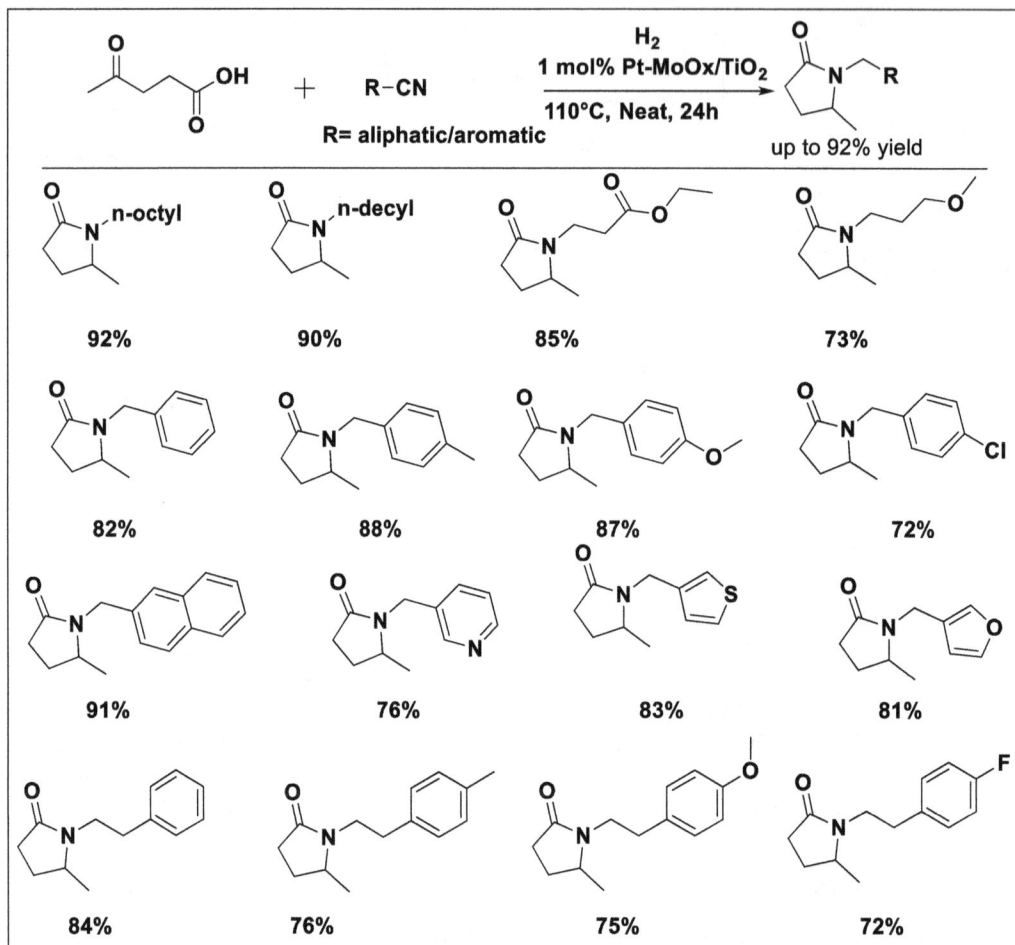

SCHEME 1.13   Synthesis of N-substituted γ-lactams

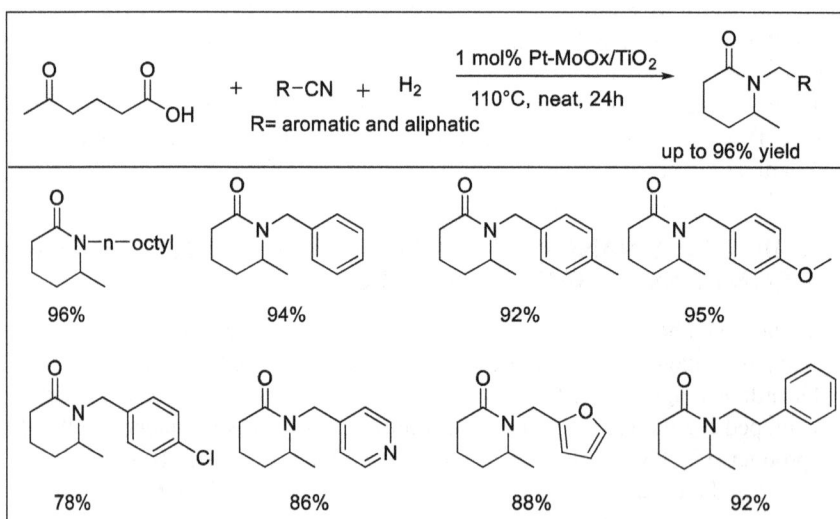

SCHEME 1.14   Synthesis of δ-lactams from 4-acetylbutyric acid and nitriles

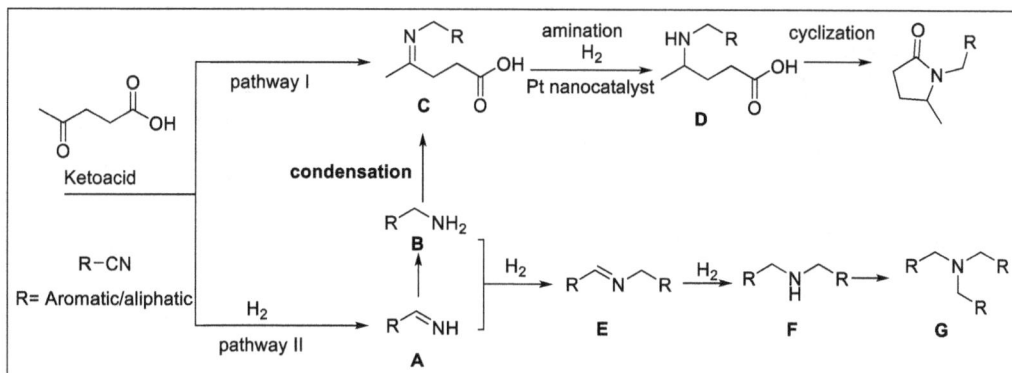

FIGURE 1.8 Plausible mechanism of reaction

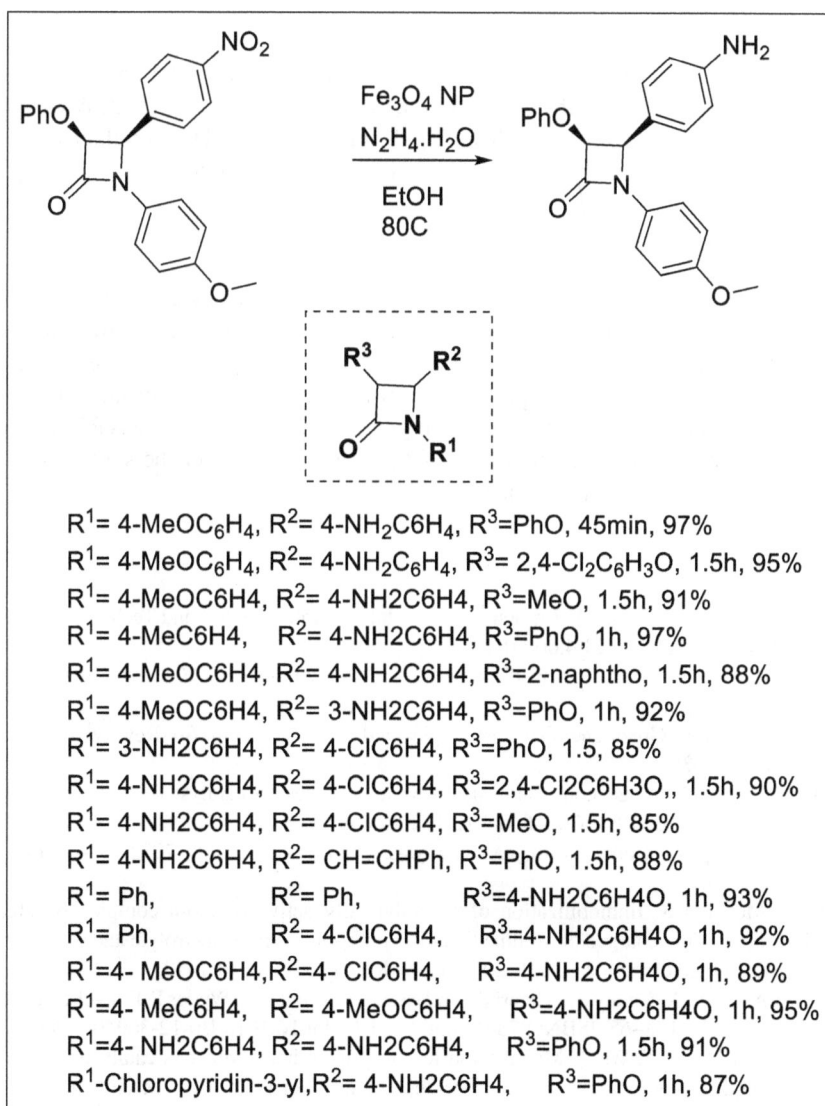

R^1= 4-MeOC$_6$H$_4$, R^2= 4-NH$_2$C$_6$H$_4$, R^3=PhO, 45min, 97%
R^1= 4-MeOC$_6$H$_4$, R^2= 4-NH$_2$C$_6$H$_4$, R^3= 2,4-Cl$_2$C$_6$H$_3$O, 1.5h, 95%
R^1= 4-MeOC6H4, R^2= 4-NH2C6H4, R^3=MeO, 1.5h, 91%
R^1= 4-MeC6H4, R^2= 4-NH2C6H4, R^3=PhO, 1h, 97%
R^1= 4-MeOC6H4, R^2= 4-NH2C6H4, R^3=2-naphtho, 1.5h, 88%
R^1= 4-MeOC6H4, R^2= 3-NH2C6H4, R^3=PhO, 1h, 92%
R^1= 3-NH2C6H4, R^2= 4-ClC6H4, R^3=PhO, 1.5, 85%
R^1= 4-NH2C6H4, R^2= 4-ClC6H4, R^3=2,4-Cl2C6H3O,, 1.5h, 90%
R^1= 4-NH2C6H4, R^2= 4-ClC6H4, R^3=MeO, 1.5h, 85%
R^1= 4-NH2C6H4, R^2= CH=CHPh, R^3=PhO, 1.5h, 88%
R^1= Ph, R^2= Ph, R^3=4-NH2C6H4O, 1h, 93%
R^1= Ph, R^2= 4-ClC6H4, R^3=4-NH2C6H4O, 1h, 92%
R^1=4- MeOC6H4,R^2=4- ClC6H4, R^3=4-NH2C6H4O, 1h, 89%
R^1=4- MeC6H4, R^2= 4-MeOC6H4, R^3=4-NH2C6H4O, 1h, 95%
R^1=4- NH2C6H4, R^2= 4-NH2C6H4, R^3=PhO, 1.5h, 91%
R^1-Chloropyridin-3-yl,R^2= 4-NH2C6H4, R^3=PhO, 1h, 87%

SCHEME 1.15 Synthesis of β-lactam containing aryl amino group

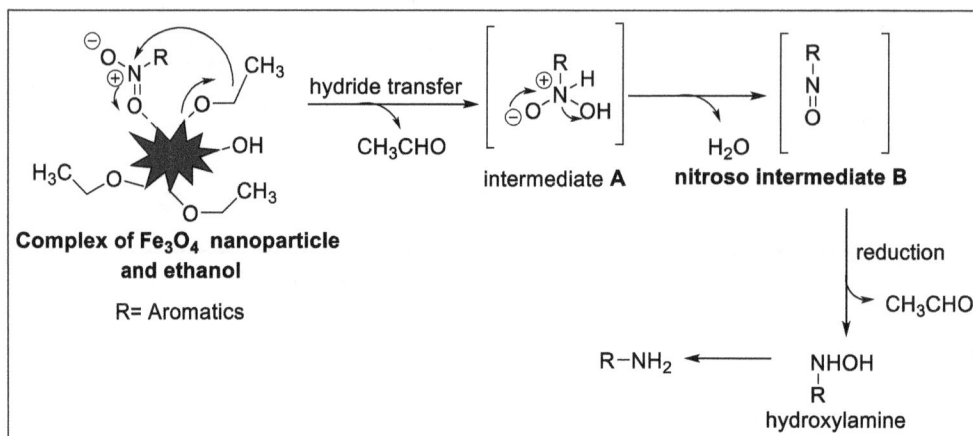

FIGURE 1.9   Plausible mechanism of reaction

The potential general mechanism involved hydride transfer by the reduction of nitro groups to amines. Fe_3O_4 NPs coordinated with the O atom of the nitro group and intermediate A was generated via hydride transfer from the solvent (i.e., ethanol) to the nitro group, and the simultaneous release of water formed nitroso intermediate B, which again underwent reduction to form amine (Figure 1.9).

1.6   CONCLUSIONS

This chapter highlighted the recent advances in the use of metal NPs as catalysts for applications in various chemical reactions. NPs including Au and Au-like/Co nanoparticles, Au–TiO_2 NPs, and PVP stabilized NPs were exploited in the synthesis of lactams (i.e., cyclic amides). The application of Cu and Pt-based NPS, and Fe_3O_4 NPs the synthetic transformation of lactam ring and the synthesis of various lactams with good to excellent yields and highly stable reusable catalyst were discussed. In the literature, a limited number of NPS have been used for the synthesis of lactams (i.e., cyclic amides) instead of other heterocycles.

REFERENCES

1. Kakaei K, Esrafili MD, Ehsani A. Introduction to catalysis. Interface Sci and Technol. 2019. 27: 1–21. doi.10.1016/B978-0-12-814523-4.00001-0.
2. Kozuch S, Martin JML. "Turning over" definitions in catalytic cycles. ACS Catal. 2012 2: 2787–94. doi.10.1021/cs3005264.
3. Anastas P, Eghbali N. Green chemistry: Principles and practice. Chem. So. Rev. (2010). 39: 301–12. doi.10.1039/b918763b.
4. Cole-Hamilton DJ. Homogeneous catalysis: New approaches to catalyst separation, recovery, and recycling. Science. 2003. 299: 1702–6. doi.10.1126/science.1081881.
5. Philippot K, Serp P. Concepts in nanocatalysis. Nanomater Catal. 2012.1–54. doi. 10.1002/9783527656875.ch1.
6. Schwab E, Mecking S. Immobilization of a catalytically active rhodium complex by electrostatic interactions of multiply charged phosphine ligands with a soluble polyelectrolyte and recovery by ultra-filtration. 2001. Organometallics. 2001. 20:5504–6. doi.10.1021/om0107542.
7. Hagemeyer A, Volpe A. Catalysts: Materials. In Bassani F, Liedl GL, Wyder P, Encycl Condens Matter Phys. Elsevier. 2005. 158–65. ISBN: 978-0-12369-401-0, doi.10.1016/B0-12-369401-9/00541-6.
8. Yang W, Vogler B, Lei Y, Wu T. Metallic ion leaching from heterogeneous catalysts: An overlooked effect in the study of catalytic ozonation processes. Environ Sci Water Res Technol. 2017. 3:1143–51. doi.10.1039/c7ew00273d.

9. Chaturvedi S, Dave PN, Shah NK. Applications of nano-catalyst in new era. J Saudi Chem Soc. 2012. 16:307–25. doi.10.1016/j.jscs.2011.01.015.

10. Prinsen P, Luque R. Introduction to nanocatalysts. In Nanoparticle Design and Characterization for Catalytic Applications in Sustainable Chemistry, RSC Catalysis Series. 2019. 1–36. eISBN: 978-1-78801-629-2 https://doi.org/10.1039/9781788016292-00001.

11. Niu Z, Li Y (2014) Removal and Utilization of Capping Agents in Nanocatalysis. *Chem. Mater.* 26: 72–83. https://doi.org/10.1021/cm4022479.

12. Campisi S, Schiavoni M, Chan-Thaw CE, Villa A (2016) Untangling the Role of the Capping Agent in Nanocatalysis: Recent Advances and Perspectives. *Catalysts* 6: 1–21. doi.10.3390/catal6120185.

13. Wojcieszak R, Genet MJ, Eloy P, Gaigneaux EM. Supported Pd nanoparticles prepared by a modified water-in-oil microemulsion method. Stud Surf Sci Catal. 2010. 175:789–92. doi.10.1016/S0167-2991(10)75161-2.

14. Mody V, Siwale R, Singh A, Mody H. Introduction to metallic nanoparticles. J Pharm Bioallied Sci. 2010 2: 282–9. doi.10.4103/0975-7406.72127.

15. Shan S, Luo J, Kang N, Wu J, Zhao W, Cronk H, Zhao Y, Skeete Z, Li J, Joseph P, Yan S, Zhong C-J. (2015). Metallic nanoparticles for catalysis applications. In Tewary VK, Zhang Y, Modeling, Characterization, and Production of Nanomaterials: Electronics, Photonics and Energy Applications. Woodhead Publishing; 2015. p. 253–88. ISBN: 978-1-78242-228-0. doi.10.1016/B978-1-78242-228-0.00010-7.

16. Loos M. (2015) Nanoscience and Nanotechnology. In Carbon Nanotube Reinforced Composites: CNR Polymer Science and Technology. Elsevier, Oxford. 2015. 1–36. doi. 10.1016/B978-1-4557-3195-4.00001-1.

17. McEwan L, Julius M, Roberts S, Fletcher JCQ. A review of the use of gold catalysts in selective hydrogenation reactions. Gold Bull. 2010. 43: 298–306. doi.10.1007/bf03214999.

18. Daniel MC, Astruc D. Gold nanoparticles: Assembly, supramolecular chemistry, quantum-size-related properties, and applications toward biology, catalysis, and nanotechnology. Chem Rev. 2004104:293–346. doi.10.1021/cr030698+.

19. Ma Z, Dai S. Development of novel supported gold catalysts: A materials perspective. Nano Res. 2011. 4: 3–32. doi.10.1007/s12274-010-0025-5.

20. Haruta M, Kobayashi T, Sano H, Yamada N. Novel gold catalysts for the oxidation of carbon monoxide at a temperature far below 0°C. Chem Lett. 1987. 16:405–8. doi.10.1246/cl.1987.405.

21. Haruta M, Yamada N, Kobayashi T, Iijima S. Gold catalysts prepared by coprecipitation for low-temperature oxidation of hydrogen and of carbon monoxide. J Catal. 1989. 115:301–9. doi.10.1016/0021-9517(89)90034-1.

22. Ishida T, Murayama T, Taketoshi A, Haruta M. Importance of size and contact structure of gold nanoparticles for the genesis of unique catalytic processes. Chem Rev. 2020. 120:464–525. doi.10.1021/acs.chemrev.9b00551.

23. Yang XF, Wang AQ, Wang YL, Zhang T, Li J. Unusual selectivity of gold catalysts for hydrogenation of 1, 3-hutadiene toward *Cis*-2-butene: A joint experimental and theoretical investigation. J Phys Chem. 2010. 114:3131–9. doi.10.1021/jp9107415.

24. Bond GC, Thompson DT. Gold-catalysed oxidation of carbon monoxide. Gold Bulletin. 2000. 33:41–50. doi.10.1007/BF03216579

25. Lin S, Vannice MA. Gold dispersed on TiO_2 and SiO_2: Adsorption properties and catalytic behavior in hydrogenation reactions. Catal Lett. 1991. 10:47–61. doi.10.1007/BF00764736.

26. Jia J, Haraki K, Kondo JN, Domen K, Tamaru K. Selective hydrogenation of acetylene over Au/AhOa catalyst. J Phys Chem B. 2000. 104: 11153–6. doi.10.1021/jp001213d.

27. Bailie JE, Abdullah HA, Anderson JA, Rochester CH, Richardson NV, Hodge N. et al. Hydrogenation of but-2-enal over supported Au/ZnO catalysts. Phys Chem Chem Phys. 2001. 3: 4113–21. doi.10.1039/b103880j.

28. Mukherjee P, Patra CR, Ghosh A, Kumar R, Sastry M. Characterization and catalytic activity of gold nanoparticles synthesized by autoreduction of aqueous chloroaurate ions with fumed silica. Chem Mater. 2002. 14:1678–84. doi.10.1021/cm010372m.

29. Okumura M, Nakamura SI, Tsubota S, Nakamura T, Haruta M. Deposition of gold nanoparticles on silica by CVD of gold acethylacetonate. Stud Surf Sci. 1998. 118:227–24. doi.10.1016/s0167-2991(98)80192-4.

30. Lian H, Jia M, Pan W, Li Y, Zhang W, Jiang D. Gold-base catalysts supported on carbonate for low-temperature CO oxidation. Catal Commun. 2005. 6:47–51. doi.10.1016/j.catcom.2004.10.012.

31. Polshettiwar V, Basset JM, Astruc D. Nanoscience makes catalysis greener. Chem Sus Chem. 2012. 5:6–8. doi.10.1002/cssc.201100850.

32. Polshettiwar V, Varma RS. Green chemistry by nano-Catalysis. Green Chem. 2010. 12:743–54. doi.10.1039/B921171C.

33. Hashmi ASK, Hutchings GJ. Gold catalysis. Angew Chem Int Ed Engl. 2006. 45:7896–936. doi.10.1002/anie.200602454.

34. Takale BS, Bao M, Yamamoto Y. Gold nanoparticle (AuNPs) and gold nanopore (AuNPore) catalysts in organic synthesis. Org Biomol Chem. 2014. 12:2005–27. doi.10.1039/c3ob42207k.

35. Jia X, Li P, Liu X, Lin J, Chu Y, Yu J. et al. Green and facile assembly of diverse fused N-heterocycles using gold-catalyzed cascade reactions in water. Molecules. 2019. 24:988. doi.10.3390/molecules24050988.

36. Abad A, Concepcion P, Corma A, Garcia HA. Collaborative effect between gold and a support induces the selective oxidation of alcohols. Angew Chem Int Ed Engl. 2005. 44:4066–9. doi.10.1002/anie.200500382.

37. Corma A, Domine ME. Gold supported on a mesoporous CeO_2 matrix as an efficient catalyst in the selective aerobic oxidation of aldehydes in the liquid phase. Chem Commun. 2005. 32:4042–4. doi.10.1039/B506685A.

38. Bond GC, Sermon PA, Webb G, Buchanan DA, Wells PB. Hydrogenation over supported gold catalysts. J Chem Soc Chem Commun. 1973. 13:444–5. doi.10.1039/C3973000444B.

39. Hughes MD, Xu YJ, Jenkins P, McMorn P, Landon P, Enache DI. et al. Tunable gold catalysts for selective hydrocarbon oxidation under mild conditions. Nature. 2005. 437:1132–5. doi.10.1038/nature04190.

40. Hashimoto M, Obora Y, Sakaguchi S, Ishii Y. Beckmann rearrangement of ketoximes to lactams by triphosphazene catalyst. J Org Chem. 2008. 73:2894–7. doi.10.1021/jo702277g.

41. Larock RC. Comprehensive organic transformations: A guide to functional group preparations. J Nat Prod. 2000. 63:735–6. doi.10.1021/np9907275.

42. Smith PAS. The Schmidt Reaction: Experimental conditions and mechanism. J Am Chem Soc. 1948. 70:320–3. doi.10.1021/ja01181a098.

43. Naota T, Murahashi S. Ruthenium-catalyzed transformations of amino alcohols to lactams. Synlett. 1991. 10:693–4.

44. Soule JF, Miyamura H, Kobayashi S. Selective lactam formation from amino alcohols using polymer-incarcerated gold and gold/cobalt nanoparticles as catalysts under aerobic oxidative conditions. Asian J Org Chem. 2012. 1:319–21. doi.10.1002/ajoc.201200093.

45. Klitgaard SK, Egeblad K, Mentzel UV, Popov AG, Jensen T, Taarning E. et al. Oxidations of amines with molecular oxygen using bifunctional gold–titania catalysts. Green Chem. 2008. 10:419–23. doi.10.1039/b714232c.

46. Muzzio M, Yu C, Lin H, Yom T, Boga DA, Xi Z. et al. Reductive amination of ethyl levulinate to pyrrolidones over AuPd nanoparticles at ambient hydrogen pressure. Green Chem. 2019. 21:1895–9. doi.10.1039/c9gc00396g.

47. Preedasuriyachai P, Chavasiri W, Sakurai H. Aerobic oxidation of cyclic amines to lactams catalyzed by PVP-stabilized nanogold. Synlett. 2011. 8:1121–4. doi.10.1055/s-0030-1259937.

48. Zaera F. Nanostructured materials for applications in heterogeneous catalysis. Chem Soc Rev. 2013. 42: 2746–2762. doi.10.1039/c2cs35261c.

49. Evano G, Blanchard N, Toumi M. Copper-mediated coupling reactions and their applications in natural products and designed biomolecules synthesis. Chem Rev. 2008. 108:3054–131. doi.10.1021/cr8002505.

50. Ahmed A, Elvati P, Violi A. Size-and phase-dependent structure of copper (II) oxide nanoparticles. RSC Adv. 2015. 5:35033–41. doi.10.1039/c5ra04276c.

51. Ranu BC, Dey R, Chatterjee T, Ahammed S. Copper nanoparticle-catalyzed carbon-carbon and carbon-heteroatom bond formation with a greener perspective. Chem Sus Chem. 2012. 5:22–44. doi.10.1002/cssc.201100348.

52. Kutaszewicz R, Grzeszczyk B, Gorecki M, Staszewska-Krajewska O, Furman B, Chmielewski M. Bypassing the stereoselectivity issue: Transformations of Kinugasa adducts from chiral alkynes and non-chiral acyclic nitrones. Org Biomol Chem. 2019. 17:6251–8. doi.10.1039/c9ob00940j.

53. Hosseini A, Schreiner PR. Synthesis of exclusively 4-substituted β-lactams through the Kinugasa reaction utilizing calcium carbide. Org Lett. 2019. 21:3746–9. doi.10.1021/acs.orglett.9b01192.

54. Kumar Y, Singh P, Bhargava G. Cu(I) mediated Kinugasa reactions of α,β-unsaturated nitrones: A facile, diastereoselective route to 3-(hydroxy/bromo)methyl-1-aryl-4-(-styryl)azetidin-2-ones. New J Chem. 2016. 40:8216–9. doi.10.1039/c6nj01747a.

55. Ameri RJ, Jarrahpour A, Ersanli CC, Atioglu Z, Akkurt M, Turos E. Synthesis of some novel indeno[1,2-b]quinoxalin spiro-β-lactam conjugates. Tetrahedron. 2017. 73:1135–42. doi.10.1016/j.tet.2017.01.009.

56. Zarei MA. Convenient synthesis of 2-aAzetidinones via 2-fluoro-1-methylpyridinium p-toluenesulfonate. Monatshefte fur Chemie. 2013. 144:1021–5. https://doi.org/10.1007/s00706-012-0918-y.

57. Deketelaere S, Van Nguyen T, Stevens CV, Dhooghe M. Synthetic approaches toward monocyclic 3-amino-β-lactams.Chemistry Open. 2017. 6:301–19. doi.10.1002/open.201700051.

58. Zarei MA. Straightforward approach to 2-azetidinones from imines and carboxylic acids using dimethyl sulfoxide and acetic anhydride. Tetrahedron Lett. 2014. 55:5354–7. doi.10.1016/j.tetlet.2014.07.089.

59. Seitz DJ, Wang T, Vineberg GJ, Honda T, Ojima I. Synthesis of a next-generation taxoid by rapid methylation amenable for C-labeling. J Org Chem. 2018. 83:2847–57. doi.10.1021/acs.joc.7b03284.

60. Marco-Contelles J. β-lactam synthesis by the Kinugasa reaction. Angew Chem In Ed Eng. 2004. 43:2198–200. doi.10.1002/anie.200301730.

61. Malig TC, Yu D, Hein EJ. A revised mechanism for the Kinugasa reaction. J Am Chem Soc. 2018. 140:9167–73. doi.10.1021/jacs.8b04635.

62. Basak A, Chandra K, Pal R, Ghosh SC. Kinugasa reaction under click chemistry conditions. Synlett. 2007. 10:1585–88. doi.10.1055/s-2007-980383.

63. Ye MC, Zhou J, Tang Y. Trisoxazoline/Cu(II)-promoted Kinugasa reaction. Enantioselective Synthesis of β-Lactams. J Org Chem. 2006. 71:3576–82. doi.10.1021/jo0602874.

64. Chen Z, Lin L, Wang M, Liu X, Feng X. Asymmetric synthesis of trans-β-lactams by a Kinugasa reaction on water. Chem Eur J. 2013. 19:7561–7. doi.10.1002/chem.201204373.

65. Hudson R. Copper ferrite (CuFe$_2$O$_4$) nanoparticles. Synlett. 2013. 24:1309–10. doi.10.1055/s-0033-1338949.

66. Shakibaei GI, Ghahremanzadeh R, Bazgir A. Recyclable bimetallic CuFe$_2$O$_4$ nanoparticles: An efficient catalyst for one-pot three-component synthesis of novel dicyanomethyl-2-oxoindolin-3-ylthiocarboxylic acids in a green solvent. Monatshefte fur Chemie. 201. 145:1009–15. doi.10.1007/s00706-014-1159-z.

67. Feng J, Su L, Ma Y, Ren C, Guo Q, Chen X. CuFe$_2$O$_4$ magnetic nanoparticles: A simple and efficient catalyst for the reduction of nitrophenol. Chem En. J. 2013. 221:16–24. doi.10.1016/j.cej.2013.02.009.

68. Zhang R, Liu J, Wang S, Niu J, Xia C, Sun W. Magnetic CuFe$_2$O$_4$ nanoparticles as an efficient catalyst for C-O cross-coupling of phenols with aryl halides. Chem Cat Chem. 2011. 3:146–9. doi.10.1002/cctc.20

69. Panda N, Jena A, Mohapatra S, Letters SRT. Copper ferrite nanoparticle-mediated N-arylation of heterocycles: A ligand-free reaction. Tetrahedron Lett. 2011. 52:1924–27.

70. Zarei M. CuFe$_2$O$_4$ nanoparticles catalyze the reaction of alkynes and nitrones for the synthesis of 2-azetidinones. New J Chem. 2020. 44:17341–5. doi.10.1039/d0nj02660c.

71. Ranu BC, Dey R, Chatterjee T, Ahammed S. Copper nanoparticle-catalyzed carbon-carbon and carbon-heteroatom bond formation with a greener perspective. Chem Sus Chem. 2012. 5: 22–44. doi.10.1002/cssc.201100348.

72. Zhang R, Miao C, Shen Z, Wang S, Xia C, Sun W. Magnetic nanoparticles of ferrite complex oxides: A cheap, efficient, recyclable catalyst for building the C-N bond under ligand-free conditions. ChemCatChem. 2012. 4:824–30. doi.10.1002/cctc.201100461.

73. Jammi S, Sakthivel S, Rout L, Mukherjee T, Mandal S, Mitra R. et al. CuO nanoparticles catalyzed C–N, C–O, and C–S cross-coupling reactions: Scope and mechanism. J Org Chem. 2009. 74:1971–6. doi.10.1021/jo8024253.

74. Xu HJ, Liang YF, Cai ZY, Qi HX, Yang CY, Feng YS. Cu(I)-nanoparticles-catalyzed selective synthesis of phenols, anilines, and thiophenols from aryl halides in aqueous solution. J Org Chem. 2011. 76:2296–300. doi.10.1021/jo102506x.

75. Zhang Z, Dong C, Yang C, Hu D, Long J, Wang L. et al. Stabilized copper(I) oxide nanoparticles catalyze azide-alkyne click reactions in water. Adv Synt. Catal. 2010. 352:1600–4. doi.10.1002/adsc.201000206.

76. Zhu H, Zhang C, Yin Y. Novel synthesis of copper nanoparticles: Influence of the synthesis conditions on the particle size. Nanotechnology. 2005. 16:3079–83. doi.10.1088/0957-4484/16/12/059.

77. Rai M, Yadav A. Plants as potential synthesiser of precious metal nanoparticles: Progress and prospects. IET Nanobiotechnol. 2013. 7:117–24. doi.10.1049/iet-nbt.2012.0031.

78. Khan M, Khan M, Adil SF, Tahir MN, Tremel W, Alkhathlan HZ. Et al. Green synthesis of silver nanoparticles mediated by *Pulicaria glutinosa* extract. Int J Nanomed. 2013. 8:1507–16. doi.10.2147/IJN.S43309.

79. Duran N, Marcato PD, Duran M, Yadav A, Gade A, Rai M. Mechanistic aspects in the biogenic synthesis of extracellular metal nanoparticles by peptides, bacteria, fungi, and plants. Appl Microbiol Biotechnol. 2011. 90:1609–24. doi.10.1007/s00253-011-3249-8.

80. Kulkarni VD, Kulkarni PS. Green synthesis of copper nanoparticles using *Ocimum sanctum* leaf extract. Int J Chem Stud. 2013. 1:1–4.

81. Gunalan S, Sivaraj R, Venckatesh R. *Aloe narbadensis miller* mediated green synthesis of monodisperse copper oxide nanoparticles: Optical properties. Spectrochim Acta A Mol Biomol Spectrosc. 2012. 97:1140–44. doi.10.1016/j.saa.2012.07.096.

82. Padil VVT, Cernik M. Green synthesis of copper oxide nanoparticles using *Gum karaya* as a biotemplate and their antibacterial application. Int J Nanomedicine. 2013. 8:889–98. doi.10.2147/IJN.S40599.

83. Abboud Y, Saffaj T, Chagraoui A, El Bouari A, Brouzi K, Tanane O. et al. Biosynthesis, characterization and antimicrobial activity of copper oxide nanoparticles (CONPs) produced using brown alga extract (*Bifurcaria bifurcata*). Appl Nanosci. 2014. 4:571–6. doi.10.1007/s13204-013-0233-x.

84. Honary S, Barabadi H, Gharaei-Fathabad E, Naghibi F. Green synthesis of copper oxide nanoparticles using Penicillium aurantiogriseum, Penicillium *citrinum* and Penicillium *wakasmanii*. Digest J Nanomater Biostruct. 2012. 7:999–1005.

85. Siddiqi KS, Husen A. Current status of plant metabolite-based fabrication of copper/copper oxide nanoparticles and their application: a review. Biomater. Res. 24: 1–15. doi.10.1186/s40824-020-00188-1

86. Halder M, Mominul IM, Ansari Z, Ahammed S, Sen K, Manirul IS. Biogenic nano-CuO-catalyzed facile C–N cross-coupling reactions: Scope and mechanism. ACS Sustainable Chem Eng. 2016. 5:648–57. https://doi.org/10.1021/acssuschemeng.6b02013.

87. Wong YC, Parthasarathy K, Cheng CH. Cobalt-catalyzed regioselective synthesis of pyrrolidinone derivatives by reductive coupling of nitriles and acrylamides. J Am Chem Soc. 2009. 131:18252–3. doi.10.1021/ja9088296.

88. Hu T, Li C. Synthesis of lactams via copper-catalyzed intramolecular vinylation of amides. Org Lett. 2005. 7:2035–8. doi.10.1021/ol0505555.

89. MacFaul PA, Arends IWCE, Ingold KU, Wayner DDM. Oxygen activation by metal complexes and alkyl hydroperoxides. Applications of mechanistic probes to explore the role of alkoxyl radicals in alkane functionalization. J Chem Soc Perkin Trans. 1997. 2:135–46. doi.10.1039/a606160e.

90. Barton DHR, Gloahec VN Le, Patin H, Launay F. Radical chemistry of tert-butyl hydroperoxide (TBHP). Part 1. Studies of the Fe(III)–TBHP Mechanism. New J Chem. 1998. 22:559–63. doi.10.1039/A709266K.

91. Gomez-Mejiba SE, Zhai Z, Akram H, Deterding LJ, Hensley K, Smith N. et al. Immuno-spin trapping of protein and DNA radicals: "Tagging" free radicals to locate and understand the redox process. Free Radic Biol Med. 2009. 46:853–65. doi.10.1016/j.freeradbiomed.2008.12.020.

92. Rossi B, Prosperini S, Pastori N, Clerici A, Punta C. New advances in titanium-mediated free radical reactions. Molecules. 2012. 17:14700–32. doi.10.3390/molecules171214700.

93. Priyadarshini S, Amal PJ, Lakshmi Kantam M. Copper catalyzed oxidative cross-coupling of aromatic amines with 2-pyrrolidinone: A facile synthesis of N-aryl-γ-amino-γ-lactams. Tetrahedron. 2014. 70:6068–74. doi.10.1016/j.tet.2014.04.070.

94. Xia Q, Chen W. Iron-catalyzed N-alkylation of azoles via cleavage of an Sp3 C–H bond adjacent to a nitrogen atom. J Org Chem. 2012. 77:9366–73. doi.10.1021/jo301568e.

95. Li Z, Bohle DS, Li CJ. CU-catalyzed cross-cehydrogenative coupling: A versatile strategy for C-C bond formations via the oxidative activation of Sp3 C-H bonds. Proc Natl Acad Sci USA. 2006. 103:8928–33. doi.10.1073/pnas.0601687103.

96. Zhang C, Tang C, Jiao N. Recent advances in copper–catalyzed dehydrogenative functionalization via a single electron transfer (SET) Process. Chem Soc Rev. 2012. 41:3464–84. doi.10.1039/c2cs15323h.

97. Jonsson M, Lind J, Eriksen T, Merenyi G. Redox and acidity properties of 4-substituted aniline radical cations in water. J Am Chem Soc. 1994. 116:1423–7. doi.10.1021/ja00083a030.

98. Hunt L. The ammonia oxidation process for nitric acid manufacture. Platinum Metals Rev. 1958. 2:129–34.

99. Somorjai GA, Davis SM. Surface science studies of catalysed reactions on platinum surfaces. Platinum Metals Rev. 1983. 27:54–65.

100. Jeyaraj M, Gurunathan S, Qasim M, Kang MH, Kim JH. A comprehensive review on the synthesis, characterization, and biomedical application of platinum nanoparticles. Nanomaterials. 2019. 9:1719. doi.10.3390/nano9121719.

101. Du XL, He L, Zhao S, Liu YM, Cao Y, He HY. et al. Hydrogen-independent reductive transformation of carbohydrate biomass into γ-valerolactone and pyrrolidone derivatives with supported gold catalysts. Angew Chem Int Ed Engl. 2011. 50:7815–19. doi.10.1002/anie.201100102.

102. Wei Y, Wang C, Jiang X, Xue D, Liu ZT, Xiao J. Catalyst-Free Transformation of Levulinic Acid into Pyrrolidinones with Formic Acid. Green Chem. 2014. 16:1093–96. doi.10.1039/c3gc42125b.

103. Touchy AS, Hakim Siddiki SMA, Kon K, Shimizu KI. Heterogeneous Pt Catalysts for Reductive Amination of Levulinic Acid to Pyrrolidones. ACS Catal. 2014. 4:3045–50. doi.10.1021/cs500757k.

104. Vidal JD, Climent MJ, Concepcion P, Corma A, Iborra S, Sabater,MJ. Chemicals from Biomass: Chemoselective Reductive Amination of Ethyl Levulinate with Amines. ACS Catal. 2015. 5:5812–21. doi.10.1021/acscatal.5b01113.

105. Zhang J, Xie B, Wang L, Yi X, Wang C, Wang G. et al. Zirconium Oxide Supported Palladium Nanoparticles as a Highly Efficient Catalyst in the Hydrogenation–Amination of Levulinic Acid to Pyrrolidones. ChemCatChem. 2017. 9:2661–7. doi.10.1002/cctc.201600739.

106. Huang YB, Dai JJ, Deng XJ, Qu YC, Guo QX, Fu Y. Ruthenium-Catalyzed Conversion of Levulinic Acid to Pyrrolidines by reductive Amination. Chem Sus Chem. 2011. 4:1578–81. doi.10.1002/cssc.201100344.

107. Gao G, Sun P, Li Y, Wang F, Zhao Z, Qin Y. et al. Highly Stable Porous-Carbon-Coated Ni Catalysts for the Reductive Amination of Levulinic Acid via an Unconventional Pathway. ACS Catal. 2017. 7:4927–35. doi.10.1021/acscatal.7b01786.

108. Xie C, Song J, Wu H, Hu Y, Liu H, Zhang Z. et al. Ambient Reductive Amination of Levulinic Acid to Pyrrolidones over Pt Nanocatalysts on Porous TiO_2 Nanosheets. J Am Chem Soc. 2019. 141:4002–9. doi.10.1021/jacs.8b13024.

109. Vidal JD, Climent MJ, Corma A, Concepcion DP. One-Pot Selective Catalytic Synthesis of Pyrrolidone Derivatives from Ethyl Levulinate and Nitro Compounds. Chem Sus Chem. 2017. 10:119–28. doi.10.1002/cssc.201601333.

110. Ernest ML. Production of 5-Methyl-N-(Methyl Aryl)-2-Pyrrolidone, 5-Methyl-N-(Methyl Cycloalkyl)-2-Pyrrolidone and 5-Methyl-N-Alkyl-2-Pyrrolidone by Reductive Amination of Levulinic Acid Esters with Cyano Compounds. *United States Patent Application Publication*. 2003. US6841520B2

111. Siddiki SMAH, Touchy AS, Bhosale A, Toyao T, Mahara Y, Ohyama J. et al. Direct Synthesis of Lactams from Keto Acids, Nitriles, and H_2 by Heterogeneous Pt Catalysts. Chem Cat Chem. 2018. 10:789–95. doi.10.1002/cctc.201701355.

112. Goksu H, Sert H, Kilbas B, Sen F. Recent Advances in the Reduction of Nitro Compounds by Heterogenous Catalysts. Curr Org Chem. 2016. 21:794–820. doi.10.2174/1385272820 666160525123907.

113. Orlandi M, Brenna D, Harms R, Jost S, Benaglia M. Recent Developments in the Reduction of Aromatic and Aliphatic Nitro Compounds to Amines. Org Process Res Dev. 2018. 22:430–45. doi.10.1021/acs.oprd.6b00205.

114. Dehghani S, Sadjadi S, Bahri-Laleh N, Nekoomanesh-Haghighi M, Poater A. Study of the Effect of the Ligand Structure on the Catalytic Activity of Pd Ligand Decorated Halloysite: Combination of Experimental and Computational Studies. Appl Organomet Chem. 2019. 33:e4891. doi.10.1002/aoc.4891.

115. Moslehi A, Zarei M. Application of Magnetic Fe_3O_4 Nanoparticles as a Reusable Heterogeneous Catalyst in the Synthesis of β-Lactams Containing Amino Groups. New J Chem. 2019. 43:12690–7. doi.10.1039/c9nj02759a.

2 Recent Advances in Nanocatalyzed Synthesis of Seven-Member N-Heterocyclic Compounds with Special Reference to Azepines, Benzoazepines, Benzodiazepines, and Their Derivatives

A Brief Review

R. M. Borade,[1] S. B. Kale,[2] S. U. Tekale,[3] C. S. Patil,[3]
S. B. Ubale,[3] Keshav Lalit Ameta,[4] and R. P. Pawar[5]

[1] Department of Chemistry, Government Institute of Forensic Science,
Aurangabad, Maharashtra, India
[2] Department of Applied Science, Government Polytechnic, Aurangabad,
Maharashtra, India
[3] Department of Chemistry, Deogiri College, Aurangabad,
Maharashtra, India
[4] Department of Chemistry, School of Liberal Arts and Sciences, Mody
University of Science and Technology, Lakshmangarh, Rajasthan, India
[5] Department of Chemistry, Shiv Chattrapati College, Aurangabad,
Maharashtra, India

2.1 INTRODUCTION

Heterocyclic motifs demonstrate noteworthy chemistry with important applications in medicinal, organic chemistry, pharmaceuticals, and related industries.[1, 2] They show the major diversity of organic molecules with chemical, biomedical and industrial significance. These compounds are usually found in many natural products, such as vitamins, hormones, antibiotics, alkaloids, herbicides, pigments, and dyes. In addition, the diversity of heterocyclic rings originates from the scaffolds of various drugs and bioactive molecules.[3–5] In this context, the most bioactive molecules commonly contain five-, six-, or seven-member heterocyclic rings with one, two, or three heteroatoms.

DOI: 10.1201/9781003141488-2

Seven-member rings are normally found in various natural products and pharmaceutical drug molecules; however, practical methods for their synthesis in the laboratory are relatively low compared with those for five- or six-member rings molecules. Currently, there is constant attention on the synthesis of seven-member heterocyclic compounds that have one, two, or three nitrogen atoms and the applications of these compounds in drug discovery. This chapter will describe the use of various nanomaterials as a heterogeneous catalyst, which are efficient and modular routes for the preparation of useful seven-membered heterocyclic intermediates in drug discovery and development. Therefore, the development of flexible methodologies for their synthesis is an important and required task. In this chapter, the merit and demerits of the use of nanomaterials as a catalyst in the synthesis of seven-membered heterocyclic compounds will be discussed.

2.2   SEVEN-MEMBERED SYSTEMS THAT CONTAIN ONE HETERO ATOM

2.2.1   AZEPINES AND DERIVATIVES

In the family of heterocyclic drugs that contain one nitrogen (N) atom, azepine and its derivatives are very important pharmacophore fragments that are present in various natural products and in a wide range of bioactive compounds,[6–8] which are shown in Figures 2.1. For example, seven-membered aza-ring systems are found in the structure of Balanol,[9] a potent inhibitor of protein kinases, or in (-)-cobactin T,[10,11] a siderophore growth promoter that is isolated from mycobacteria. An N-sulfonylhydroazepine motif is found in synthetic relacatib,[12] a potent inhibitor of human cathepsin K. Stemoamide is one of the typical Stemona alkaloids that is isolated from *Stemona tuberosa* Lour and used for the treatment of respiratory diseases.[13] (-)-Securinine can be used for the treatment of serious diseases, such as amyotrophic lateral sclerosis and poliomyelitis.[14] The 2H-azepine alkaloid chalciporone is responsible for the pungent taste of the common mushroom *Chalciporus piperatus*.[15] Azepine and its derivatives are present in some pharmaceutical and a few agrochemical products. Therefore, the development of efficient methodologies for the synthesis of azepine-containing heterocycles is highly attractive. Currently, synthetic access to (hydro) azepine systems that start from simple and robust building blocks remains challenging, especially when

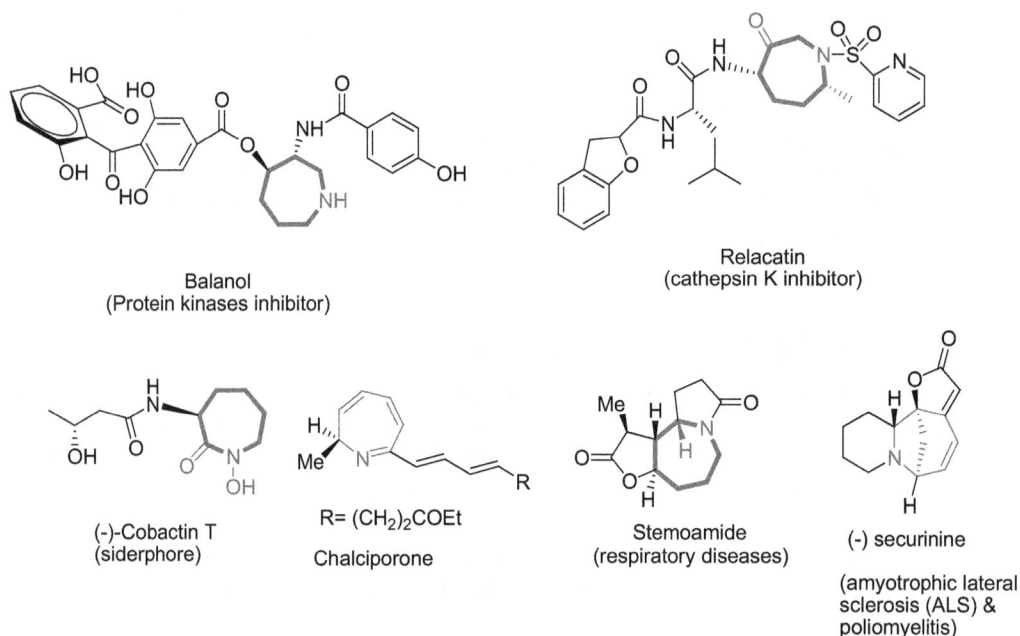

Balanol
(Protein kinases inhibitor)

Relacatin
(cathepsin K inhibitor)

(-)-Cobactin T
(siderphore)

R= (CH₂)₂COEt

Chalciporone

Stemoamide
(respiratory diseases)

(-) securinine

(amyotrophic lateral
sclerosis (ALS) &
poliomyelitis)

FIGURE 2.1   Bioactive azepine derivatives

targeting densely functionalized motifs. From the tailor-made synthesis of azetidine, derivatives were developed using diastereoselective protocols to reach broad spectrum azepines in notable yields that used the super capacity of a range of nanocatalysts, quasi-nontoxic metal oxides to favor nucleophilic addition reactions onto unsaturated carbon–carbon (C–C) bond construction reaction.

2.2.2 BENZAZEPINES AND DERIVATIVES

Benzazepines, which are seven-membered azaheterocyclic fused aromatic ring motifs, has received more attention due to their broad range of biological activity and are used as building blocks in the synthesis of various natural products, drug discovery, and developments.[16-30] For the total synthesis of natural products, such as the synthesis of alkaloids with a benzazepine skeleton, for example, aphanorphine,[31-34] cephalotaxine,[35, 36] and lennoxamine,[37, 38] have been reported because of their outstanding chemical, structural, and useful pharmacological activities. In addition, a hydrobenzazepine core is quite common in drug structures, as exemplified by the commercial benazepril drug,[39] which is an angiotensin-converting enzyme inhibitor that is used to treat renal insufficiency or hypertension as shown in Figures 2.2 and 2.3.

Orimi et al. reported the synthesis of potassium fluoride supported on a clinoptilolite (KF/CP) nanocatalyst with readily available source materials and found an effective catalyst for the preparation of benzazepine derivatives 5 via a four-component reaction of isoquinoline 1, α-haloalkanes 2, isatin or its derivatives 3, and activated acetylenic compound 4 that used water as a green solvent.[40] In this report the authors mentioned the synthesis of KF supported on a KF/CP catalyst was easy and was performed with source materials without any activation. CP has a large internal surface, naturally abundant occurring zeolite, which has much more capacity to exchange the cations, for instance, K$^+$, effectively. Therefore, by trapping anions, fluoride anions (F$^-$) were free and could be used as an appropriate candidate to act as a base. For the optimization of catalyst

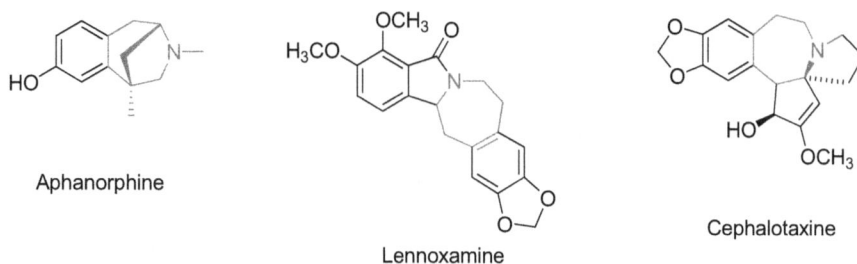

FIGURE 2.2 Alkaloids containing bioactive benzapine derivatives

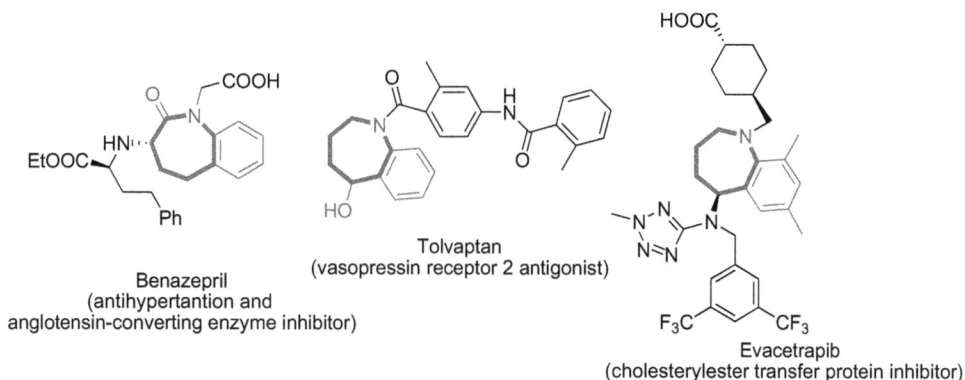

FIGURE 2.3 Bioactive benzazepine derivatives

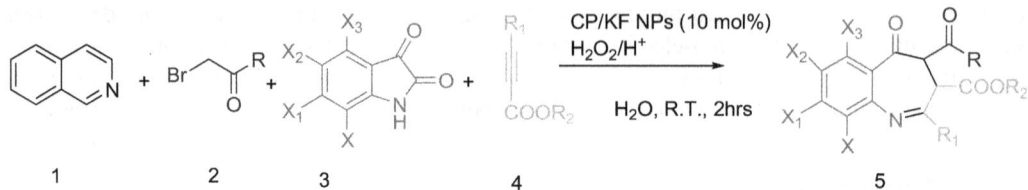

SCHEME 2.1   Synthesis of benzazepine (5) in acidic solution of H_2O_2 using KF/CP composite nanocatalyst

TABLE 2.1
Various benzazepine derivatives (5) synthesized in acidic solution of H_2O_2 using KF/CP nanocomposite

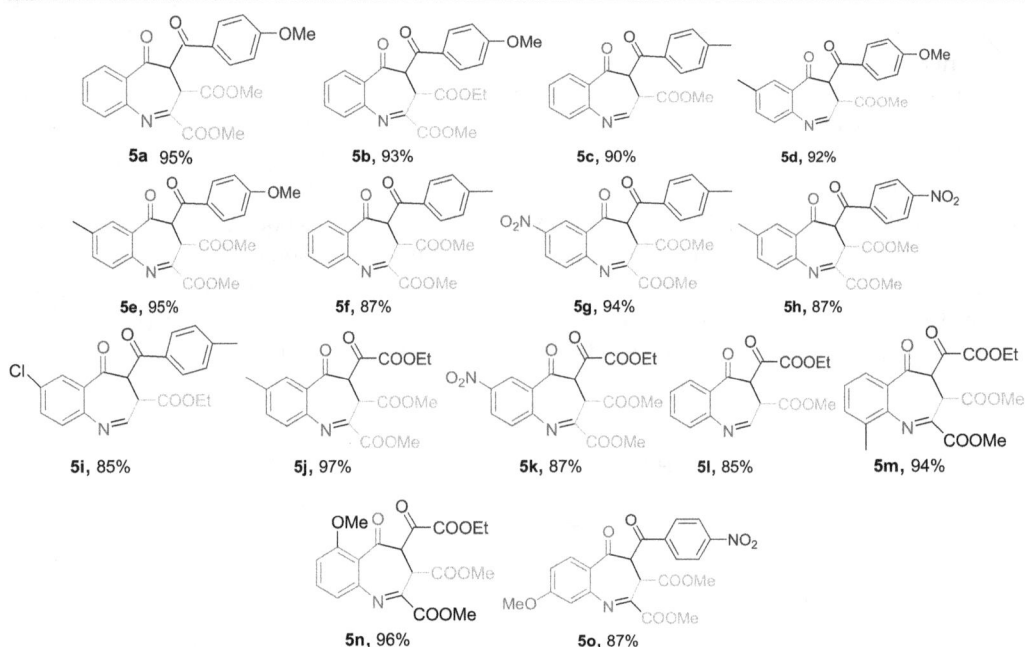

load, and the selection of the best solvent and temperature conditions, a number of reactions were carried out with reactant condensation processes for ethyl bromopyruvate **2j** isoquinoline 1, 5-methyl isatin **3j**, and dimethyl acetylenedicarboxylate **4j** in an acidic solution of hydrogen peroxide (H_2O_2) to find the best reaction conditions. After performing a set of reactions, it was confirmed that a KF/CP–NPs nanocomposite (NC) with a 10 mol% load gave the best results at room temperature (RT) in water as the solvent (Scheme 2.1). For a general protocol, the optimized conditions were maintained to prepare various derivatives of benzazepine **5** and summarized in Table 2.1.

2.3   SEVEN-MEMBERED SYSTEMS THAT CONTAINS TWO HETEROATOMS

2.3.1   BENZODIAZEPINES AND DERIVATIVES

Benzodiazepines (BZDs) represent one of the important and highly explored classes of seven-membered aromatic heterocycles that contain a two-ring N that are critical for numerous applications in the pharmaceutical industry and the organic synthesis of complex molecules.[41] Due to their diverse spectrum of biological activities, they are considered privileged structures in medicinal chemistry. Further, they are key synthons for the synthesis of various fused ring compounds.[42,43] Therefore, the further development of BZDs has gained significant attention from organic and medicinal chemists in an attempt to discover new and effective BZD-based therapeutic agents.[44]

BZDs have been prescribed in many parts of the world; first as anxiolytics and then as hypnotics.[45] They are extensively indicated for various central nervous system disorders, such as anxiolytics (e.g., chlordiazepoxide and diazepam), anticonvulsants (e.g., clonazepam and clobazam), muscle relaxants, anesthesia (i.e., midazolam), insomnia, some motor disorders, and in psychoses (e.g., olanzapine and clozapine).[46] The BZDs are classified as short-acting, intermediate-acting and long-acting, which depends on their duration of action.[47] Some of the marketed BZD-based drugs are shown in Figure 2.4.

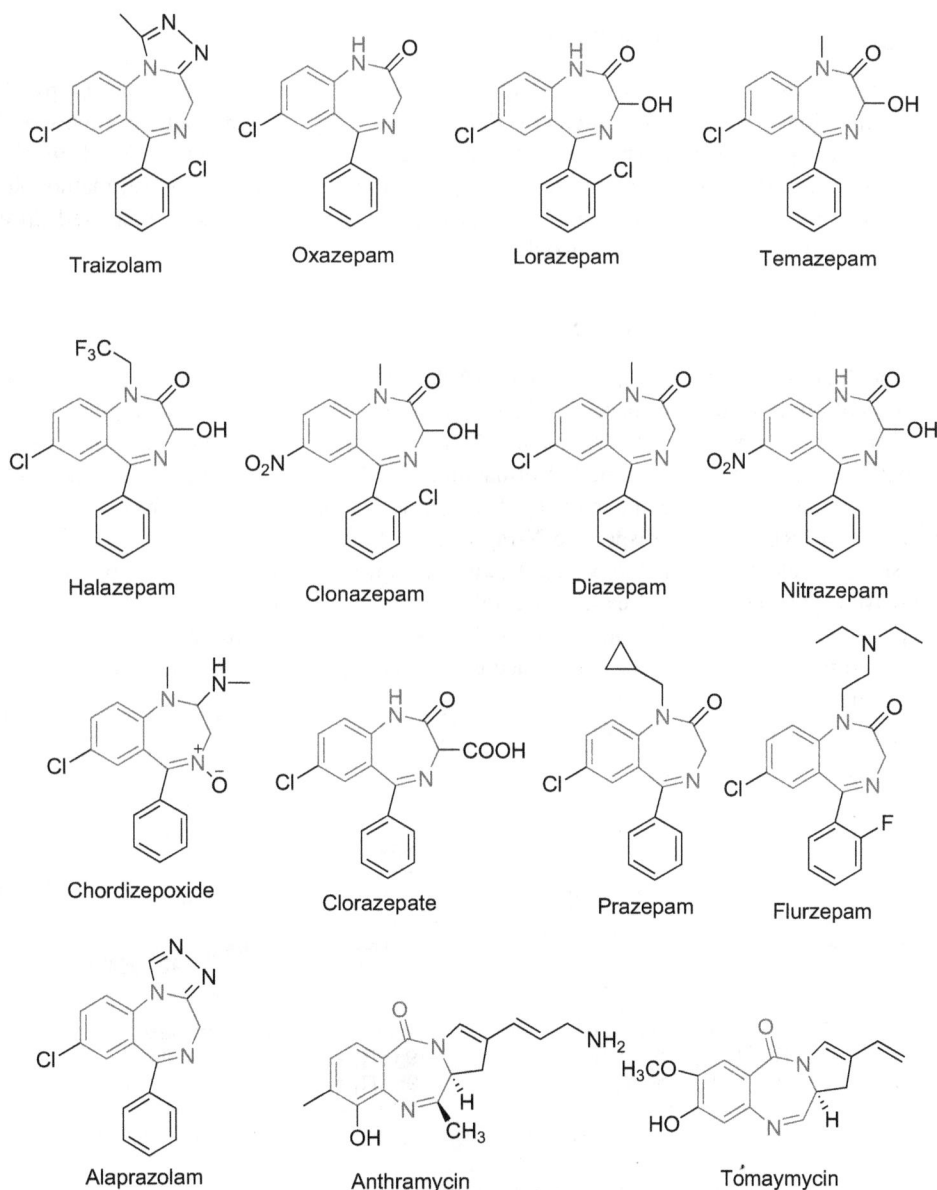

FIGURE 2.4   Some of the BZD-based drugs available in the market

The BZDs exert their effect by binding to the central BZD receptors, which are located at the post and presynaptic membranes. However, certain side effects are associated with the short and long term use of BZDs, such as confusion, drowsiness, amnesia, and ataxia.[48]

Following the guidance provided by structure–activity relationship studies, compounds with high potency and an expanded spectrum of activity, improved absorption, and distribution properties were biologically evaluated against various disease areas. BZD derivatives possessed various pharmacological activities, such as antimicrobial, anticancer, anti-anxiolytic, antidepressant, anticonvulsant, antitubercular, anti-inflammatory, analgesic, antihistaminic, and anti-anxiety.[49–51] Various BZD-based compounds have different groups or substituents attached to their core structural motif at positions 1, 2, 5, or 7 respectively.[52] These different side groups affect the binding properties of molecules with the relevant target proteins or receptors, and therefore, modulate their pharmacological properties, the potency of the biological response, and pharmacokinetic profile.[53]

2.3.2 SYNTHETIC APPROACHES OF BENZODIAZEPINES

BZD and its derivatives have been successfully employed in the treatment of various psychotic disorders, infections, and microbial infections that are caused by resistant bacteria. Emerging bacterial resistance represents an alarming situation and requires better treatments. Therefore, significant effort has been devoted by various researchers into the development of novel methodologies for the synthesis of BZDs. In this chapter, the synthetic approaches of BZD that used different nanocatalysis methodologies were discussed.

2.3.3 METHODS FOR THE SYNTHESIS OF 1, 5-BENZODIAZEPINE DERIVATIVES

Ghasemzadeh et al. reported CuI nanoparticles (NPs) as highly efficient heterogeneous catalysts for the one-pot synthesis of some benzo[b][1,5]diazepine derivatives **9** by multicomponent condensation of aromatic diamines **6**, Meldrum's acid **7** and isocyanides **8** (Scheme 2.2)[54] by coprecipitation that used acetonitrile and dimethylformaamide (DMF) organic solvents, both solvents do not fulfill the conditions of green chemistry. The synthesized CuI NPs were characterized by X-ray diffraction (XRD), energy dispersive X-ray (EDX), Fourier-transform infrared spectroscopy (FTIR), scanning electron microscopy (SEM), and transmission electron microscopy (TEM) analysis and were pure and showed excellent catalytic activity with good yields (92%–98%). The recovery and reuse of CuI NPs was carried out by simple filtration followed by washing with methanol and ethyl acetate and reported a decrease in catalytic activity from 97% to 88% yield after the fifth run.

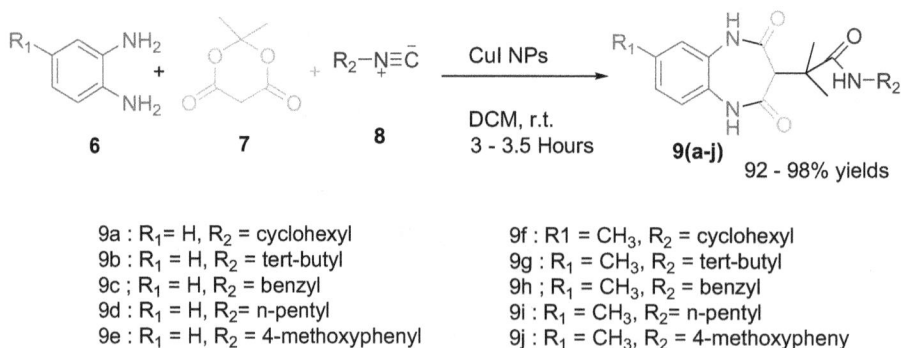

9a : R_1= H, R_2 = cyclohexyl
9b : R_1 = H, R_2 = tert-butyl
9c ; R_1 = H, R_2 = benzyl
9d : R_1 = H, R_2= n-pentyl
9e : R_1 = H, R_2 = 4-methoxyphenyl

9f : R1 = CH_3, R_2 = cyclohexyl
9g : R_1 = CH_3, R_2 = tert-butyl
9h ; R_1 = CH_3, R_2 = benzyl
9i : R_1 = CH_3, R_2= n-pentyl
9j : R_1 = CH_3, R_2 = 4-methoxypheny

SCHEME 2.2   Preparation of benzo[b][1,5]diazepines using CuI NPs catalyst

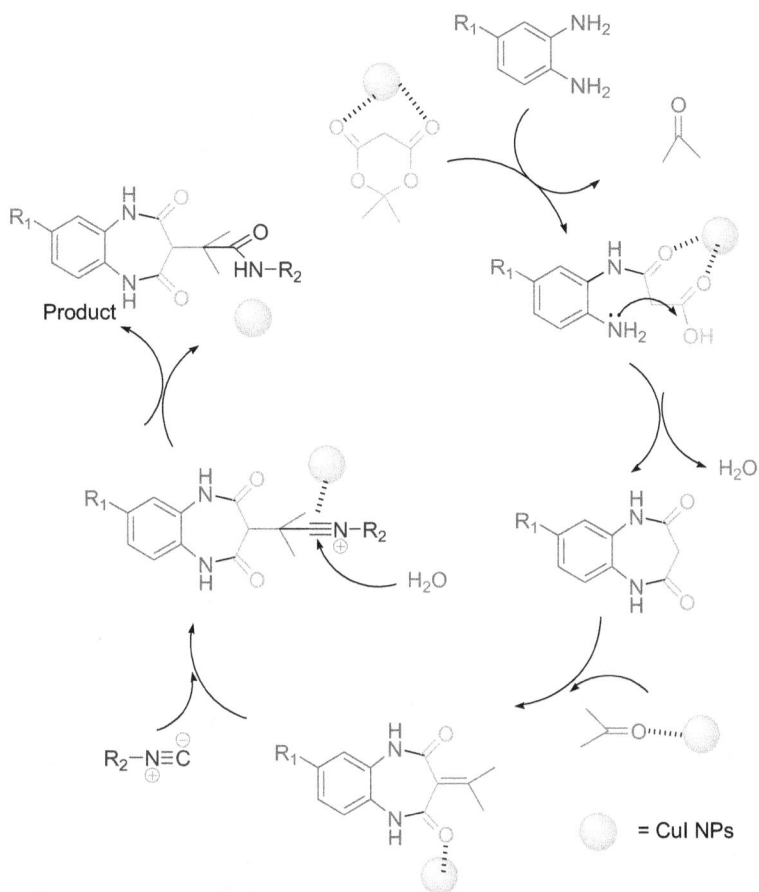

FIGURE 2.5 Proposed reaction pathway for the synthesis of 1,5-benzodiazepin-2-ones by CuI NPs

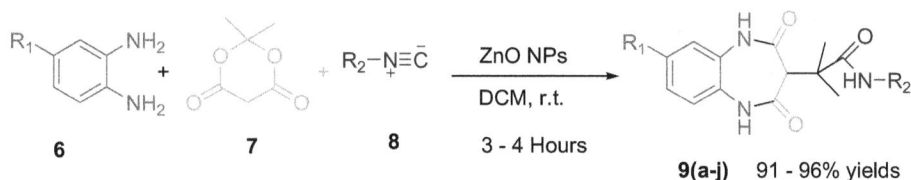

SCHEME 2.3 Preparation of benzo[b][1,5]diazepines using ZnO NPs catalyst

The possible mechanism is shown in Figure 2.5, which shows that the CuI NPs act as Lewis's acid for the initiation of the reaction by interacting with the electronegative oxygen of the carbonyl group of Meldrum's acid to give a condensed product as an intermediate, followed by a reaction with isocyanides to give the desired benzo[b][1,5]diazepine products

Ghasemzadeh and Ghomi reported the fabrication of zinc oxide (ZnO) NPs by coprecipitation and investigated the catalytic applicability in the one-pot synthesis of benzo[b][1,5]diazepine derivatives **9** through MCRs of 1,2-phenylenediamines **6**, isocyanides **8**, and Meldrum's acid **7** (Scheme 2.3).[55] This work agreed with the previously cited research work by the same research group in which CuI NPs were replaced by ZnO NPs.

Naeimi and Foroughi reported the hydrothermal synthesis of zinc sulfide (ZnS) NPs semiconductor material, which was characterized by FTIR, XRD, photoluminescence (PL), SEM, and TEM.

The FTIR and XRD techniques were used to investigate the structure of ZnS NPs, SEM and TEM were used to determine the surface morphology and structure, and particle size analysis. PL was used for the identification of the photochemical properties of prepared ZnS NPs. Prepared ZnS NPs was tested as heterogeneous catalysts for the synthesis of 4-substituted-1, 5-BZD derivatives **12** via one-pot three-component reaction of *o*-phenylenediamine (OPD) **6**, dimedone **10** and aldehyde **11** in ethanol (EtOH) as the green solvent under reflux conditions. ZnS NPs were efficient heterogeneous catalysts for the synthesis of 4-substituted-1, 5-BZD derivatives because of their low Curie temperature, high coercively, and high surface area.[56]

First, optimized reaction conditions, such as the quantity of catalyst, solvent, and reaction temperature were considered by a representative model reaction of dimedone **10**, OPD **6** and benzaldehyde **11** in equal ratios to manufacture the BZDs under various reaction conditions for an appropriate time (Scheme 2.4).

From the outcome of various reactions, 100 mg of ZnS NPs was sufficient for use as a catalyst, and EtOH was the best solvent under reflux conditions for the synthesis of 1, 5-BZD derivatives. The possibility of recycling the catalyst was examined through the reaction of OPD **6**, dimedone **10**, and 4-chlorobenzaldehyde **11** catalyzed by ZnS NPs under optimized conditions. On completion of the reaction, the catalyst was centrifuged, filtered, and washed several times with ethyl acetate. In addition, the recycled catalyst was saved for the following reaction.

In 2015, Gasemzadehh et al. reported the preparation of iron oxide (ferrite) Fe_3O_4 NPs and employed them as a heterogeneous catalyst for the synthesis of tetrahydro-2,4-dioxo-1H-benzo[b][1,5]diazepine-3-yl-2-methylpropanamides **9** using a one-pot three-component reaction of aromatic diamines **6**, Meldrum's acid **7**, and isocyanides **8** in dichloromethane at room temperature (RT). The products were obtained in a short time with excellent yields. Further, the recovered catalyst was reused successfully in six subsequent reactions without significant loss of catalytic activity (Scheme 2.5).[57] The main advantage of this catalyst is that it can be separated using an external magnet because Fe_3O_4 NPs exhibit excellent magnetic properties.

Shaabani et al. presented the catalytic activity results of Fe3O4@wool as a nanocatalyst in the synthesis of tetrahydro-1H-1, 5-benzodiazepine-2-carboxamide and 4, 5, 6, 7-tetrahydro-1H-1, 4-diazepine-5-carboxamide derivatives (Scheme 2.6).[58] In this report, the composite nanocatalyst (Fe3O4@wool) was synthesized, characterized, and investigated for catalytic utility. Some supported magnetic metal oxides have received significant attention from researchers due to their potential applications in chemical processes as catalysts. Simple separation (i.e., using an external

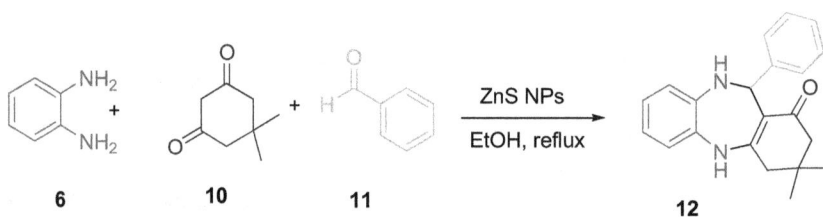

SCHEME 2.4 Optimized reaction conditions

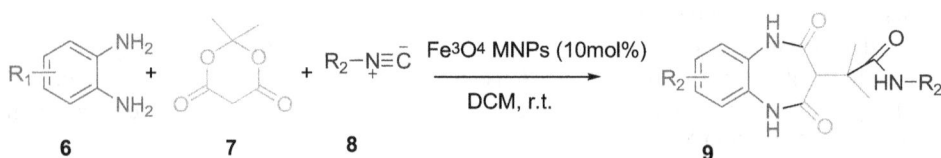

SCHEME 2.5 Preparation of benzo[b][1,5]diazepines using Fe_3O_4 NPs catalyst

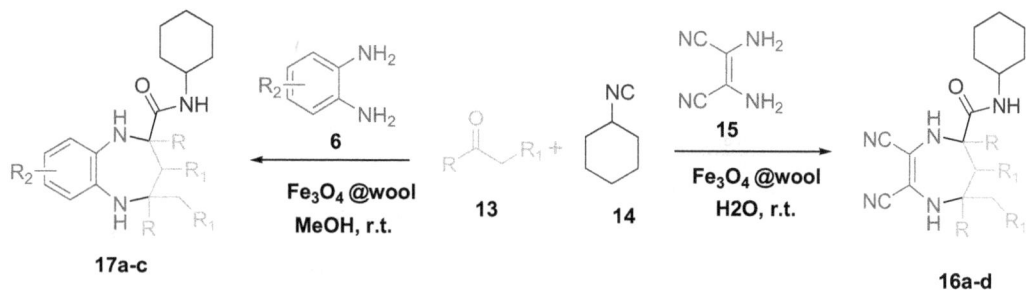

SCHEME 2.6   Preparation of wool-supported Fe_3O_4 NPs catalyst

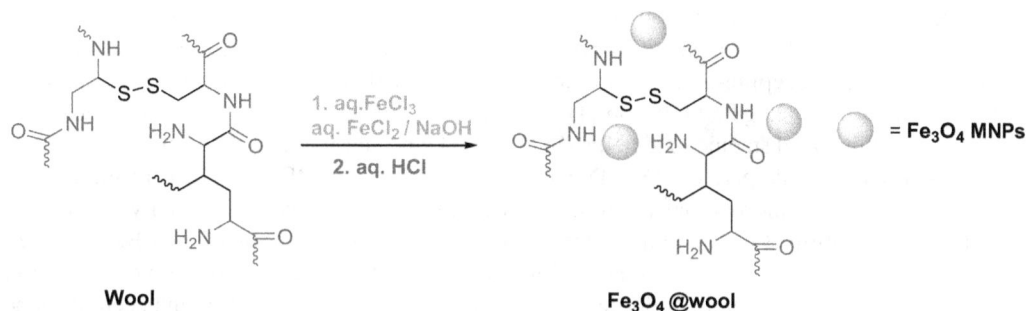

SCHEME 2.7   Synthesis of tetrahydro-1H-1, 5-benzodiazepine-2-carboxamide and 4, 5, 6, 7-tetrahydro-1H-1, 4-diazepine-5-carboxamide derivatives

magnet), high catalytic activity, high chemical stability, reusability, and environmental friendliness are some important advantages of these heterogeneous nanocatalysts. Since unsupported NPs are usually unstable and coagulation of the NPs during the reaction is frequently unavoidable, aggregation and agglomeration of Fe_3O_4 NPs into less active large particles and bulk Fe_3O_4 during the reaction decreases its catalytic activities. Wool is a chiral natural biopolymer that is composed of repetitive units of amino acids cross-linked by sulfur–sulfur (S–S) bonds. Keratin is the main component of wool and is insoluble in any solvent; therefore, this biopolymer could be used as natural solid support. As mentioned previously, wool contains numerous amino acids units with amide (–NH–CO–), amine (–NH_2), and –S–S– functional groups and the metal oxide NPs uptake by wool fibers can be carried by these functional groups; due to the structurally ordered amino acid chains, the aggregation of Fe_3O_4 could be prevented and improve catalytic activity.

Preparation of wool-supported Fe_3O_4 NPs was carried out in an aqueous solution of iron (III) chloride ($FeCl_3$) and iron (II) chloride ($FeCl_2$) in a molar ratio of Fe(III)/Fe(II)=2 at pH 11–12 by coprecipitation. In a magnetically stirred suspension of 1.00 g wool pieces in 100 cm^3 of deionized water, 0.31 g of $FeCl_3$ and 0.12 g of $FeCl_2$ were successively dissolved in the solution with stirring. A solution of sodium hydroxide (NaOH) was added dropwise for 4 h into the resulting mixture under vigorous stirring at RT to give black Fe_3O_4@wool. It showed magnetic properties in situ by placing a magnet near the Fe_3O_4@wool. The catalyst was isolated in the magnetic field and the supernatant was removed from Fe_3O_4@wool by decanting and the residue was washed with water several times. Then, the Fe_3O_4@wool catalyst was added to the aqueous acid (HCl) solution with stirring to neutralize the anionic charges on the NPs (Scheme 2.7). Fe_3O_4@wool was again separated and washed with water several times and dried at 80°C.

The optimization of catalyst load, temperature, and solvent for the synthesis of BZD and diazepine derivatives that used the synthesized catalyst and found (0.22 g Fe_3O_4@wool) in

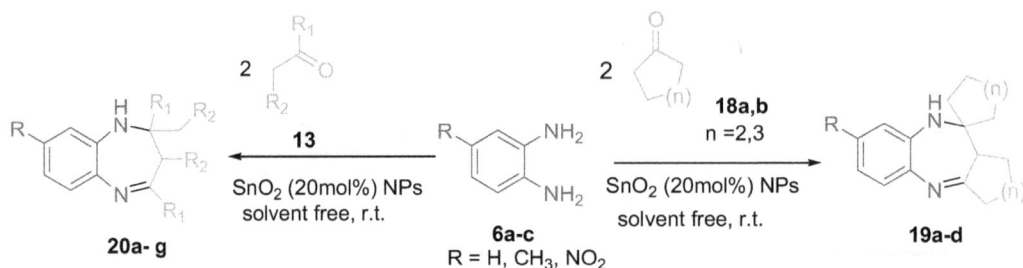

SCHEME 2.8 Synthesis of 1, 5-BZDs by condensation of OPD with various ketones catalyzed by SnO$_2$ NPs

methanol and water as the preferred solvents at RT, respectively. Finally, the synthesis of the various tetrahydro-1H-1,5 benzodiazepine-benzodiazepine-2-carboxamide **16** and 4,5,6,7-tetrahydro-1H-1,4-diazepine-5-carboxamide derivatives **17** that used the synthesized catalysts was carried out (e.g., 0.22 g Fe$_3$O$_4$@wool, H$_2$O solvent, RT) under optimized reaction conditions.

Singh et al. fabricated stannic oxide NPs (SnO$_2$ NPs) by advanced thermal decomposition under microwave irradiation. Prepared SnO$_2$ NPs were characterized by XRD and TEM for the investigation of structural and morphological properties (Scheme 2.8).[59] The catalytic activity of prepared SnO$_2$ NPs was confirmed by applying a one-pot multicomponent synthesis of 1, 5-BZDs **19, 20** strategies under solvent-free conditions at RT. First, an optimization study was performed to confirm the ability of SnO$_2$ NPs as catalysts during synthesis of 1, 5-BZDs using OPD **6** and acetophenone **13** as a model reaction, by varying the amount of SnO$_2$ NPs catalyst and found that 20 mol% of SnO$_2$ NPs gave a good outcome (i.e., 90% yields) and with no catalyst, no product was formed. Therefore, a high surface area and better dispersion of NPs in the reaction mixture cause better activities of SnO$_2$ NPs. Catalyst SnO$_2$ NPs showed good reusability after three cycles; however, was not sufficient to examine catalytic reusability.

Korbekandi et al. fabricated and characterized nicotine-based organocatalyst supported silica NPs (Fe(III)- NicTC@nSiO$_2$) by different techniques. The synthesized catalyst was tested as an efficient catalyst by exploring the synthesis of functionalized 1, 5-BZD (**12a-k**) in water as a green solvent at RT. The optimization conditions studied showed that the use of Fe(III)-NicTC@nSiO$_2$ (3 mol%) was a sufficient catalyst for the smooth condensation of OPD, **6**, (1 mmoL), dimedone (**10**, 1 mmoL), and aldehyde (**11**,1mmoL) with water as the green solvent after 10 min of stirring provided best results (Scheme 2.9). In addition, chemoselectivity of the nanocatalyst was reported and it was demonstrated with high chemoselectivity. In addition to this selectivity, the synthesis of mono and bis-1, 5-BZDs was demonstrated. Using a 1:1:1 M ratio of starting materials in the presence of the catalyst, the corresponding mono-1, 5-BZDs (**12l** and **12m**) was formed with excellent selectivity and yields. However, when, a 2:2:1 M ratio of starting materials was used, the desired bis-1, 5-BZDs were efficiently produced.[60]

The catalytic applications of metal–organic frameworks (MOFs) that possess Lewis's acid sites as the metallic centers in their structures for the cyclocondensation of acetone with different 1,2-diamines have been explored. They are valuable heterogeneous catalysts for the synthesis of biologically active 1,5-BZDs. In addition, calix[4]arenes with acidic groups were successfully employed as acid catalysts for the synthesis of heterocycles by Isaeva et al. In their research, the catalytic properties of novel nanoporous materials composed of metal organic framework of para-sulfonatocalixarene (MIL/K-SO$_3$H) and a metal organic framework of para-tert-butylthiacalix-[4]-arene (MIL/Ks-CN) were utilized by developing a highly efficient microwave-assisted one-pot synthesis of 1,5-BZDs via the encapsulation of para-sulfonatocalixarene (K-SO$_3$H) and para-tert-butylthiacalix-[4]-arene (Ks-CN) with strong (–SO$_3$H) and weak (–CN) acidic functionalities, respectively, in the MOF (NH$_2$-MIL-101(Al)) cavities, MIL/K-SO$_3$H as shown in Figure 2.6.

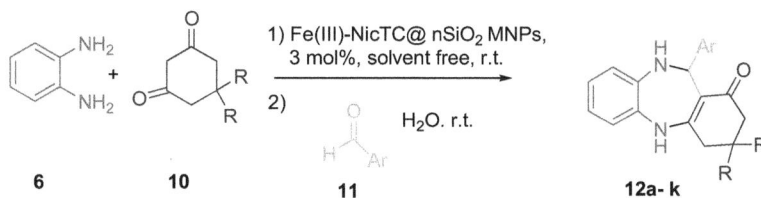

SCHEME 2.9 Solvent-free synthesis of 1, 5-BZDs using (Fe(III)-NicTC@nSiO₂) NPs catalyst

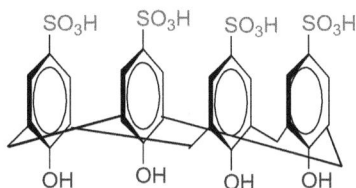

FIGURE 2.6 Structural framework of catalyst MIL/K-SO₃H

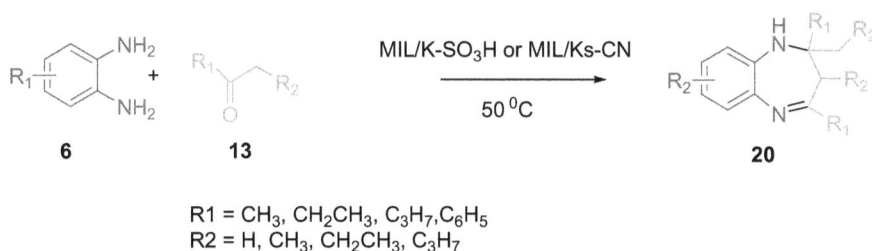

R1 = CH₃, CH₂CH₃, C₃H₇,C₆H₅
R2 = H, CH₃, CH₂CH₃, C₃H₇

SCHEME 2.10 1, 5-BZDs synthesis using MIL/K-SO₃H or MIL/Ks-CN as metal–organic frameworks

MIL/K-SO₃H and MIL/Ks-CN composite materials were prepared from an aluminium(III) 2-aminoterephthalate metal organic framework (NH₂-MIL-101(Al)) matrix and calix[4]arene using microwave-assisted synthesis. Catalytic use of the novel composite materials was investigated during condensation of 1, 2-phenylenediamine (**6**) and ketone **13** (e.g., acetone, ethylmethylketone, diethylketone, and acetophenone) at 50°C for the synthesis of substituted 1, 5-BZDs (**20**) (Scheme 2.10). The catalytic activity depended on the nature of the functional groups in the calix[4]arene structure. The MIL/Ks-CN catalyst showed higher activity compared with MIL/K-SO₃H, whose activity was comparable with that of MIL-100(Al) material. The decrease in surface acidity was because of the catalytic activity of the MIL/K-SO₃H, which was related to the strong H bond between the proton of the SO₃H group and amino (NH₂) group in this composite. The efficiencies of the MIL/K-SO₃H and MIL/Ks-CN catalysts were compared with zeolites and the results showed that the MIL/Ks-CN composite had superior results compared with all zeolites, whereas the activity of the MIL/K-SO₃H system was lower.[61]

Maleki reported the synthesis of 2,3,4,5-tetrahydro-1H-1,5-benzodiazepine-2-carboxamide derivatives and 4,5,6,7-tetrahydro-1H-1,4-diazepine-5-carboxamide derivatives **24** that used simple and readily available chemicals 1,2-diamine **6**, a linear **21, 22** or cyclic ketone **23** and an isocyanide **8** in the presence of a catalytic amount of ferrite–silica (Fe₃O₄–SiO₂) NC particles in EtOH as the green solvent at ambient temperature with excellent yields. In this work, diazepine derivatives were prepared from one of the starting materials is isocyanide, which was why this reaction is known as an isocyanide-based MCRs (I-MCRs) reaction (Scheme 2.11).[62]

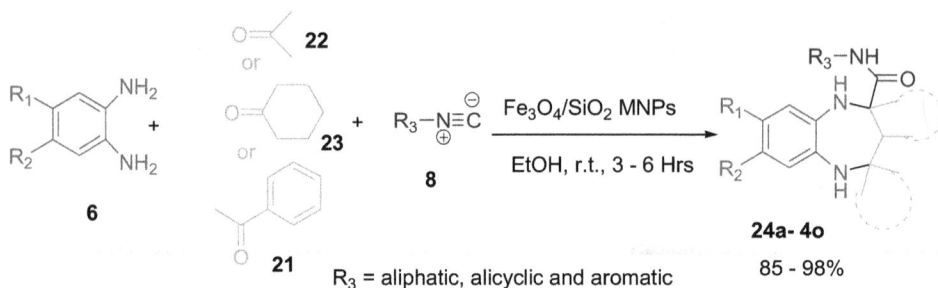

SCHEME 2.11   Synthesis of diazepine-2-carboxamide derivatives catalyzed by Fe_3O_4/SiO_2NPs

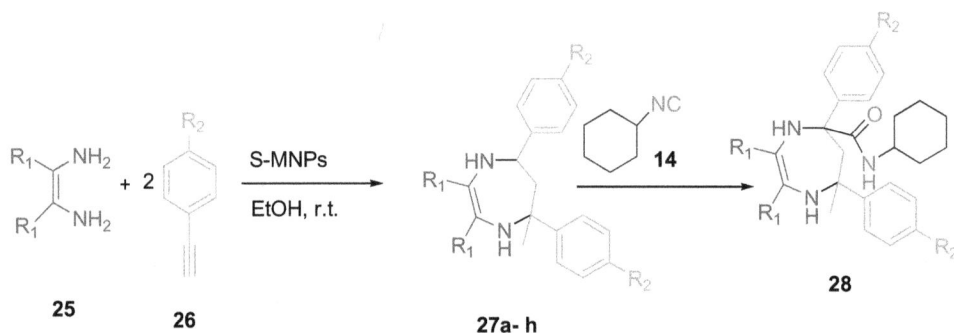

SCHEME 2.12   Synthesis of diazepines and diazepine carboxamides in the presence of the supported Fe_3O_4/ SiO_2 (S–MNPs) nanocatalyst

The preparation of Fe_3O_4–SiO_2 NC particles was carried out by coprecipitation using readily available Fe_3O_4 NPs and tetraethylorthosilicate (TEOS). The prepared Fe_3O_4–SiO_2 NC particles were characterized by TEM analysis for the size and structural identification of the catalyst.

The utility of the catalyst was confirmed using different substituted OPD **6**, ketone **21** and isocynide **8** to give the corresponding product 24 with good to excellent yields of the product.

The reusability of this catalyst was confirmed by a simple reaction and was very active after several cycles without a remarkable loss of catalytic performance. The speciality of this catalyst was mentioned as non-toxic, economically efficient, environmentally benign, and could be separated from the reaction mixture by an external magnet to avoid centrifugation and filtration by traditional methods.

Maleki reported the catalytic application of the previously mentioned nanocatalyst (i.e., Fe_3O_4– SiO_2) NC in a one-pot multicomponent synthesis for diazepine derivatives with excellent yields was described. The reactions of various 1,2-diamines **25**, terminal alkynes **26**, and an isocyanide **14** occur in the presence of a catalytic amount of magnetically recoverable Fe_3O_4–SiO_2 NC supported magnetic nanoparticles (S–MNPs) in EtOH as a green reaction solvent at ambient temperature (Scheme 2.12).[63]

In 2015, Maleki et al. reported the preparation, characterization, and catalytic application of an environmentally benign, clean biopolymer-based heterogeneous Fe_3O_4–chitosan NPs in the synthesis of 1,5-BZD derivatives **29** were carried out using 1,2-diamines **6** and aldehydes or ketones **21** in EtOH as the green solvent at ambient temperature with good yields (Scheme 2.13).[64] The Fe_3O_4–chitosan NC was recovered easily by applying an external magnetic field and reused without any major loss of catalytic performance after a number of cycles.

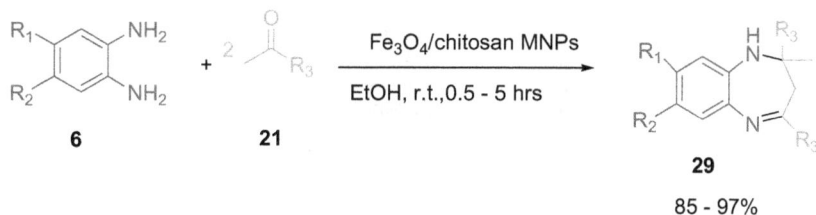

SCHEME 2.13   Synthesis of 1, 5-BZDs derivatives in the presence of Fe_3O_4/chitosan nanocatalyst

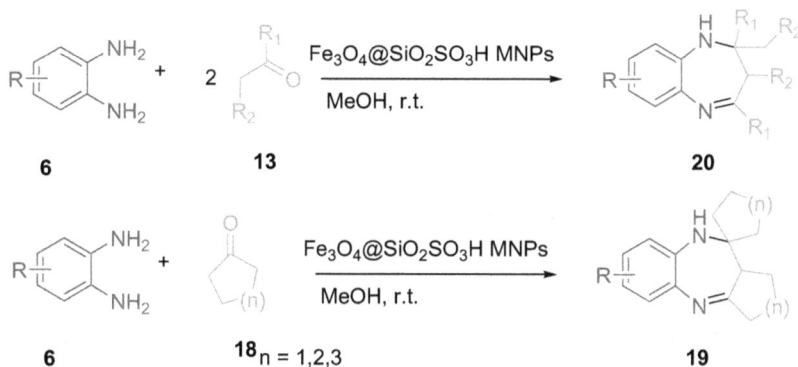

SCHEME 2.14   Synthesis of 1, 5-BZDs using Fe3O4@SiO2SO3H MNPs

To explore the generality of this protocol, extensively described the synthesis of 1, 5-diazepines, as the main part of a seven-membered heterocyclic compound, under similar reaction conditions. In this context, diversified 1,5-BZD derivatives **29a–p** were successfully synthesized using aromatic 1, 2-diamines **6**, and various ketones **21** in the presence of a catalytic amount of nano Fe_3O_4–chitosan NC in EtOH at RT. The process was found to be excellent in terms of yields and time using ketones substituted with electron-donating as well as electron-withdrawing moieties.

Sathe et al. invented the catalytic power of sulfonic acid supported on ferrite–silica super magnetic NPs (Fe3O4@SiO2SO3H MNPs) via a one-pot synthesis of 1, 5-BZD derivatives. This catalyst was a composite of Fe_3O_4 NPs and sulfated silica, which acted as an acid catalyst for the one-pot condensation of substituted OPD **6** with various ketones **12** and **18** in methanol occurred at RT to manufacture the corresponding 1,5-BZD derivatives **19** and **20** with good to excellent yield (70%–98%, Scheme 2.14). The catalyst quantity was optimized to 20 mol% of $Fe_3O_4@SiO_2SO_3H$ MNPs and the solvent effect was studied by performing the reaction with various ketones in different solvents, in which methanol showed the greatest performance. The reaction showed broad substrate scope and was applied to various aliphatic cyclic, acyclic, and aromatic ketones to produce a range of functionalized BZD derivatives.[65]

Maleki et al., in 2018, reported a green and efficient procedure for the synthesis of various substituted 1, 5-BZD derivatives **12** by a one-pot three-component reaction between OPD **6**, dimedone **10,** and aldehyde derivatives **11** in the presence of copper ferrite ($CuFe_2O_4$) MNPs as a heterogeneous nanocatalyst under ball-milling conditions at RT (Scheme 2.15).[66] $CuFe_2O_4$ MNPs were prepared by thermal decomposition of copper nitrate ($Cu(NO_3)_2$) and $Fe(NO_3)_3$ in water in the presence of NaOH and calcinated at 700°C for 5 h. For the optimization of reaction conditions, a model reaction of OPDA **6** (1 mmol), 4-chlorobenzaldehyde **11d** (1 mmol), and 5, 5- dimethylcyclohexane-1,3-dione **10** (1 mmol) were obtained under ball-milling conditions at RT. Using 0.046 g (20 mol %) of

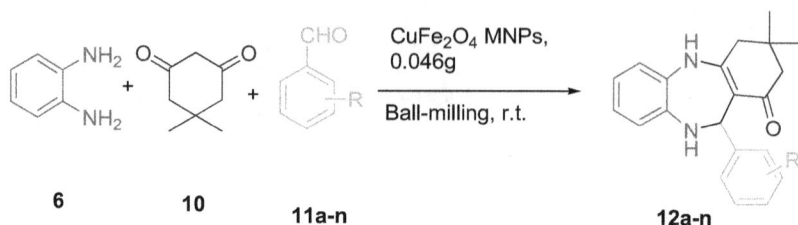

SCHEME 2.15   Synthesis of 1, 5-BZDs derivatives using CuFe$_2$O$_4$ MNPs

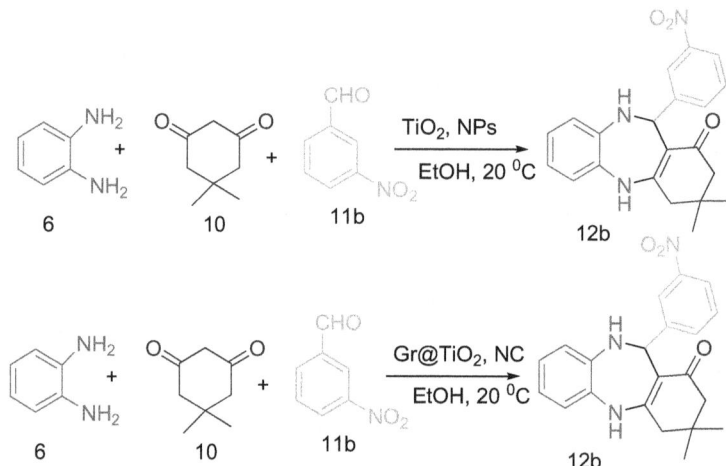

SCHEME 2.16   Optimization of reaction conditions

CuFe$_2$O$_4$ MNPs was sufficient to complete the reaction after 25 min to give **12d** (98% yield). Then, to examine the scope and generality of these conditions for the synthesis of a variety of 4-substituted 1, 5-BZD derivatives were studied under the optimized reaction conditions.

Shoeb et al. reported the relative study of mesoporous titanium dioxide (TiO$_2$) NPs and graphene-mesoporous TiO$_2$ NCs (Gr@TiO$_2$ NCs) as a heterogeneous catalyst in the synthesis of pharmaceutically important BZD derivatives. Mesoporous TiO$_2$ NPs and Gr@TiO$_2$ NCs catalysts were synthesized via a wet chemical method. In the study of catalytic activity of TiO$_2$ NPs and Gr@TiO$_2$ NCs in the synthesis of BZDs by the reaction of dimedone **10**, OPD **6** and aromatic aldehydes **11** were compared, and with the addition of Gr, the catalytic activity of TiO$_2$ was appreciably enhanced (Gr@TiO$_2$ NCs). Therefore, potentially there were only strong π–π interactions between the aromatic derivatives and GR sheet, and the Gr@TiO$_2$ NCs had a better catalytic performance for the synthesis of BZD derivatives **12** compared with mesoporous TiO$_2$ NPs (Scheme 2.16).[67]

The authors optimized the reaction conditions for h the catalysts, such as the quantitative load of catalysts, reaction temperature, and suitable solvents by considering model reactions of OPD **6**, dimedone **10,** and m-nitro benzaldehyde **11b** to give the corresponding BZD product **12b** (Scheme 2.16).

After conducting a set of experiments, the optimized conditions for the reaction used 0.14 g Gr@TiO$_2$ NCs stirred in EtOH at 20°C with a short reaction time (10 min) to produce a high yield (98%) of product **12b**. In addition, they investigated the individual catalytic potential of TiO$_2$ NPs and Gr@TiO$_2$ NCs in the model reaction mentioned previously. Individually, TiO$_2$ NPs catalyzed the reaction at the same time and temperature; however, the yield of the reaction was very low, and in the presence of Gr@TiO$_2$ NCs yield was improved, because the incorporation of Gr into Gr@TiO$_2$ NCs

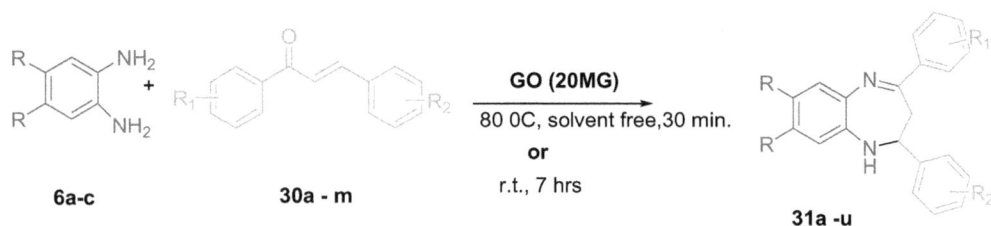

SCHEME 2.17 Synthesis of 1,5-BZD derivatives from chalcone

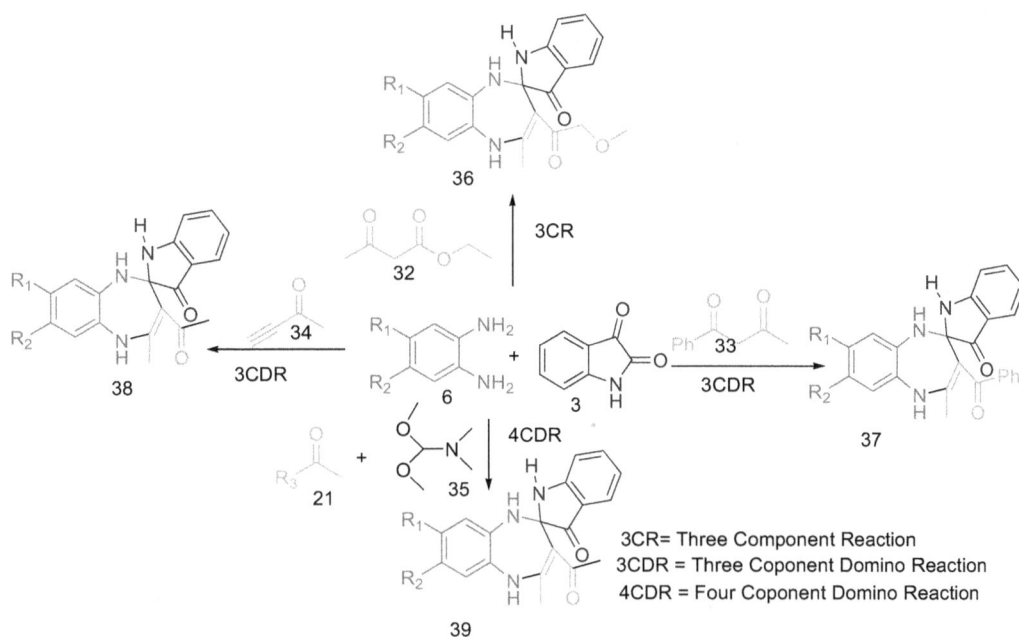

3CR= Three Component Reaction
3CDR = Three Coponent Domino Reaction
4CDR = Four Coponent Domino Reaction

SCHEME 2.18 Multicomponent domino reactions

was due to the specific surface area and active center of Ti, which was well dispersed among the catalyst, which led to a remarkable improvement in the catalytic performance.

Jamatia et al. reported that graphite oxide (GO) catalyzed the synthesis of 1,5-BZDs **31** at RT and under solvent-free reaction conditions at 80°C from substituted aromatic diamines **6** and various chalcone derivatives **30**. The main advantages of this protocol were the metal-free carbocatalyst, reusability of the catalyst, high substrate variation, solvent-free, mild reaction conditions, and higher yield (Scheme 2.17).[68]

They proposed metal-free synthesis of BZD derivatives, to explore GO as a potential catalyst. GO was prepared and characterized by various spectral techniques to confirm the formation of GO nanoplatelets.

For the optimization of catalyst load, reaction solvent, temperature conditions, and the catalytic role of GO for the synthesis of biologically active 1,5-BZDs **31a** that started from OPD **6a**, (1 mmoL) and α,β-unsaturated ketone (**30a**, 1mmol) was studied.

Zhang et al. reported the synthesis of bioactive 1, 5-BZD derivatives by multicomponent domino reactions that were catalyzed by value-added p-toluenesulfonic acid MNPs (Fe_3O_4@SiO_2-PTSA) (Scheme 2.18). In addition, the magnetic nanocatalyst was used in the synthesis of a number of 1,5-dihydrospiro[benzo[b][1,4]diazepine-2,3'- indole derivatives with good to excellent yields

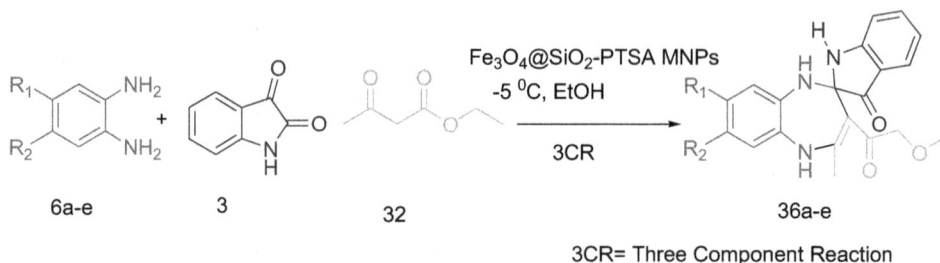

SCHEME 2.19   Substrate range of three-component synthesis of 3a-e compounds

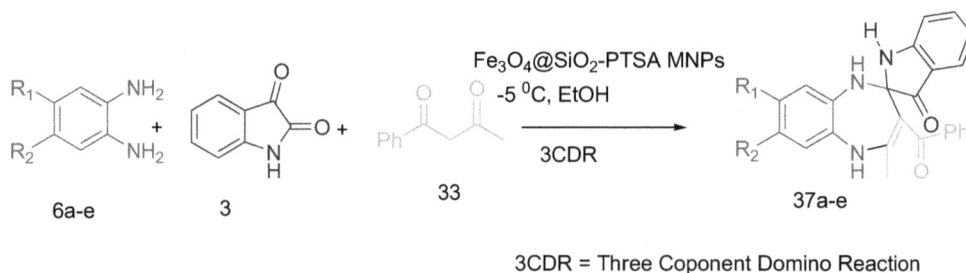

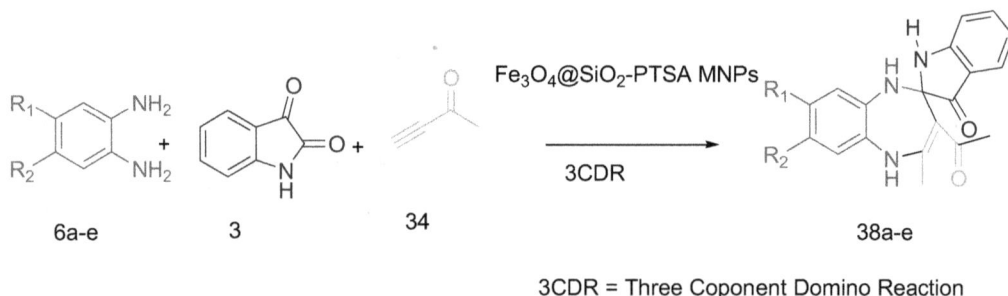

SCHEME 2.20   Substrate variation for the domino synthesis of 1, 5-BZDS

(Scheme 2.19). In a one-pot synthesis strategy, two new N heterocycle (E.G., indole and diazepine) rings and four new chemical bonds (E.G., one C–C, two C=N, and one C=C) were constructed by a series of multicomponent domino reactions. This was the first reported method for the synthesis of functional 1, 5-BZD derivatives that used an indole ring.[69]

After the successful synthesis of BZDs by a three-component reaction as discussed previously, the next reaction tried to execute the same type of reaction with benzoyl acetone **33** instead of ethyl acetoacetate **32** (Scheme 2.20).

Four-component domino reactions (4CDR) have been effectively carried out by the condensation of OPD **6**, isatin **3,** and ketones **21** or **40** with N,N-dimethylformamide dimethyl acetal **35** to give compound **39** with an excellent yield of 97%. Then, compound **39** was successfully synthesized from compounds **3** and 1, 2-phenylenediamine **6** with an outstanding yield of 96% (Scheme 2.21). Due to the straightforward process and high yield of the previous steps, the formation of targeted molecule 6 was achieved as the key step for this protocol. For optimization of the reaction conditions for this protocol, which included the catalysts load, solvents selection, and temperature, 10 mol% of the catalyst Fe$_3$O$_4$@SiO$_2$-PTSA MNPs were sufficient for an excellent yield, EtOH gave the best results at RT.

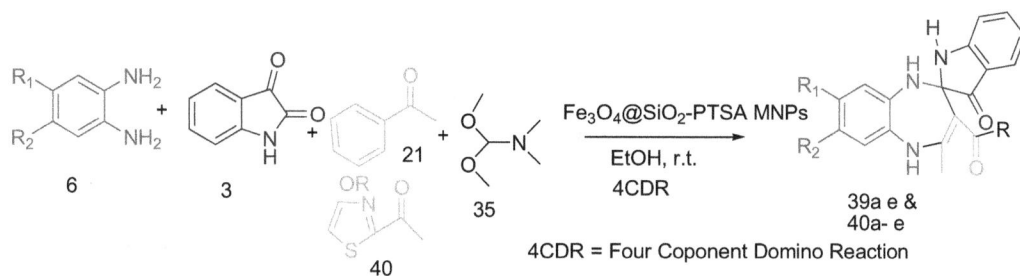

SCHEME 2.21   One-pot synthesis of 1,5-dihydrospiro[benzo[b][1,4]diazepine-2,3'-indole] derivatives

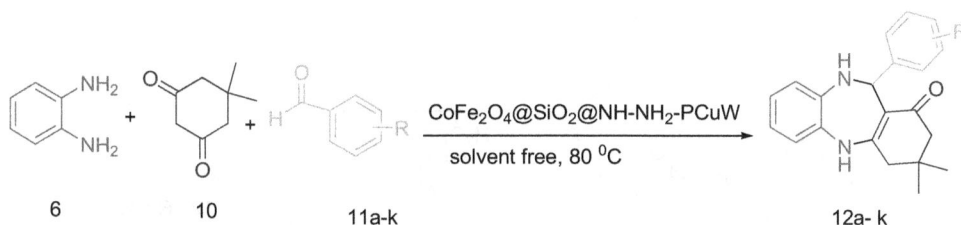

SCHEME 2.22   Synthesis of benzodiazepine derivatives 4a–k in the presence of CoFe2O4@SiO2@NH-NH2-PCuW under solvent-free conditions

The merit of these protocols have been discussed, along with the green reaction process, recyclable magnetic catalysts, mild reaction conditions, short reaction times, and high yields of products.

2.3.4   METHODS FOR THE SYNTHESIS OF 1,4-BENZODIAZEPINES

Savari et al. reported the manufacture and characterization and investigated the catalytic performance of $CoFe_2O_4$@SiO_2@NH-NH_2-PCuW NC (diamine modified silica coated cobalt ferrite polyoxometalate nanocomposite) as a magnetic heterogeneous nanocatalyst that had Bronsted and Lewis acid properties for the synthesis of 1, 4-BZDs.The authors prepared $CoFe_2O_4$@SiO_2@NH-NH_2-PCuW by the reaction of heteropoly acid ($H_3PW_{11}CuO_{39}$) with diamine modified silica-coated magnetic nanoparticles (MNPs) in an EtOH–water solvent system. The catalytic activity of the developed NC catalyst was confirmed in the synthesis of 1, 4-BZD derivatives **12** via the three-component condensation of OPD **6**, dimedone **10,** and various aldehydes **11** under solvent-free conditions (Scheme 2.22).[70]

Singh et al. explored the synthesis and catalytic utility of lanthanum oxide [La_2O_3] and lanthanum hydroxide [$La(OH)_3$] NPs as heterogeneous bases for the three-component reaction of aldehyde **11**, dimedone **10,** and OPD **6** for the synthesis of 1,4-BZD derivative **12** (Scheme 2.23).[71] Both synthesized catalysts showed a pure phase formation by XRD pattern. The basicity of La_2O_3 and $La(OH)_3$ were measured by CO_2–temperature-programmed desorption (TPD) experiment at RT. These compounds are basic and show considerable CO_2 uptake and show two major peaks with peak temperatures at 350°C and 500°C. This experiment suggested that there were two different basic sites with varying strengths and a broad peak was present in La_2O_3 NPs and had an ample choice of sharing in basic site strength. Surface area measurements that used Brunauer–Emmett–Teller (BET) revealed a low surface area for both the materials. TEM measurements indicated agglomerated particles with heterogeneous size distribution. The multicomponent reaction proceeded smoothly in aqueous media and organic solvents. The heterogeneous catalyst was successfully recycled 11 times without losing catalytic activity.

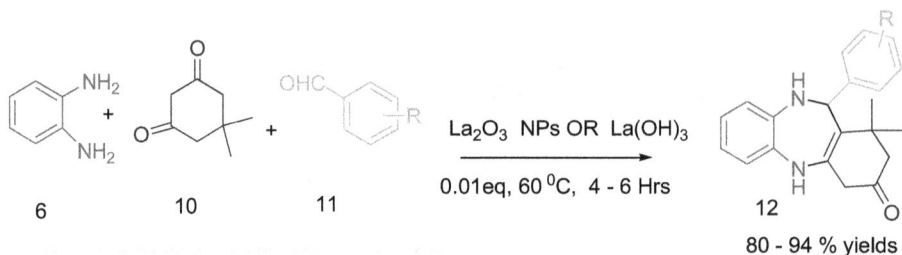

SCHEME 2.23 Synthetic strategy for preparation of 1,4-BZD derivatives

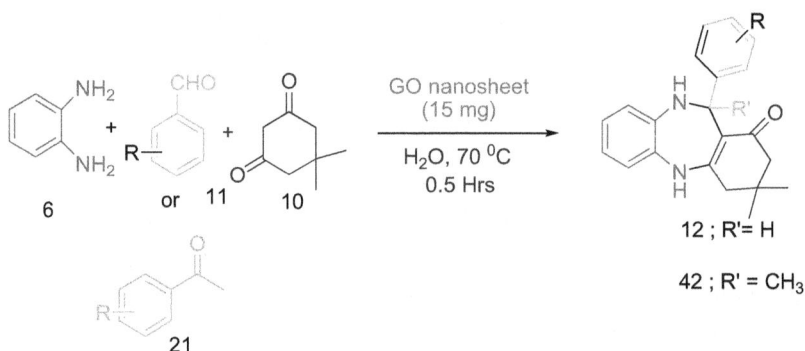

SCHEME 2.24 Optimization of reaction conditions

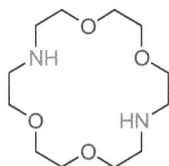

FIGURE 2.7 Structure of K 22

Kausar et al. reported carbon nanomaterials, particularly Gr-based materials (i.e., GO) nanosheets that were used as carbocatalysis in a one-pot, three-component reaction for the synthesis of biologic-ally relevant dibenzo[1,4]diazepine scaffold **12** and **41** from the reaction between OPD **6**, aldehydes **11,** ketones **21,** and 1,3-dicarbonyls **10** in aqueous medium effectively with high selectivity.[72]

GO nanosheets were prepared by the oxidation of Gr powder that used an improved Hummer's method. Characterization of the prepared GO nanosheets was carried out with field emission scanning electron microscopy (FESEM), TEM, XRD, and FTIR spectral analysis. The structural properties of the synthesized GO nanosheets were carried out with XRD analysis and FTIR. The surface morphological properties were investigated by the FESEM and TEM images of the GO nanosheets and confirmed that GO was composed of a few layers, which resulted in a high surface area, which is an essential criterion for efficient catalytic activity.

Three-component synthesis of BZD derivatives via OPD, dimedone, and benzaldehyde has been carried out. The outcome of the reaction showed that GO nanosheets were low-weight (15 mg) in water at 70°C and gave excellent yield (95%) within 30 min (Scheme 2.24).

In contrast, Kryptofix **22** (K 22) as a precise class of aza-crown ether are known for their high binding affinity and selectivity toward transition metals (Figure 2.7).

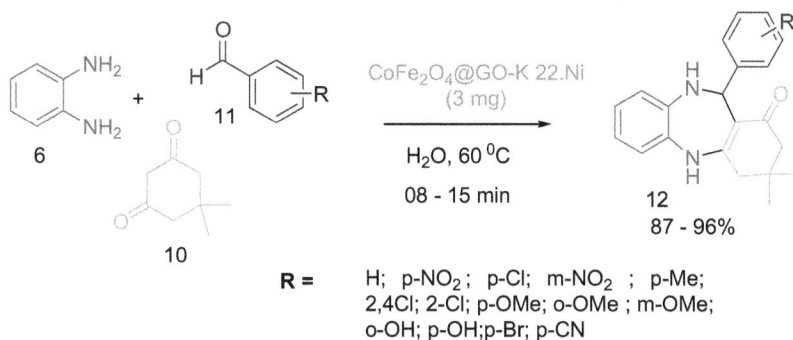

SCHEME 2.25   Synthesis of 1,4-BZD derivatives in the presence of CoFe2O4@GO–K 22.Ni nanocatalyst

The unique structure and properties of K 22 have made them a favorable candidate for a broad array of applications over the last few decades. They have been extensively used in several disciplines, such as supramolecular chemistry, biochemistry, materials science, catalysis, separation, and biomedicine applications and have are versatile when selectively binding a range of metal ions for the development of the new concept of host–guest chemistry.[73–78] Therefore, Mozafari and Ghadermazi reported the fabrication of GO-based nickel (Ni) NPs incorporated into a Kryptofix **22** conjugated magnetic nano GO composite (CoFe$_2$O$_4$@GO–K 22.Ni), by the grafting Kryptofix **22** moieties onto the magnetic nano GO surface, followed by the reaction of the NC with nickel nitrate (Ni(NO$_3$)$_2$) solution. The Kryptofix **22** host material unit cavities can stabilize the Ni NPs effectively and prevent their aggregation and separation from the surface. Fabricated NC catalysts were characterized by FTIR, FE-SEM, thermo-gravimetric analysis (TGA), inductively coupled plasma (ICP), EDX, XRD, vibrating sample magnetometer (VSM), and BET to determine their structural, morphological, thermal, elemental composition, and magnetic properties. The surface area, pore volume and size were found by BET analysis, which are important conditions for a good catalyst. CoFe$_2$O$_4$@GO–K 22.Ni NC catalyst was efficiently applied for the synthesis of 1, 4-BZD derivative **12** (Scheme 2.25). [79] The main advantages of this method were the mild reaction conditions, inexpensive catalyst, environmentally benign, and shorter reaction time. This organometallic catalyst could be easily separated from a reaction mixture and was successfully examined for six runs with a slight loss of catalytic activity.

In 2016, Shaabani reported the fabrication of two catalysts from the Nobel metals, gold and silver with copper bimetallic (Au-Cu and AgCu) NPs supported on guanidine-grafted and were characterized by various instrumental techniques to investigate the structural, morphological, and surface properties. The synthesized bimetallic NPs supported on guanidine-grafted reduced GO nanosheets (e.g., AuCu@G-rGO and AgCu@G-rGO) nanocatalysts reported excellent catalytic property for a one-pot tandem reductive/multicomponent reactions (MCRs) with 2-nitroanilines **43** for the synthesis of tetrahydro-1H-benzo[b][1,4]diazepine-2-carboxamide **47** and 1H-tetrazolyl-benzo[b][1,4]diazepine derivatives**48** (Scheme 2.26).[80]

In the previous protocol, an Au-containing bimetallic nanocatalyst showed the best results for high yields and better selectivity compared with an Au-containing bimetallic nanocatalyst.

De et al. investigated the catalytic utility of zeolite-Y nanopowder in a one-pot three-component MCR for the synthesis of spiro dibenzo[1,4]diazepine derivatives **49** by reacting isatins **3**, cyclic-1,3-diketones **10** and 1,2-phenylenediamines **6**. The zeolite-Y nanopowder catalyst was synthesized by a hydrothermal method that used NaOH, tetramethylammonium hydroxide, aluminum isopropoxide and demineralised (DM) water. The synthesized catalyst was characterized by XRD, high resolution transmission electron microscopy (HRTEM), EDS, and BET analysis for the structural, morphological, and elemental compositions and stoichiometry and the surface properties, respectively.

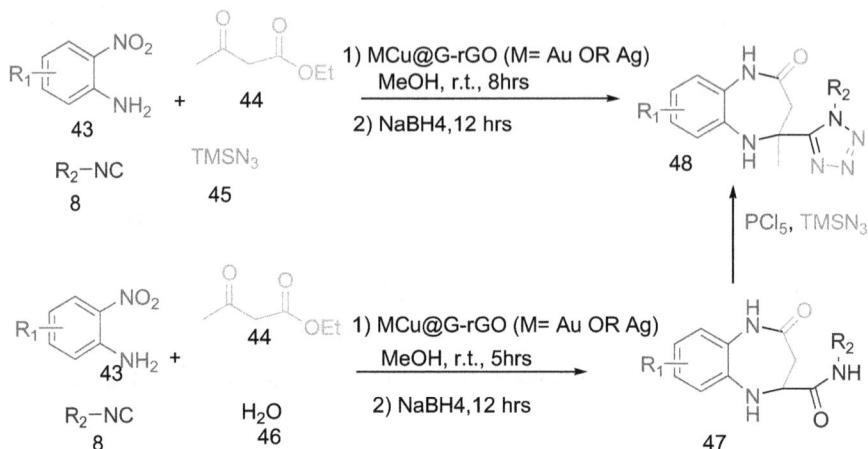

SCHEME 2.26 Synthesis of tetrahydro-1H-benzo[b][1,4]diazepine-2-carboxamide and 1H-tetrazolyl-benzo[b][1,4]diazepine derivatives using tandem reductive/MCRs strategy

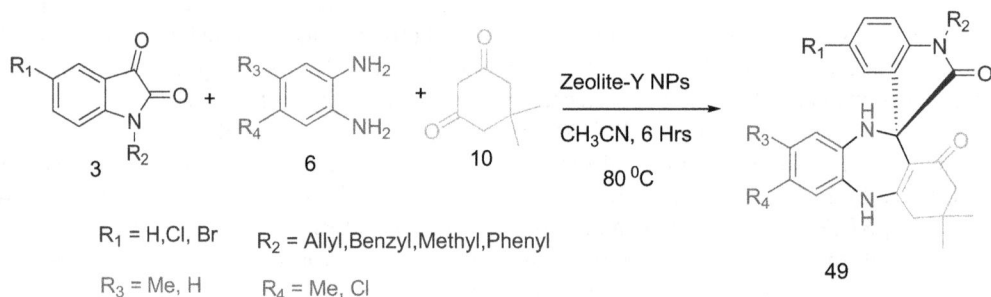

R$_1$ = H,Cl, Br   R$_2$ = Allyl,Benzyl,Methyl,Phenyl

R$_3$ = Me, H   R$_4$ = Me, Cl

SCHEME 2.27 Synthesis of Spiro dibenzo[1,4]diazepine derivatives

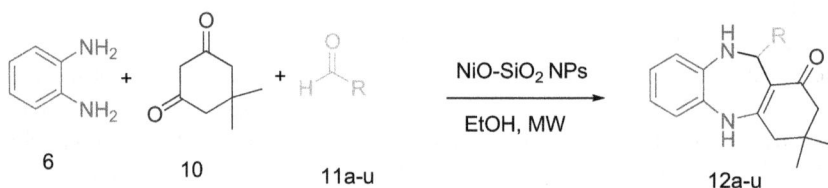

SCHEME 2.28 Synthesis of one-pot multicomponent 1, 4-benzodiazepine derivatives

X-ray photoelectron spectroscopy (XPS) analysis was carried out to investigate the actual electronic environment and oxidation state of the elements (Scheme 2.27).[81]

Nasir et al. studied the synthesis of heterogeneous versatile NiO-SiO$_2$ nanocatalysts by a sol-gel auto-combustion method and used it as a catalyst for the synthesis of one-pot multicomponent 1, 4-BZD derivatives (12**a-u**) from a mixture of OPD **6**, aromatic aldehydes **11,** and dimedone **10** under microwave irradiation (Scheme 2.28).[82]

The experiment was carried out by conventional and microwave irradiation methods. In general, the materials that have high dielectric constants and absorb microwave irradiation were used for microwave applications. One drawback of this protocol was noted, which was the conventional synthesis method required less time for completion of the reaction over the microwave strategy.

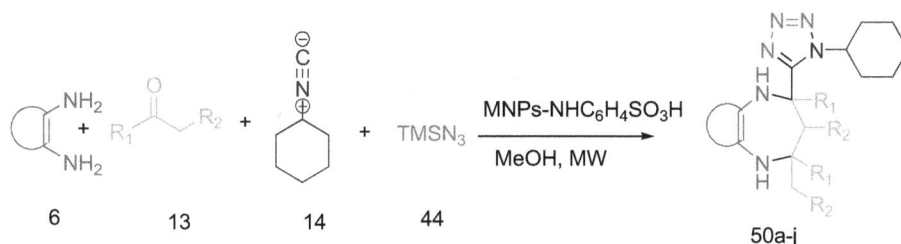

SCHEME 2.29 Synthesis of MNPs-NHC$_6$H$_4$SO$_3$H

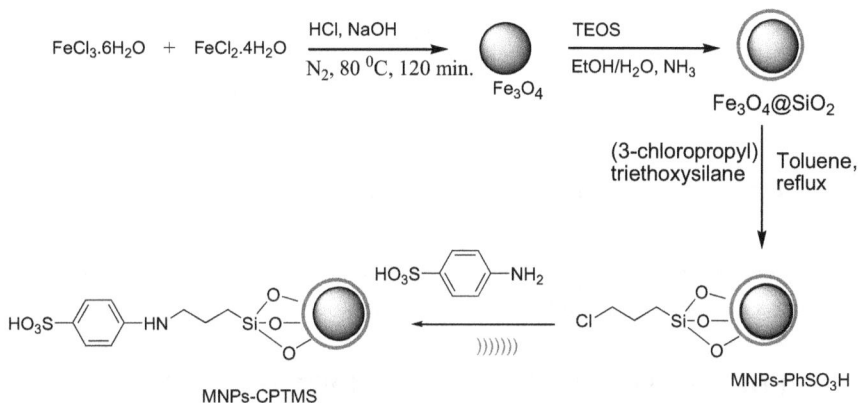

SCHEME 2.30 Synthesis of 1,4-diazepine derivatives in the presence of MNPs-NHC$_6$H$_4$SO$_3$H under microwave irradiation

Safaei-Ghomi et al. presented their results on the catalytic activity of Fe$_3$O$_4$@SiO$_2$- NHC$_6$H$_4$SO$_3$H MNPs in the microwave irradiation/assisted heterogeneous catalysis for the synthesis of 1,4-diazepines that contained a tetrazole ring **50**.[83] These compounds possess more importance in many applications, mostly in medicinal chemistry and drug discovery (Scheme 2.29). In this report, the preparation and characterization of magnetic NC materials (Fe$_3$O$_4$@SiO$_2$-NHC$_6$H$_4$SO$_3$H MNPs) were depicted. First, magnetic nano ferrite material particles (Fe$_3$O$_4$ MNPs) were synthesized by chemical coprecipitation that started with from FeCl$_3$ and FeCl$_2$, then SiO$_2$-coated MNPs (Fe$_3$O$_4$@SiO$_2$ MNPs) were prepared by the addition of tetraethylorthosilicate (TEOS). After vigorous stirring at RT for16 h, the core/shell MNPs (Fe$_3$O$_4$@SiO$_2$ MNPs) were isolated by magnetic decantation to remove the unbounded silica particles and dried at RT under a vacuum and finally washed with deionized water, EtOH, and acetone. In the next step preparation of Fe$_3$O$_4$@SiO$_2$-Cl MNPs were reported by the treatment of (3-Chloropropyl)trimethoxysilane on Fe$_3$O$_4$@SiO$_2$ MNPs in an inert N atmosphere. Finally, MNPs-NHC$_6$H$_4$SO$_3$H as the final catalyst was prepared by the chemical treatment of sulfanilic acid in triethylamine solvent in an atmosphere. After 2 days a brown solid catalyst was obtained (Scheme 2.30). The prepared MNPs-NHC$_6$H$_4$SO$_3$H catalyst was characterized by XRD, FTIR, SEM, and VSM for structural, morphological, and magnetic properties, respectively.

For optimization studies for the synthesis of 1, 4-diazepines, the model reaction of acetone **13**, 2, 3-diaminomalononitril **6**, cyclohexylisocyanid **14,** and trimethylsiliazide **44** was used as standard reagents. Different reaction conditions were performed, and the best results were obtained under microwave irradiation (400 W) in methanol, and the reaction gave a satisfactory result in the presence of MNPs-NHC$_6$H$_4$SO$_3$H (0.008 g). In this study, microwave irradiation was utilized as green and complementary technique for the synthesis of a 1, 4-diazepines containing tetrazole ring **50**.

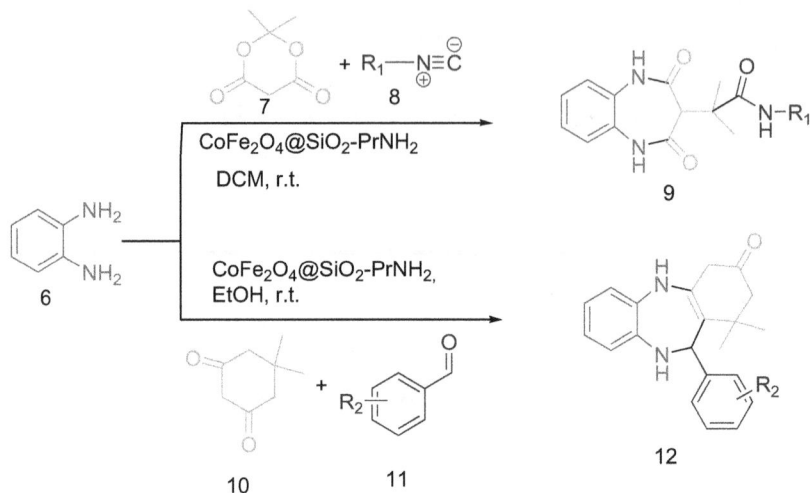

SCHEME 2.31 $CoFe_2O_4@SiO_2$-$PrNH_2$ NC catalyzed synthesis of BZDs

The efficiency of MNPs-NHC$_6$H$_4$SO$_3$H catalysts was confirmed in the synthesis of 1, 4-diazepine derivatives using a number of substituted ketones and diamines.

2.4   SYNTHETIC APPROACHES FOR FUSED BENZODIAZEPINES

Miri et al. reported a novel, simple, and efficient method for the synthesis of BZD derivatives that was catalyzed by $CoFe_2O_4@SiO_2$-$PrNH_2$ MNPs. The fabricated NC $CoFe_2O_4@SiO_2$-$PrNH_2$ MNPs acted as an efficient catalyst for the synthesis of BZD using MCRs between 1, 2-phenylenediamine **6** with dimedone **10** and different aldehydes **11,** or with Meldrum's acid 7 and isocyanide **8** substrates (Scheme 2.31). Various reaction conditions were optimized by performing the MCRs at RT with different catalysts. The NC $CoFe_2O_4@SiO_2$-$PrNH_2$ catalyst provided the best results and the optimized reaction conditions were applied to a wide range of substrates to yield a diversity-oriented library of BZD.[84]

2.5   CONCLUSIONS AND FUTURE PERSPECTIVES

The discovery of bioactive natural products that contain a seven-membered ring has helped to establish valuable synthesis methods for their construction. Particular focus has been placed on the synthesis of azepine and diazepine derivatives because these are important skeletal units that are found in numerous natural products and compounds with important chemical, biological, and medicinal activities.

BZDs have an advantageous structural framework in progressive medicinal chemistry and have a large spectrum of biological activities and wide applications in several areas. Their potential has increased interest from organic and medicinal chemists to design a library of medicinally active compounds. In the last two decades, significant developments have been made in the improvement of the synthesis strategies for BZDs compared with the conventional approach. Currently, the scope of one-pot MCRs has been explored to design easy, straightforward, and efficient protocols for the synthesis of BZD derivatives. MCRs are frequently used as potent protocols for the synthesis of biologically important organic compounds, These processes are fast and trouble-free in conjunction with their scaffold diversity, which has been used by the pharmaceutical industry to design and discover biologically relevant compounds.

The previous remarks and discussion reflect that there is significant and extended scope in the development of MCRs protocols to extend the substrate range of seven-membered rings. This chapter summarized the catalytic uses of various nanocatalysts in the synthesis of many pharmaceutically active seven-membered compounds, such as various derivatives of azepines, analogs of benzoazepines, and diazepines can be obtained via one-pot MCRs as a competent synthetic approach. The applications of nanocatalysts are increasing in catalysis as they are designed at the nanolevel, especially for heterogeneous catalysts. Nanosized supported NPs or NCs have attracted much attention due to their versatile physical surface and catalytic properties and applications in catalysis, especially the oxides of transition metals. These nano oxides exhibit good catalytic activity due to their large surface area, inherent adsorptive properties, and active sites. Recently, MNCs have increased their demands in catalysis, especially for heterogeneous catalysis. MNCs could assist researchers in the design of catalysts with good activity, stability, selectivity, and reusability due to their isolation using an external magnet. Most of the heterogeneous systems require filtration or a centrifugation step or a complicated workup for the final reaction mixture to recover the catalyst. These active magnetic nanocatalytic systems possess several advantages over conventional catalyst systems. Magnetic nanocatalysts are small and have a large surface area to volume ratio. Since the available surface area of the active component of the catalyst is large, the contact between the reactant molecules and catalyst is enhanced to a significant extent to facilitate the heterogeneous catalytic system. The easy control over size, shape, and morphology makes it possible to rationally design materials that are needed for a particular catalytic application. Tuning the properties of metals is possible at the nanoscale, which would be impossible with their macroscopic counterparts. Their magnetic nature allows them to be separated using an external magnet: therefore, facilitating recyclability and reusability.

This smart synthetic method is much more prolific for the synthesis of many seven-membered drug-like azepines, analogs of benzoazepines, and diazepines scaffolds as pharmaceutically interesting heterocycles. This chapter should motivate more interesting research in this field and could provide useful information on the synthesis of seven-membered heterocyclic compounds for the improvement of clinically viable agents for the treatment of various diseases.

REFERENCES

1. Gomtsyan A. Heterocycles in drugs and drug discovery. Chemistry of Heterocyclic Compounds. 2012. 48:7–10. doi.10.1007/s10593-012-0960-z.
2. Taylor AP, Robinson RP, Fobian YM, Blakemore DC, Jones LH, Fadeyi O. Modern advances in heterocyclic chemistry in drug discovery. Org Biomol Chem. 2016, 14:6611–37.
3. Baumann M, Baxendale IR. An overview of the synthetic routes to the best selling drugs containing 6-membered heterocycles. Beilstein J Org Chem. 2013. 9:2265–319. doi.10.3762/bjoc.9.265.
4. Taylor RD, MacCoss M, Lawson AD. Rings in drugs. J Med Chem. 2014. 57:5845–59. doi:10.1021/jm4017625
5. Carreira EM, Fessard TC. Four-membered ring-containing spirocycles: Synthetic strategies and opportunities. Chem Rev. 2014. 114(16): 8257–322. doi.10.1021/cr500127b.
6. Zha GF, Rakesh KP, Manukumar HM, Shantharam CS, Long S. Pharmaceutical significance of azepane based motifs for drug discovery: a critical review. Eur J Med Chem. 2019. 162:465–94. doi.10.1016/j.ejmech.2018.11.031.
7. Vitaku E, Smith DT, Njardarson JT. Analysis of the structural diversity, substitution patterns, and frequency of nitrogen heterocycles among U.S. FDA approved pharmaceuticals. J Med Chem. 2014. 57:10257–274. doi.10.1021/jm501100b.
8. Riley DL, van Otterlo WAL. Oxepines and azepines. In: Majumdar KC and Chattopadhyay SK, editors. Heterocycles in natural products synthesis. Wiley-VCH; 2011. p. 535–68.
9. Kulanthaivel P, Hallock YF, Boros C, Hamilton SM, Janzen WP, Ballas LM, Loomis CR. et al. Balanol: a novel and potent inhibitor of protein kinase C from the fungus *Verticillium balanoides*. J Am Chem Soc. 1993. 115:6452–3. doi:10.1021/ja00067a087.

10. Maurer PJ, Miller MJ. Mycobactins: synthesis of (-)-cobactin T from ε-hydroxynorleucine. J Org Chem. 1981. 46:2835– 6.

11. Yang SM, Lagu B, Wilson LJ. Mild and efficient Lewis acid-promoted detritylation in the synthesis of N-hydroxy amides: a concise synthesis of (-)-cobactin T. J Org Chem. 2007. 72:8123–6.

12. Kumar S, Dare L, Vasko-Moser JA, James IE, Blake SM, Rickard DJ. et al. A highly potent inhibitor of cathepsin K (relacatib) reduces biomarkers of bone resorption both in vitro and in an acute model of elevated bone turnover in vivo in monkeys. Bone. 2007. 40(1):122–31. doi:10.1016/j.bone.2006.07.015.

13. Lin WH, Ye Y, Xu RS. Chemical studies on new Stemona alkaloids, IV. Studies on new alkaloids from *Stemona tuberose*. J Nat Prod. 1992. 55(5):571–6. doi.10.1021/np50083a003.

14. Beutler JA, Karbon EW, Brubaker AN, Malik R, Curtis DR, Enna SJ. Securinine alkaloids: A new class of GABA receptor antagonist. Brain Res. 1985. 330:135–40. doi.10.1016/0006-8993(85)90014-9.

15. Sterner O, Steffan B, Steglich W. Novel azepine derivatives from the pungent mushroom *Chalciporus piperatus*. Tetrahedron. 1987. 43(6):1075–82. doi.10.1016/S0040-4020(01)90044-4.

16. Hoyt SB, London C, Gorin D, Wyvratt MJ, Fisher MH, Abbadie C. et al. Discovery of a novel class of benzazepinone Na(v)17 blockers: potential treatments for neuropathic pain. Bioorg Med Chem Lett. 2007. 17(16): 4630–4. doi.10.1016/j.bmcl.2007.05.076.

17. Smith BM, Smith JM, Tsai JH, Schultz JA, Gilson CA, Estrada SA. et al. Discovery and SAR of new benzazepines as potent and selective 5-HT2C receptor agonists for the treatment of obesity. Bioorg Med Chem Lett. 2005. 15(5):1467–70. doi.10.1016/j.bmcl.2004.12.080.

18. Seto M, Miyamoto N, Aikawa K, Aramaki Y, Kanzaki N, Iizawa Y. et al. Orally active CCR5 antagonists as anti-HIV-1 agents. Part 3: synthesis and biological activities of 1-benzazepine derivatives containing a sulfoxide moiety. Bioorg Med Chem. 2005. 13(2):363–86. doi.10.1016/j.bmc.2004.10.021.

19. Seto M, Aramaki Y, Okawa T, Miyamoto N, Aikawa K, Kanzaki N. et al. Orally active CCR5 antagonists as Anti-HIV-1 agents: synthesis and biological activity of 1-benzothiepine 1,1-dioxide and 1-benzazepine derivatives containing a tertiary amine moiety. Chem Pharm Bull. 2004. 52:577–590. doi.10.1248/cpb.52.577.

20. Kondo K, Kan K, Tanada Y, Bando M, Shinohara T, Kurimura M. et al. Characterization of Orally Active Nonpeptide Vasopressin V2 Receptor Agonist. Synthesis and Biological Evaluation of Both the (5R)- and (5S)-Enantioisomers of 2-[1-(2-Chloro-4-pyrrolidin-1-yl-benzoyl)-2,3,4,5-tetrahydro-1H-1-benzazepin- 5-yl]-N-isopropylacetamide. J Med Chem. 2002. 45:3805–8. doi.10.1021/jm020133q.

21. Kawase M, Saito S, Motohashi N. Chemistry and biological activity of new 3-benzazepines. Int J of Antimicrobial Agent. 2000. 14(3):193–201. doi.10.1016/S0924-8579 (99)00155-7.

22. McNulty J, Nair JJ, Codina C, Bastida J, Pandey S, Gerasimoff J. et al. Selective apoptosis-inducing activity of crinum type Amaryllidaceae alkaloids. Phytochem. 2007. 68(7):1068–74. doi.10.1016/j.phytochem.2007.01.006.

23. Chang JH, Kang H, Jung I, Cho C. Total Synthesis of (±)-Galanthamine via a C3-Selective Stille Coupling and IMDA Cycloaddition Cascade of 3,5-Dibromo-2-pyrone. Org Lett. 2010. 12(9):2016–18. doi.10.1021/ol100617u.

24. Enders D, Lenzenm A, Raabe G. Asymmetric synthesis of the 1-epi aglycon of the cripowellins A and B. Angew Chem Int Ed. 2005. 44(24):3766–9. doi.10.1002/anie.200500556.

25. Cedron JC, Estevez-Braun A, Ravelo AG, Gutierrez D, Flores N, Bucio MA. et al. Bioactive montanine derivatives from halide-induced rearrangements of haemanthamine-type. Alkaloids absolute configuration by VCD. Org Lett. 2009. 11(7):1491–4. doi.10.1021/ol900065x.

26. Soto S, Vaz E, Dell'Aversana C, Alvarez R, Altucci L, de Lera AR. New synthetic approach to paullones and characterization of their SIRT1 inhibitory activity. Org Biomol Chem. 2012. 10:2101–12. doi.10.1039/C2OB06695E.

27. Ali A, Reddy GSK, Nalam MNL, Anjum SG, Cao H, Schiffer CA. et al. Structure-based design, synthesis, and structure-activity relationship studies of HIV-1 protease inhibitors incorporating phenyloxazolidinones. Med Chem. 2010. 53(21):7699–708. doi.10.1021/jm1008743.

28. Hughes RA, Harris T, Altmann E, Mcallister D, Vlahos R, Robertson A. et al. 2-methoxyestradiol and analogs as novel antiproliferative agents: analysis of three-dimensional quantitative structure-activity relationships for DNA synthesis inhibition and estrogen receptor binding. Mol Pharmacol. 2002. 61(5):1053–69.doi.10.1124/mol.61.5.1053.

29. Tashima T, Toriumi Y, Mochizuki Y, Nonomura T, Nagaoka S, Furukawa K. et al. Design, synthesis, and BK channel-opening activity of hexahydrodibenzazepinone derivatives. Bioorg Med Chem. 2006. 14(23):8014–31. doi.10.1016/j.bmc.2006.07.042.

30. Miki T, Kori M, Fujishima A, Mabuchi H, Tozawa R, Nakamura M. et al. Syntheses of fused heterocyclic compounds and their inhibitory activities for squalene synthase. Bioorg Med Chem. 2002. 10(2):385–400. doi.10.1016/S0968-0896(01)00289-9.

31. Bower JF, Szeto P, Gallagher T. Cyclic sulfamidates as versatile lactam precursors. An evaluation of synthetic strategies towards (–)-aphanorphine. Org Biomol Chem. 2007. 5:143–50. doi.10.1039/B614999E.

32. Bower JF, Szeto P, Gallagher T. Cyclic sulfamidates as lactam precursors: An efficient asymmetric synthesis of (-)-aphanorphine. Chem Commun. 2005. 46: 5793–5795. doi.10.1039/B510761J.

33. Zhai H, Luo S, Ye C, Ma Y. A facile asymmetric route to(–)- aphanorphine. J Org Chem. 2003. 68(21):8268–71. doi.10.1021/jo0348726.

34. Fuchs JR, Funk RL. Intramolecular electrophilic aromatic substitution reactions of 2-amidoacroleins: a new method for the preparation of tetrahydroisoquinolines, tetrahydro-3-benzazepines, and hexahydro-3-benzazocines. Org Lett. 2001. 3(21):3349–51. doi.10.1021/ol016592n.

35. Worden SM, Mapitse R, Hayes CJ. Towards a total synthesis of (–)-cephalotaxine: construction of the BCDE-tetracyclic core. Tetrahedron Lett. 2002. 43(34):6011–14. doi.10.1016/S0040-4039(02)01219-4.

36. Tietze LF, Modi A. Multicomponent domino reactions for the synthesis of biologically active natural products and drugs. Med Res Rev. 2000. 20(4):304–22. doi.10.1002/1098-1128(200007)20:4<304::AID-MED3>3.0.CO;2-8.

37. Couty S, Liegault B, Meyer C, Cossy J. Synthesis of 3-(arylmethylene)isoindolin-1-ones from ynamides by Heck–Suzuki–Miyaura domino reactions. Application to the synthesis of lennoxamine. Tetrahedron. 2006. 62(16):3882–95. doi.10.1016/j.tet.2005.11.089.

38. Comins DL, Schilling S, Zhang Y. Asymmetric Synthesis of 3-Substituted Isoindolinones: Application to the Total Synthesis of (+)-Lennoxamine. Org Lett. 2005. 7:95–8. doi.10.1021/ol047824w.

39. Hou FF, Zhang X, Zhang GH, Xie D, Chen PY, Zhang WR. et al. Efficacy and safety of benazepril for advanced chronic renal insufficiency. N Engl J Med. 2006. 354:131–40. doi.10.1056/NEJMoa053107.

40. Orimi FG, Mirza B, Hossaini Z. Production of benzazepine derivatives via four-component reaction of isatins: study of antioxidant activity. Mol Divers. 2020. 25:2171–82. doi. 10.1007/s11030-020-10110-5.

41. Sternbach LH. The benzodiazepine story. J Med Chem. 1979. 22(1):1–7. doi.10.1021/jm00187a001.

42. Walser A, Fryer IR. Dihydro-1, 4-Benzodiazepinones and Thiones. In: Fryer IR, Chemistry of Heterocyclic Compounds. A Series of Monographs. 1991. 50:631–848. doi.10.1002/9780470187371.ch8.

43. Qadir M. Recent structure activity relationship studies of 1, 4-benzodiazepines. Open J Chem. 2015. 8:8–12. doi.10.17352/pjmcr.000002.

44. Bernardy NC, Friedman MJ. Psychopharmacological strategies in the management of posttraumatic stress disorder (PTSD): what have we learned? Curr Psychiatry Rep. 2015. 17(20). doi.10.1007/s11920-015-0564-2.

45. Kaufmann CN, Spira AP, Depp CA, Mojtabai R. Long-term use of benzodiazepines and non benzodiazepine hypnotics 1999–2014. Psychiatr Serv. 2018. 69:235–8. doi.10.1176/appi.ps.201700095.

46. Paton C. Benzodiazepines and disinhibition: a review. Psychiat Bull. 2002. 26:460–2. doi. 10.1192/pb.26.12.460.

47. Batlle E, Lizano E, Vinas M, Pujol MD. 1, 4-benzodiazepines and new derivatives: description, analysis, and organic synthesis. Medicinal Chemistry. 2019. 63–90. doi.10.5772/intechopen.79879.

48. Goodman L, Gilman A. The pharmacological basis of therapeutics. Anesth Analg. 1941. 20:232–300. doi.10.1213/00000539-194101000- 00064.

49. Barbui C, Cipriani A, Patel V, Ayuso-Mateos JL, Ommeren MV. Efficacy of antidepressants and benzodiazepines in minor depression: Systematic review and meta-analysis. Br J Psychiatry. 2011. 198: 1–16. doi.10.1192/bjp.bp.109.076448.

50. File SE. The history of benzodiazepine dependence: A review of animal studies. Neuro Sci Bio Behav Rev. 1990. 14:135–46. doi.10.1016/s0149- 7634(05)80214-3.

51. Sawada N, Uchida H, Suzuki T, Watanabe K, Kikuchi T, Handa T. Persistence and compliance to antidepressant treatment in patients with depression: A chart review. BMC Psychiatry. 2009. 9:38. doi.10.1186/1471-244x-9-38.

52. Wick JY. The history of benzodiazepines. Consult Pharm. 2013. 28:538–48. doi.10.4140/tcp.n.2013.538.

53. Lopez-Munoz F, Alamo C, Garcia-Garcia P. The discovery of chlordiazepoxide and the clinical introduction of benzodiazepines: Half a century of anxiolytic drugs. J Anxiety Disord. 2011. 25:554–62. doi.org/10.1016/j.

54. Ghasemzadeh MA, Safaei-Ghomi J. CuI Nanoparticles as a Remarkable Catalyst in the Synthesis of Benzo[b][1,5]diazepines: an Eco-friendly Approach. Acta Chim Slov. 2015. 62:103–10. doi:10.17344/acsi.2014.775.

55. Ghasemzadeh MA, Ghomi JS. Synthesis and characterization of ZnO nanoparticles: Application to one-pot synthesis of benzo[b][1,5]diazepines. Cogent Chem. 2015, 1:1095060.doi:10.1080/23312009.2015.1095060.

56. Naeimi H, Foroughi H. ZnS nanoparticles as an efficient recyclable heterogeneous catalyst for one-pot synthesis of 4-substituted-1, 5-benzodiazepines. New J Chem. 2015. 39:1228–36. doi:10.1039/C4NJ01893A.

57. Gasemzadehh MA, Ghasemi-Seresht N. Facile and efficient synthesis of benzo[b][1,5]diazepines by three-component coupling of aromatic diamines, Meldrum's acid, and isocyanides catalyzed by Fe_3O_4 nanoparticles. Res Chem Intermed. 2015. 41:8625–36. doi.10.1007/s11164-014-1915-z

58. Shaabani A, Hezarkhani Z, Faroghi MT. Wool-SO_3H and nano-Fe_3O_4@wool as two green and natural-based renewable catalysts in one-pot isocyanide-based multicomponent reactions. Monatsh Chem. 2016. 147: 963–73. doi.10.1007/s00706-016-1717-7.

59. Singh RK, Saini M, Kumar S. Rapid and efficient synthesis of 1, 5-benzodiazepines promoted by stannic oxide nanoparticles under solvent-free conditions. Indian J Heterocyclic Chem. 2015. 25:151–6.

60. Korbekandi MM, Nasr-Esfahani N, Mohammadpoor-Baltork I, Moghadam M, Tangestaninejad S, Mirkhani V. Preparation and application of a new supported nicotine-based organocatalyst for synthesis of various 1,5-benzodiazepines.Catal Lett. 2019. 149:1057–66. doi.org/10.1007/s10562-019-02668-z.

61. Isaeva VI, Timofeeva MN, Panchenko VN, Lukoyanov IA, Chernyshev VV, Kapustin GI et al. Design of novel catalysts for synthesis of 1,5-benzodiazepines from1,2-phenylenediamine and ketones: NH_2-MIL-101(Al) as integrated structural scaffold for catalytic materials based on calix[4]arenes. J Catal. 2019. 369:60–71. doi.10.1016/j.jcat.2018.10.035.

62. Maleki A. Fe_3O_4/SiO_2 nanoparticles: an efficient and magnetically recoverable nanocatalyst for the one-pot multicomponent synthesis of diazepines. Tetrahedron. 2012. 68:7827–33. doi. 10.1016/j.tet.2012.07.034.

63. Maleki A. One-pot multicomponent synthesis of diazepine derivatives using terminal alkynes in the presence of silica-supported superparamagnetic iron oxide nanoparticles. Tetrahedron Lett. 2013. 54: 2055–9.

64. Maleki A, Ghamari N, Kamalzare M. Chitosan-supported Fe_3O_4 nanoparticles: a magnetically recyclable heterogeneous nanocatalyst for the syntheses of multifunctional benzimidazoles and benzodiazepines. RSC Adv. 2014. 4: 9416–23. doi.10.1039/C3RA47366J.

65. Sathe BP, Phatak PS, Dalve VS, Rote AB, Tigote RM, Haval KP. Synthesis of 1, 5-benzodiazepines by using Fe_3O_4@ SiO_2SO_3H nanocatalyst. Int Res J Science & Eng. 2018. A5:93–2.

66. Maleki A, Firouzi-Haji R, Farahani P. Green multicomponent synthesis of benzodiazepines in the presence of $CuFe_2O_4$ as an efficient magnetically recyclable nanocatalyst under solvent-free ball milling conditions at room temperature. Org Chem Res. 2018. 4(1):86– 94. doi.10.22036/org.chem.2018.96769.1106.

67. Shoeb M, Mobin M, Ali A, Zaman S, Naqvi AH. Graphene-mesoporous anatase TiO_2 nanocomposite: A highly efficient and recyclable heterogeneous catalyst for one-pot multicomponent synthesis of benzo-diazepine derivatives. Appl Organometal Chem. 2017. 32(1): e3961. doi.10.1002/aoc.3961.

68. Jamatia R, Gupta A, Dam B, Saha M, Pal AK. Graphite oxide: a metal free highly efficient carbocatalyst for the synthesis of 1,5-benzodiazepines under room temperature and solvent free heating conditions. Green Chem. 2017. 19:1576–85. doi.10.1039/c6gc03110b.

69. Zhang KY, Li J, Wang KX, An X, Wang LZ. Atom-economical Approaches to 1,5-Benzodiazepines Containing Indole Ring via Fe_3O_4@SiO_2-PTSA-catalyzed Multicomponent Domino Reactions. Chem Select. 2020. 5:14056–61. doi.org/10.1002/slct.202003903.

70. Savari A, Heidarizadeh F, Pourreza N. Synthesis and characterization of $CoFe_2O_4$@SiO_2@NH-NH_2-PCuW as an acidic nano catalyst for the synthesis of 1,4-benzodiazepines and a powerful dye remover. Polyhedron. 2019. 166: 233–47. doi.10.1016/j.poly.2019.03.046.

71. Singh A, Palakollu V, Pandey A, Kanvah S, Sharma S. Green synthesis of 1,4-benzodiazepines over La_2O_3 and $La(OH)_3$ catalysts: possibility of Langmuir–Hinshelwood adsorption. RSC Adv. 2016. 6:103455–62. doi.10.1039/C6RA22719H.

72. Kausar N, Mukherjee P, Das AR. Practical carbocatalysis by graphene oxide nanosheets in aqueous medium towards the synthesis of diversified dibenzo[1,4]diazepine scaffolds. RSC Adv. 2016. 6: 8904–10. doi.10.1039/C6RA17520A.

73. Vogler A. Fluorescence of Kryptofix 5 metal complexes. Inorg Chem Comms. 2015. 51:78–9. doi.10.1016/j.inoche.2014.11.011.

74. Iwata R, Pascali C, Terasaki K, Ishilkawa Y, Yanai K. Minimization of the amount of Kryptofix 222 - KHCO$_3$ for applications to microscale F-radiolabeling. Appl Radiat Isot. 2017. 125:113–18. doi.10.1016/j.apradiso.2017.04.021.

75. Huang A, Weidenthaler C, Caro J.Facile and reproducible synthesis of ITQ-29 zeolite by using Kryptofix 222 as the structure directing agent. Microporous Mesoporous Mater. 2010. 130:352–6. doi.10.1016/j.micromeso.2009.10.021.

76. Movassagh B, Ranjbari S. Kryptofix 5 as an inexpensive and efficient ligand for the palladium-catalyzed Mizoroki-Heck reaction. Appl OrganometChem. 2018. 32(4):e4224. doi.org/10.1002/aoc.4224.

77. Tudose M, Caproiu M, Badea FD, Nedelcu G, Ionita P, Constantinescu T. et al. New mono- and di-branched derivatives of Kryptofix K22 with N-4-methoxyamino-3,5-dinitrobenzoyl substituents. Synthesis and properties. ARKIVOC. 2011 73:343–54.

78. Ghaedi M, Niknam K, Zamani S, AbasiLarki H, Roosta M, Soylak M. Silica chemically bonded N-propyl kriptofix 21 and 22 with immobilized palladium nanoparticles for solid phase extraction and preconcentration of some metal ions, Mater Sci Eng. 2013. 33:3180–9. doi.10.1016/j.msec.2013.03.045.

79. Mozafari R, Ghadermazi M. A nickel nanoparticle engineered CoFe$_2$O$_4$@GO–Kryptofix 22 composite: a green and retrievable catalytic system for the synthesis of 1,4- benzodiazepines in water. RSC Adv. 2020. 10(26):15052–64. doi.10.1039/D0RA01671C

80. Shaabani A, Hezarkhani Z, Nejad MK. AuCu and AgCu bimetallic nanoparticles supported on guanidine-modified reduced graphene oxide nanosheets as catalysts in the reduction of nitroarenes: tandem synthesis of benzo[b][1,4] diazepine derivatives. RSC Adv. 2016. 6:30247–57. doi.10.1039/C6RA03132C.

81. De K, Bhanja P, Bhaumik A, Mukhopadhyay C.Zeolite-Y mediated multicomponent reaction of isatins, cyclic-1,3- diketones and 1,2-phenylenediamine: An easy access to Spiro dibenzo [1,4] diazepines. ChemCatChem. 2017. 10:590–600. doi:10.1002/cctc.201701487.

82. Nasira Z, Alia A, Shakira M, Wahabb R, Shamsuzzamana L. Silica supported NiOnanocomposite prepared *via* sol-gel technique and its excellent catalytic performance for one-pot multicomponent synthesis of benzodiazepine derivatives under microwave irradiation. *New J Chem.* 2017. 41:5893–903. doi.10.1039/C6NJ04013F.

83. Safaei-Ghomi J, Paymard-Samani S, Shahbazi-Alavi H. MNPs-NHC$_6$H$_4$SO$_3$H as high-performance catalyst for the synthesis of 1,4-diazepines containing tetrazole ring under microwave irradiation. J Chin Chem Soc. 2018. 65:1119–26. doi.10.1002/jccs.201700349.

84. Miri NS, Safaei-Ghomi J. Synthesis of benzodiazepines catalyzed by CoFe$_2$O$_4$@SiO$_2$-PrNH$_2$ nanoparticles as a reusable catalyst. Int J Med Nano Res. 2018. 72:497–503. doi.10.1515/nano.0074.00001.

3 An Overview of the Synthesis of Pyrroline, Indolizine, and Quinolizinium Derivatives Using Different Nanocatalysts

R. N. Shelke,[1] A. B. Kanagare,[2] S. U. Deshmukh,[2]
S. R. Bembalkar,[2] D. N. Pansare,[2] Keshav Lalit Ameta,[3] and
R. P. Pawar[4]

[1] Department of Chemistry, Sadguru Gadage Maharaj College Karad, Maharashtra, India
[2] Department of Chemistry, Deogiri College, Aurangabad, Maharashtra, India
[3] Department of Chemistry, School of Liberal Arts and Sciences, Mody University of Science and Technology, Lakshmangarh, Rajasthan, India
[4] Department of Chemistry, Shiv Chhatrapati College, Aurangabad, Maharashtra, India

3.1 INTRODUCTION

3.1.1 PYRROLINE

Heterocyclic ring systems are the fundamental building blocks in the majority of drugs that are used to treat animal and human diseases. Among these heterocyclic rings, those that contain nitrogen (N) are the most significant. Pyrrolines, which are the dihydro derivatives of pyrroles, have received considerable attention recently since they exhibit a large range of biological activities. Pyrrolines have three structural isomer classes (Figure 3.1), which is based on the double bond: (1) 1-pyrrolines (3,4-dihydro-2H-pyrroles); (2) 2-pyrrolines (2,3-dihydro-1H-pyrroles); and (3) 3-pyrrolines (2,5-dihydro-1H-pyrroles).

Pyrrolines are considered privileged structures, which is reflected by their presence in many bioactive compounds from natural sources,[1–9] such as hemes, chlorophyll,[10] alkaloids,[11,12] and in bioactive synthetic molecules.[13–19]

1-pyrrolines are cyclic imines whose reactivity allows synthetic manipulation through a nucleophilic attack on the prochiral endocyclic imine. Therefore, stereoselective transformations can occur.[20] 2-pyrrolines possess an enamine moiety that permits the further functionalization of the ring system. 2-pyrrolidines are found frequently within the literature as 2,3-dihydropyrroles since the monohydrogenation of pyrroles leads to 2,3-dihydropyrroles. In contrast, the cyclic amine and alkene functional groups of the 3-pyrrolines react separately. When this cyclic core is employed as a precursor, further modifications often involve the covalent bond, which might be easily transformed, for example, by hydrogenation, (di)halogenation and dihydroxylation. Therefore, the 1-, 2-, and 3-pyrrolines represent appealing intermediates to produce pyrroles and pyrrolidines

DOI: 10.1201/9781003141488-3

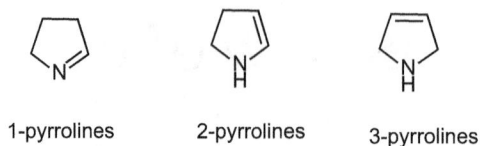

1-pyrrolines   2-pyrrolines   3-pyrrolines

FIGURE 3.1   Structural isomers of the pyrrolines

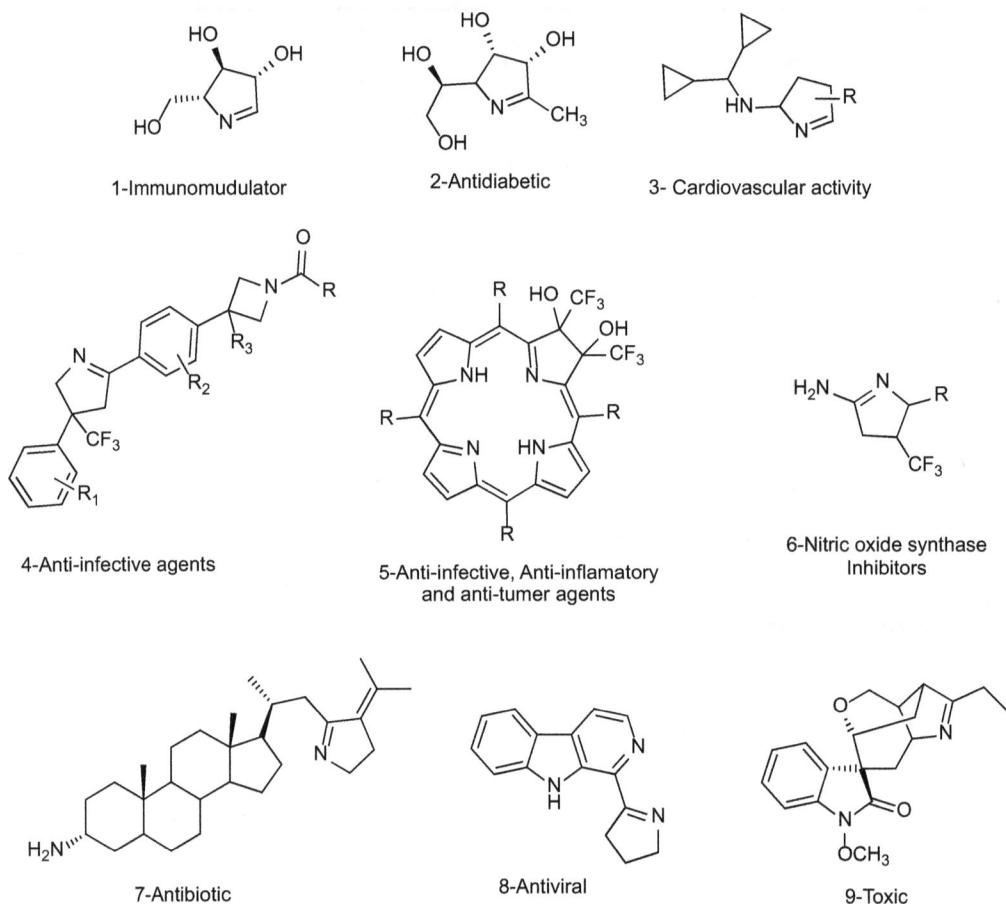

1-Immunomudulator   2-Antidiabetic   3- Cardiovascular activity

4-Anti-infective agents   5-Anti-infective, Anti-inflamatory   6-Nitric oxide synthase
                              and anti-tumer agents   Inhibitors

7-Antibiotic   8-Antiviral   9-Toxic

FIGURE 3.2   Selected examples of biologically active 1-pyrrolines

through oxidation[21] and reduction,[22,23] respectively. Due to the remarkable breadth of their reactivity, pyrrolines are useful intermediates within the preparation of more complex heterocycles.[24–37]

The 1-pyrroline core is found in numerous compounds with biological activity (Figure 3.2). Examples include the iminosugar nectrisine (1),[38] which was discovered as an immunomodulator; the iminosaccharide 2 that has glycosidase inhibitory activity,[39,40] and 1-pyrroline 3 that has antihypertensive properties,[41] b-trifluoromethylated 1-pyrrolines (4–6)[42] are gas synthase inhibitors[43] and possess anti-infective,[44–46] antitumor,[47] and anti-inflammatory activities.[48]

The five-membered, nitrogen-containing (N) pyrroline ring might be a privileged structure. This ring is present in many bioactive compounds from natural sources. This chapter aims to elucidate the most recent advances for the synthesis of pyrrolines by transition metal-catalyzed cyclizations. Only reactions during which the pyrroline ring is made by metal promotion will be described. Transformations of the pyrroline ring in other heterocycles, and therefore, the structural manipulations of the pyrroline itself are not discussed. The chapter is organized into three parts, each covers the metal-mediated synthesis of the three pyrroline isomers. Each part is subdivided according to the metal involved and concludes with a brief description of notable biological activities within the class.[49]

1-pyrrolines can be synthesized by copper (Cu) catalysis. Chiba et al[50] developed a way for the synthesis of oxymethyl substituted pyrrolines that employed Copper(II) acetate ($Cu(OAc)_2$)-mediated intramolecular aminooxygenation of alkenylimines with 2,2,6,6-tetramethylpiperidinyloxy (TEMPO) (Scheme 3.1). The addition of a Grignard reagent (i.e., p-tolylmagnesium bromide) to a variety of alkenyl carbonitriles **1** was performed in a sealed tube at 60°C, methanol (MeOH) was used to protonate the products, and dimethyl formamide (DMF) was added in a degree of 0.1 molar concentration. Then, 1 equivalent of $Cu(OAc)_2$ and 1.5 equivalents of TEMPO were added. The aminooxygenation proceeded smoothly at 60°C producing (after 2 h) diverse oxymethyl pyrrolines **2** in moderate yields (typically 50%). Various other Grignard reagents were equally successful in this process.

Stevens et al[51] synthesized a library of 10 1-pyrrolines from α,α,-dichlorinated imines **3** that employed a heteroatom transfer radical cyclization (HATRC) (Scheme 3.2). The free radical ring closure reaction was performed with copper chloride (CuCl) in the presence of N,N,N',N",N"-pentamethyldiethylenetriamine (PMDTA) as a ligand. Other ligands, such as N,N,N',N'-tetramethylethylenediamine (TMEDA) proved equally efficient. The addition of these ligands modified the solubility, and therefore, the redox potential of the Cu catalyst; therefore, improving its activity. The formation of the five-membered ring proceeded through a radical 5-exo-trig cyclization **4**. Two stereogenic centers were generated during the ring closure. The reaction displayed a superb cis/trans diastereoselectivity (i.e., diastereoisomeric ratios are in the range of 90 to 100). The diastereoselectivity was attributed to the steric hindrance caused by the ethoxy substituents of the phosphonate.

The development of a novel selective Cu-catalyzed, azide radical-mediated, [2 + 2 + 1] annulation of benzene-linked **5**, n-enynes (n = 6, 7) to give fused pyrrolines **7** (Scheme 3.3). Azidobenziodoxolone **6** was the source of the azide radical. Other azide reagents, such as trimethylsilyl azide ($TMSN_3$) and sodium azide (NaN_3) failed to produce the fused pyrrolines. This one-step synthesis of fused pyrrolines proceeded via the generation of the azide radical from azidobenziodoxolone **6** with the aid of the Cu^{2+} species as catalyst.[52]

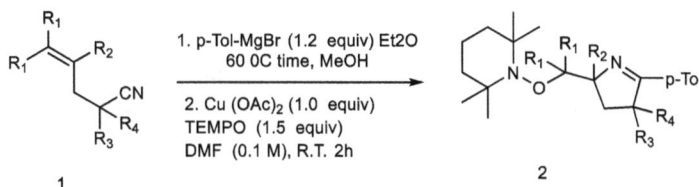

SCHEME 3.1 Cu(II)-mediated intramolecular aminooxygenation of alkenylimines toward 1-pyrrolines

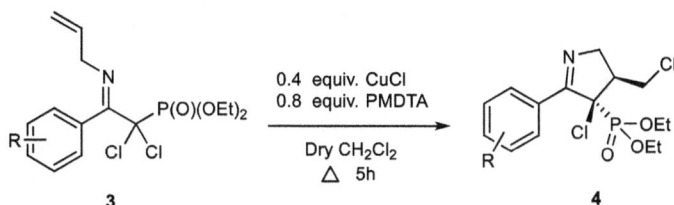

SCHEME 3.2 Cu-catalyzed HATRC toward 1-pyrrolines

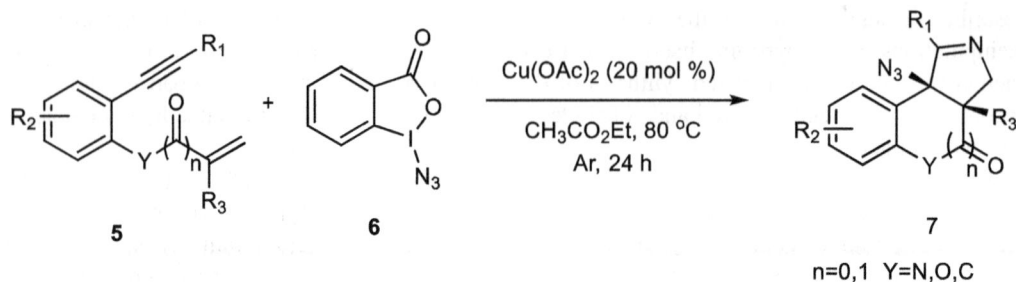

SCHEME 3.3 [2 + 2 + 1] Annulation/azidation of 1,n-enynes as an entry to fused 1-pyrrolines

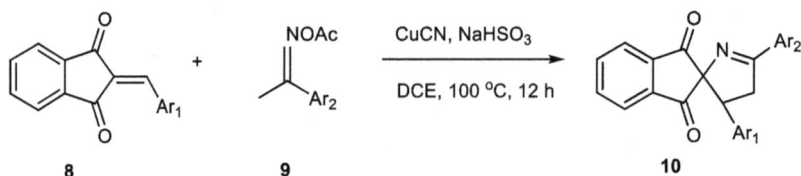

SCHEME 3.4 Cu-catalyzed heteroannulation reaction between aryl ketone-derived ketoxime acetates and 2-arylideneindane-1,3-dione

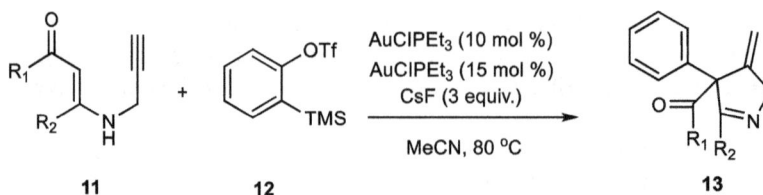

SCHEME 3.5 Au-catalyzed cyclization of N-propargylic β-enaminones **1** toward 1-pyrrolines **2** in presence of aryne precursor **3**

The development of an efficient Cu-catalyzed heteroannulation reaction between 2-arylideneindane-1,3-diones **8** and ketoxime acetates **9** for the straightforward synthesis of spiro[indane-1,3-dione-1-pyrrolines] **10** was developed (Scheme 3.4). The methodology showed broad substrate scope and tolerated functionalities in the 2-arylideneindane-1,3-diones and aromatic ketoxime acetates. Alkyl ketoxime acetates did not deliver the spiro compounds.[53]

3.1.2 Synthesis of 1-pyrrolines by Gold Catalysis

Through catalyst screening, the mixture of gold triphenylphosphine gold(I) chloride (AuCl·Pet$_3$) (10 mol%) and silver hexa fluoroantimonate (AgSbF$_6$) (15 mol%) in the presence of the aryne precursor **13** in CH$_3$CN at 80°C gave the best yields (Scheme 3.5). Evaluation of the scope of the reaction using different N-propargylic β-enaminones demonstrated that enaminone with electron-donating groups increased the yield of cyclization products.[54]

Yang et al[55] showed oxime esters as electrophilic partners for iron (Fe) catalysis (Scheme 3. 6). Reductive cleavage of the oxime nitrogen–oxygen (N–O) bond by Fe generated useful iminyl radicals,[56] Coupling of iminyl radical derivatives of ɤ,δ-unsaturated oxime **14** with silyl enol ether **15** lead to pyrroline **16** through an intramolecular C–N bond formation. The Oche and therefore the Okamoto group disclosed a Fe-catalyzed methodology to realize 1-pyrrolines **16** (Scheme 3.6),

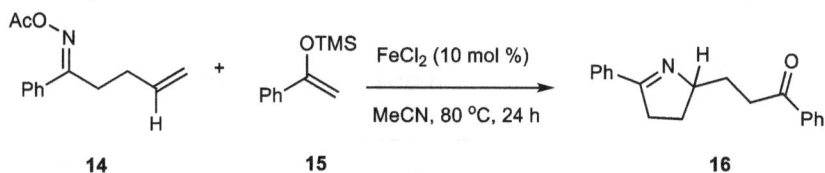

SCHEME 3.6 Fe-catalyzed coupling of O-acyloximes with silyl enol ethers.

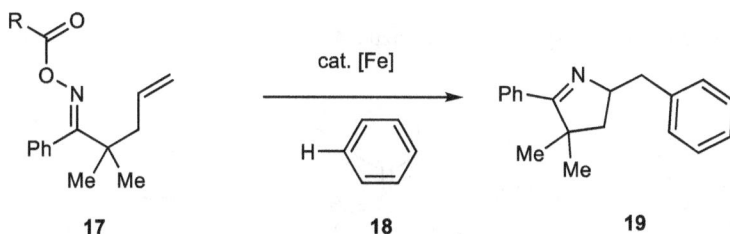

SCHEME 3.7 Synthesis of 1-pyrrolines **19**

which involved the formation of iminyl radicals from alkene-tethered oxime esters **14** and subsequent aminative cyclization and intermolecular homolytic aromatic substitution (Scheme 3.7).[57] The optimized conditions used 10 mol% of iron(II) trifluoro methanesulfonate (Fe(OTf)$_2$) and ligand L1 in the presence of aromatic compounds (150 equiv.). The mixture was heated a 120°C for 12 h. The reaction tolerated different arenes **18** with electron-rich and electron-poor substituents, polycyclic aromatic compounds and as N or sulfur-containing (S) heteroarenes. For the scope of alkene-tethered oxime ester **17**, R = picolinoyl ester **17a**-2-Py and R= pivaloyl ester **17a**-tBu could be used with the picolinoyl ester that gave better yields with substituted arenes. Oxime esters with substituted alkenes (R1≠ H and/or R2 ≠ H) provided 1-pyrrolines **19** in good yields.

3.2 INDOLIZINE

An indolizine-based oligomer was synthesized by stirring of 1-(α-alkoxybenzyl)-indolizine derivative in chloroform. The oligomer was characterized as an octamer; it had been the most component within the obtained mixture of oligomers. The oligomerization was accelerated by acid and lightweight. The green color of the oligomer under acidic conditions turned raw sienna under basic conditions. This color change might be repeated by changing the acidic/basic conditions. An indolizine framework that consisted of an electron-deficient pyridine ring and an [a]-fused electron-rich pyrrole ring (Scheme 3.8), provided a biased electron density. Because of this electronic structure, indolizine derivatives exhibit potential biological activities,[58,59] and optical properties.[60–62] Therefore, numerous indolizines have been synthesized by several methods.[63–65] Previously, an artificial method was demonstrated for functionalized indolizines from 2-ethynylpyridines that used functionalities; a nucleophilic ring N and reactive ethynyl group.[66] When a solution of indolizine in chloroform-d was stirred at room temperature (RT) for 1 day, the color of the solution changed from yellowish-brown to bluish-green. This experimental result prompted the study of this phenomenon; an indolizine-based oligomer was formed.[67] However, detailed information was not obtained due to a poor experimental environment. After the preliminary findings, any report that handled indolizine-based oligomer was not found during the last half century, which prompted a focus and reinvestigation of this phenomenon. Indolizine has gained increased attention as a key pharmacophore in a number of small molecule drug discovery research.[68,69] Distinctive substitution patterns of basic indolizine backbone allowed a variety of biological activities. Therefore, synthetic methods

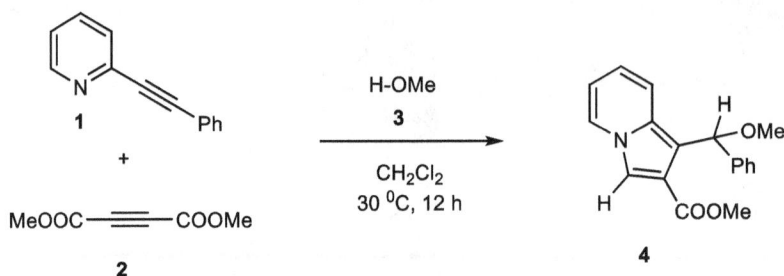

SCHEME 3.8 Three-component synthesis of indolizine **4**

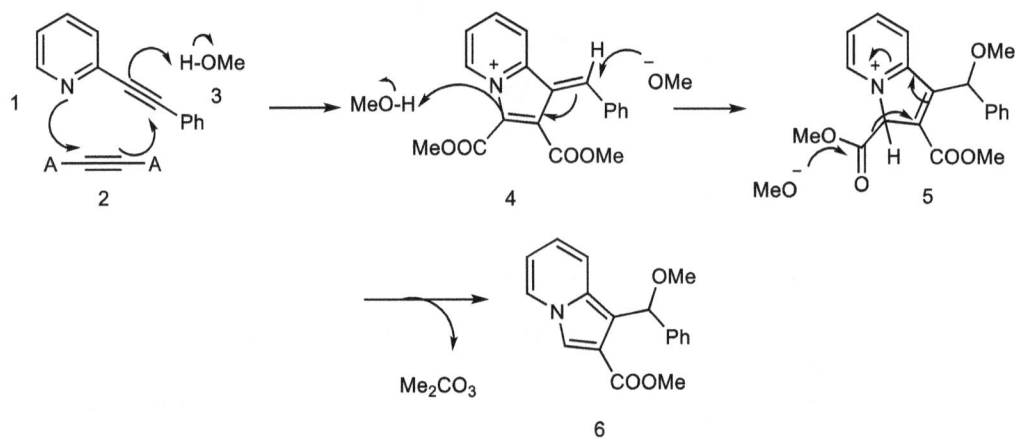

SCHEME 3.9 Potential mechanism for the formation of indolizine **4**

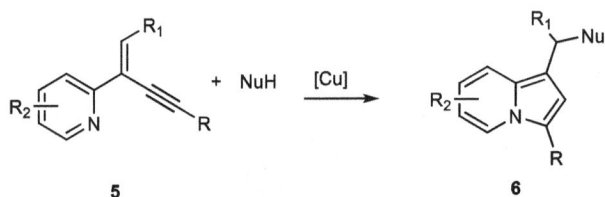

SCHEME 3.10 Synthesis of indolizine derivatives

to allow suitable functional groups to be inserted around this chemical core are highly desirable.[70,71] Therefore, a highly efficient domino Knoevenagel condensation or intramolecular aldol cyclization route for novel indolizines with polyfunctionalized pyridine units has previously been reported.[72] The synthesized indolizine chemical library has unprecedented substitution patterns on the pyridine moiety, which enabled research into their pharmacological activity. The potential mechanism for the formation of indolizine 4 is shown in Scheme 3.9. The synthesis of indolizine derivatives 6 is shown in Scheme 3.10. The synthesis of indolizine 8 is shown in Scheme 3.11.

3.2.1 GENERAL PROCEDURE FOR PREPARATION OF INDOLIZINES

To a solution of 2-phenylethynylpyridine **1a** (179 mg, 1.0 mmoL) in dichloromethane (10 mL), dimethyl acetylenedicarboxylate **2a** (213 mg, 1.5 mmol) and methanol **3a** (0.81 mL, 20 mmoL) were added, and the resultant mixture was stirred at 30°C for 1 day. After removal of the solvent,

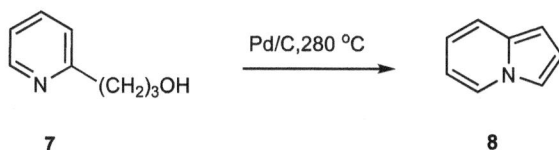

SCHEME 3.11 Synthesis of indolizine

the residue was treated with chromatography on a colloid wrapped with aluminum foil to produce indolizine **4a** (e.g., eluted with dichloromethane, 177 mg, 0.6 mmol, 60%) as pale yellow oil. Other indolizines were prepared similarly.

Efficient and atom economical access to indolizines was developed by a Cu-catalyzed cyclization of 2-(2-enynyl)pyridines with various nucleophiles through the simultaneous formation of a C–N bond and a foreign C–nucleophile bond. 1,3-dicarbonyl compounds, indoles, amides, alcohol, and even water, were used as nucleophiles during this reaction. Good to excellent yields of the corresponding indolizines were obtained under mild reaction conditions.[73]

3.2.2 INHIBITORY ACTIVITIES OF INDOLIZINE DERIVATIVES

3.2.2.1 Anticancer Activity

The indolizine derivative 1 that has 2-pyridyl amide moiety (Figure 3.1) was synthesized and discovered as a potent inhibitor of the hedgehog pathway for tumor regression with a Gli-luciferase (Gli-Luc) S12 IC_{50} value of 4.2 µM. The screening was carried out according to Gli-Luc activity in S12 cells assay.[74]

Inhibitions of tubulin polymerization and HL60 cell growth assays were reported using the synthesized indolizine compounds 2 and 3 (Figure 3.3) were determined by molecular docking analysis. Indolizines **2** and **3** exhibited potent inhibition of tubulin polymerization in vitro with IC_{50} values of 20 and 12.8 µM, respectively. Compounds 2 and 3 demonstrated strong antiproliferative activities with IC_{50} values of 1.4 and 0.6 µM, respectively, against HL60 cancer cell lines compared with positive control. The results of the molecular docking study revealed that compounds 2 and 3 interacted directly with the colchicine binding pocket on tubulin where the 3,4,5-trimethoxyphenyl group was bound to the binding site of colchicine through a hydrophobic interaction with Leu 248, Ala 250, Leu 255, and Ala 316 of tubulin, respectively. The indolizine ring of compound 2 interacted with the non-aromatic part of the sidechain of Asn 258 in β-tubulin.

For compound **3**, the cyano group interacted with Val 181 and Lys 352 sidechains and Asn 258 sidechain in β-tubulin, and the carbonyl function acted as an H bond acceptor to the amino group of Asp 251 main chain.[75]

A series of 3-cyclopropylcarbonyl-indolizines 4 (Figure 3.3) were prepared and investigated for their antiproliferative and epidermal growth factor receptor (EGFR) kinase inhibitory activity against Hep-G2 cell line (i.e., human hepatocellular liver carcinoma) using 3-(4,5-dimethylthiazol-2-yl)-2,5-diphenyl tetrazolium bromide (MTT) and the reference compound 5-fluorouracil. Compared with the 5-fluorouracil reference, the most active compounds were 4 (R=H, R_1=1,2-N-phenylamleimide), 4 (R=R_1=H, R_2=CN), 4 (R=7-CH_3, R_1=H, R_2=CN) and 4 (R=5-CH_3,8-Br, R_1=H, R_2=CN) with IC_{50} values of 0.48, 0.39, 0.29, and 0.20 mg/mL. In addition, compound 4 (R=5-CH_3, 8-Br, R_1=H, R_2=CN) exhibited potent EGFR kinase inhibitory activity with IC_{50}= 0.085 µM, which was closely related to the reference anticancer drug Iressa (IC_{50}= 0.033 µM).[76]

The synthesized benzoyl-indolizine derivatives 5 (Figure 3.3) were established as potent human farnesyltransferase (FTase) inhibitors. The p-bromophenyl derivatives 5 (R_1=CH_3, R_2=H, X=Br, Y=O, n=1) that incorporated an ester moiety on the indolizine ring showed the most potent inhibition potential with IC_{50} = 1.3 µM. The FTase inhibitors were developed for anticancer therapy.[77]

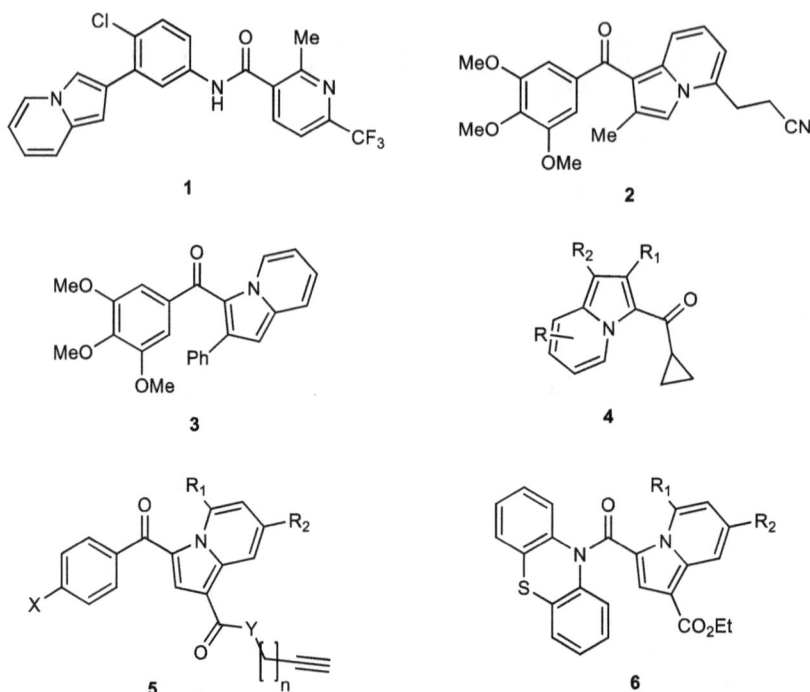

FIGURE 3.3 Indolizine derivative

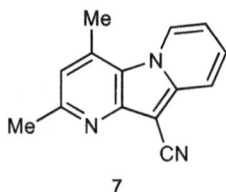

FIGURE 3.4 Pyrido-fused-indolizine derivative

The phenothiazine-based indolizine derivatives **6** (Figure 3.3) were synthesized by [3+2] cycloaddition reaction and then tested for their antiproliferative activity against 60 cell lines and as microtubule-targeting agents. Compounds 6 showed modest tubulin polymerization inhibition of 31% and 42%, respectively, at 10.40 M. The phenothiazine derivative 6 was the most potent with GI_{50} values between 0.67 and 7.90 μM on 60 cell lines, where the best activity was for a melanoma (SK-MEL-2) cell line (GI_{50} 0.67 μM) and the least was for ovarian cancer (OVCAR-4) cell line (GI_{50} 7.9 μM).[78] The pyrido-fused-indolizine derivatives 7 (Figure 3.4) were reported as potent anticancer agents. They were effective against all colorectal cancer (CRC) cell lines. Compound 7 (R=3,4-of hydrophilic (OH)) showed the highest activity against HT-29 and HCT116 with IC_{50} values 14.3 and 14.8 μM, respectively. Structure-activity relationship (SAR) established that the presence of OH groups at the 3- and 4- positions of the aromatic ring and at C4 of the indolizine moiety were fundamental for the potency against CRC cell lines. The cytotoxicity results confirmed that compound 7 (R = 3,4-OH) was not toxic at the concentrations needed to minimize the viability of the CRC cell lines by 50%.[79]

3.2.2.2 Antiviral activity

A number of indolizine-esters 1 (Figure 3.5) were synthesized by a multistep reaction and examined for their anti-HIV-1 activity. Compound **1** (Ar = Ph) (VEC-5) was established as a potent HIV-1 viral

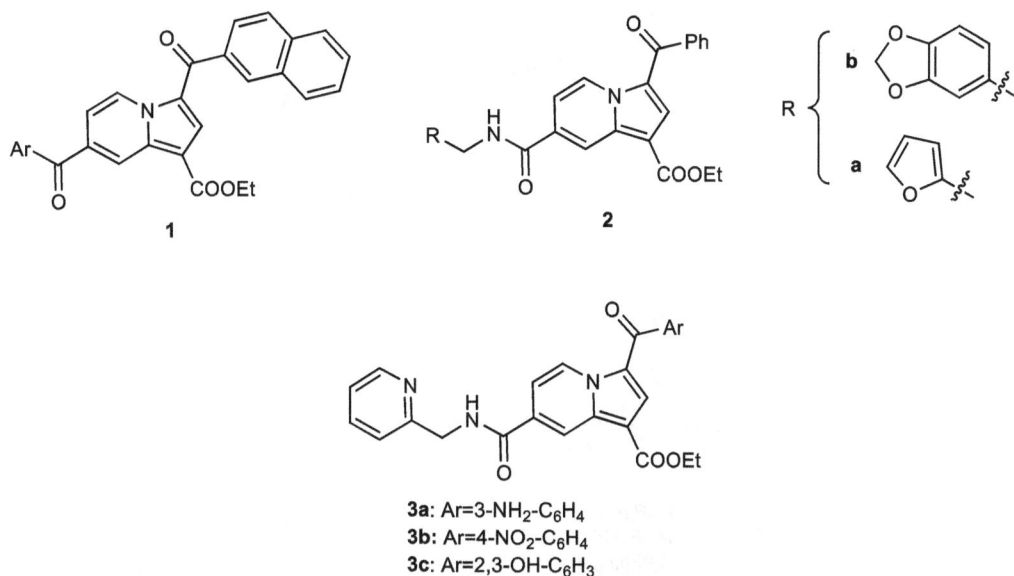

FIGURE 3.5 Indolizine-esters

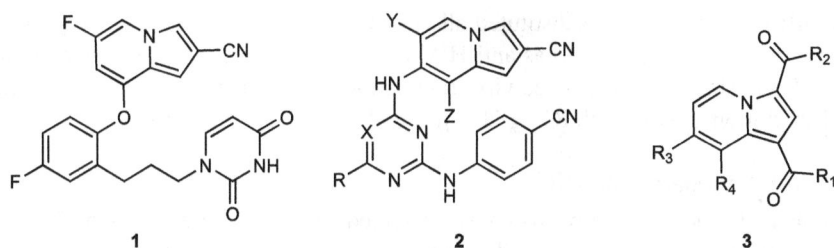

FIGURE 3.6 Indolizine derivatives

infectivity factor (VIF) inhibitor under clinical trials and was promising as a potent prodrug (with $IC_{50}= 36.1$ μM and $CC_{50}= 167.4$ μM). SAR proved that the insertion of hydrophilic groups (OH or NH_2) at the benzoyl moiety led to a remarkable decrease in antiviral activity than the unsubstituted benzoyl. However, replacing phenyl with 4-pyridyl moiety significantly improved the antiviral activity.

Therefore, compound 1 (Ar = 4-pyridyl) revealed the best inhibitory potency against HIV-1 VIF with an IC_{50} of 11.0 μM and SI of 12.5, which was far better than VEC-5, and proved that it was a highly promising candidate for HIV-1 clinical trials. The modification of the ester group led to promising results to further improve the inhibitor's activity.[80, 81] The synthesis of various indolizine heterocycles 2 and 3 (Figure 3.5) was reported and their activity as HIV-1 VIF inhibitors was evaluated. Most of the reported derivatives showed good inhibition activities for VIF-mediated A3G degradation, compared with the known VIF inhibitor VEC-5 with low cytotoxicities. The best inhibitory activity was observed in compounds 2a and 2b with IC_{50} of 19.3 and 20.1 μM, respectively. The reported results were important for the development of more potent anti-HIV drugs.[82,83] A series of indolizine derivatives that had pyrimidine or 1,3,5-triazine moieties 1 and 2 (Figure 3.6) were useful as non-nucleoside inhibitors of HIV-1 reverse transcriptase (HIV-RT). Compounds 1 and 2 were potent HIV-RT inhibitors with EC_{50} values <10 nM with greater activity than the reference Efavirenz (EC_{50} 30 μM) and had normal cytotoxicity and good solubility.[84] Numerous indolizine compounds that have general structure 3 (Figure 3.5) [R_1 = NH_2, NHalkyl, OH, OEt; R_2 = aryl, alkyl,

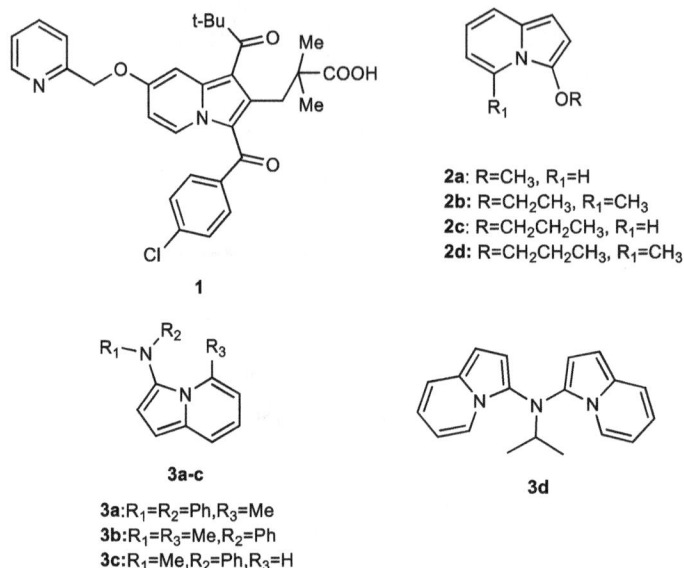

FIGURE 3.7 Indolizine derivatives

NH_2, NHCOR; R_3 = H and R_4 = substituted alkyl or CHO; or R_3 = substituted alkyl or CHO and R_4 = H] were invented and evaluated as anti-HIV-1 agents. The prepared compounds inhibited the activity of VIF and significantly reduced virus replication. Compound 3, for example, demonstrated high HIV-1 inhibition activity with IC_{50} = 20.1 μM and 50% CC_{50} 250.5 μM[85].

3.2.2.3   Anti-inflammatory activity

A large number of indolizine derivatives were patented as effective inhibitors of 5-lipoxygenase activating protein (FLAP) that inhibit leukotriene production for the treatment of asthma. Among the reported compounds, **1** (Figure 3.7) exhibited high inhibitory activity against inhibitor of 5-lipoxygenase-activating protein (LAP) with IC_{50} = 44 nM.[86] 3-alkoxyindolizine derivatives **2** (Figure 3.7) were reported as interesting inhibitors of interleukin-6 (IL-6) on lipopolysaccharide (LPS)-induced IL-6 expression using dexamethasone as a reference drug with inhibition of 100% at 1.0 μM. The compounds **2a** and **2b** revealed better IL-6 inhibitory action at 100 μM in macrophages with 66% and 74% inhibition ratio, respectively. Compounds **2** were found lead ones for further optimization as potent anti-inflammatory agents.[87]

The anti-inflammatory activity of synthesized four derivatives of 3-aminoindolizines **3a-d** (Figure 3.7.) was examined against LPS in RAW264.7 cells for the inhibition of IL-6. The four derivatives (3a-d) revealed moderate inhibition effects (45%–61% at 50 μM) compared with the reference dexamethasone (100% at 1.0 μM). The best candidate was **3b,** which showed 61% inhibition at 50 μM for IL-6, which was the lead compound for the investigation of potential anti-inflammatory drugs.[88]

3.2.2.4   Antimicrobial agents

A number of indolizine compounds 1-3 (Figure 3.8) were reported as effective antibacterial and antifungal agents. An antimicrobial assay was conducted against four fungal and 13 bacterial strains. Three derivatives **1a** (R=CO_2Me), **1b** (R=CO_2Et), and **2a** (R_1=H, R=CN) were effective against all 13 bacterial strains (e.g., Gram-positive and negative bacterial strains). Compound **3** showed minimum inhibitory concentration (MIC) values of 32–128 μg/ml against seven bacterial strains (*Escherichia coli, Bacillus subtilis, Vibrio cholera, Klebsiella pneumoniae, Staphylococcus aureus,*

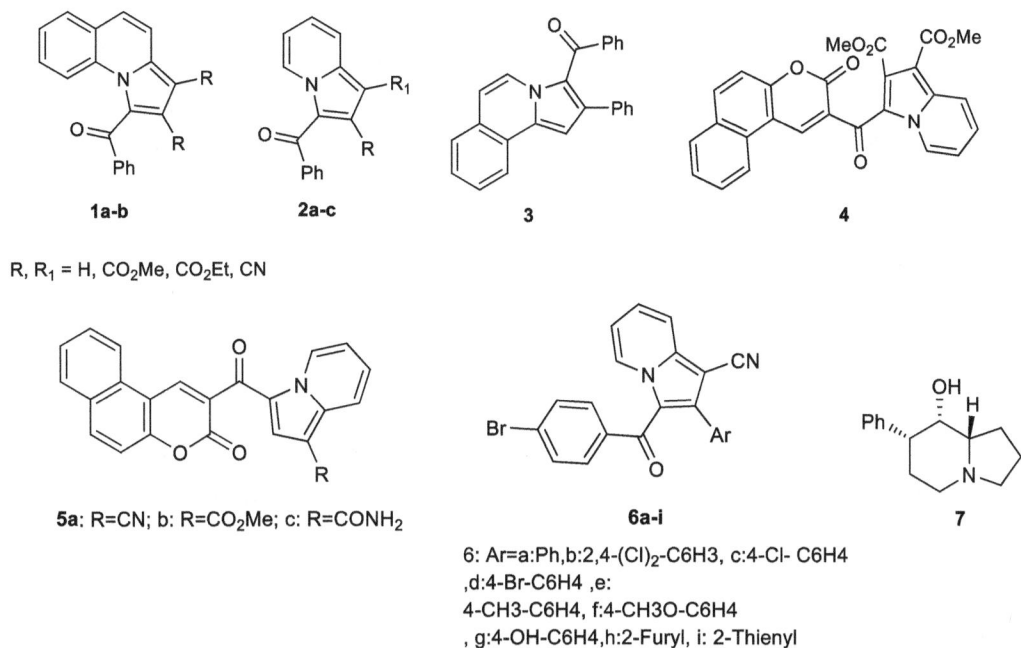

R, R$_1$ = H, CO$_2$Me, CO$_2$Et, CN

1a-b   **2a-c**   **3**   **4**

5a: R=CN; b: R=CO$_2$Me; c: R=CONH$_2$ **6a-i**   **7**

6: Ar=a:Ph,b:2,4-(Cl)$_2$-C6H3, c:4-Cl- C6H4
,d:4-Br-C6H4 ,e:
4-CH3-C6H4, f:4-CH3O-C6H4
, g:4-OH-C6H4,h:2-Furyl, i: 2-Thienyl

FIGURE 3.8   Indolizine derivatives

Shigella dysenteriae, and *Pseudomonas aeruginosa*) and showed inhibition activity toward three fungi (*Candid. albicans, Aspergillus niger* and *Candida tropicalis*) with MIC values 500–1,000 µg/mL and zone diameters 12, 30, and 10 mm, respectively.[89] The antimicrobial activity of the synthesized indolizine derivatives **4** and **5** (Figure 3.8) was evaluated. The reported results showed that most of the examined compounds had variable inhibitory activity on the growth of bacterial and fungal strains. Inhibition activity against the Gram-positive bacteria was better than the Gram-negative one. The tested compounds showed moderate inhibition activity against *Aspergillus fumigates, Geotrichum candidum,* and *C. albicans* compared with the standard itraconazole and clotrimazole drugs. Compound **4** was the most potent against *S. aureus, B. subtilis, P. aeruginosa,* and *E. coli* compared with penicillin G and streptomycin standard drugs.[90] A number of indolizine-1-carbonitrile derivatives **6** (Figure 3.8) were synthesized and evaluated for in vitro antibacterial activity against a number of Gram-positive and negative bacteria and antifungal activity against a variety of filamentous fungi and yeasts. The best in vitro antifungal activity was observed for compound 6b (Ar = 2,4-Cl$_2$C$_6$H$_3$) with MICs = 8-32 µg/mL; however compound **6g** (Ar = 4-HOC$_7$H$_4$) was the most active against bacteria with MICs = 16-256 µg/mL. In addition, compound **6g** exhibited bactericidal activities with minimum bactericidal concentrations similar to their corresponding MICs.[91]

A series of indolizine derivatives 5-7 (Figure 3.8) were synthesized and screened for their antibacterial effects. The studied microbes included several bacterial (Gram-positive and negative bacteria) and fungal strains. The synthesized indolizines 5-7 exhibited selective toxicity to Gram-positive bacteria *S. aureus* and inhibited the acido-resistant rod *Mycobacterium smegmatis.*[92]

3.2.2.5   Antitubercular activity

Several indolizine derivatives 1-4 87-90 (Figure 3.9) were synthesized and their in vitro antimycobacterial activity were screened against *Mycobacterium tuberculosis* H37Rv (MTB) by determining the MIC in triplicate. All indolizines revealed potent antimycobacterial activities and among them, three derivatives, **3** (R = 4-F), **4** (R = 4-Cl), and **4** (R = 4-F), with MIC values of 3,

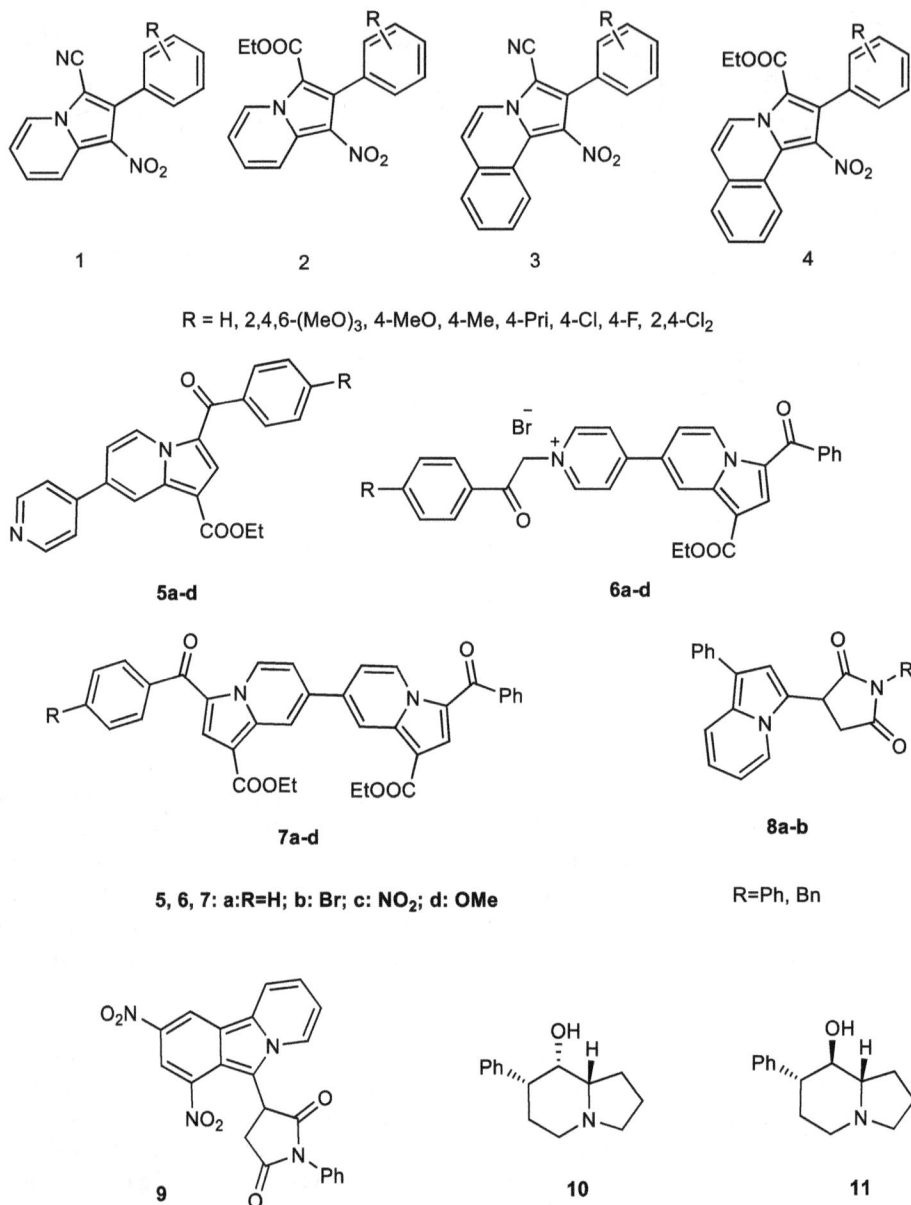

R = H, 2,4,6-(MeO)$_3$, 4-MeO, 4-Me, 4-Pri, 4-Cl, 4-F, 2,4-Cl$_2$

5a-d

6a-d

7a-d

8a-b

5, 6, 7: a:R=H; b: Br; c: NO$_2$; d: OMe

R=Ph, Bn

9

10

11

FIGURE 3.9 Structures of indolizines derivatives

3.9 and 1.0 μM, respectively, were stronger than the reference drug ethambutol (MIC 7.6 μM). Of interest, the best inhibition activity was detected in compound **4** (R= 4-F) which displayed 7.6 and 4.7 times more powerful than ethambutol and ciprofloxacin reference drugs, respectively.[93]

Then, the indolizine heterocycles 5-6 (Figure 3.9) were synthesized and evaluated for antimycobacterial effects. The mono-indolizine mono-salts **6a-d** on primary antimycobacterial screening exhibited superior potency to the second-line antitubercular drugs (e.g., cycloserine and pyrimethamine) is equal because of the first cell line anti-TB ethambutol. In particular, compound **6d** displayed a strong inhibition against *M. tuberculosis* (MIC 12.50 μM) and it had antimycobacterial activity adequate to that of anti-TB drug ethambutol (MIC 12.50 μM) and was superior to the anti-TB drugs cycloserine (MIC 25 μM) and pyrimethamine (MIC 100 μM). Therefore, the salt 6d was

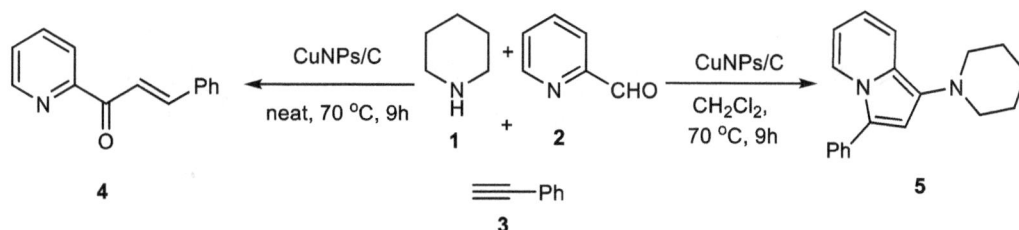

SCHEME 3.12 Multicomponent synthesis of indolizines derivatives from pyridine-2-carbaldehyde

potent against replicating and non-replicating *M. tuberculosis* and had no toxicity.[94] The synthesis of the indolizine derivatives **8a,b,** and **9** (Figure 3.9) was conducted and their tubercle bacillus H37Rv growth and InhA inhibitory activities were evaluated. The MIC values of the obtained compounds on *M. tuberculosis* H37Rv strain were 109.2, 52.6, and 46.5 μM, respectively. In contrast, compounds **8a,b** and **9** exhibited moderate InhA inhibition activities.[95]

Cu nanoparticles supported on activated catalyzed the multicomponent synthesis of indolizines from pyridine-2-carbaldehyde derivatives, secondary amines, and terminal alkynes in dichloromethane, in the absence of solvent, afford the heterocyclic chalcones (Scheme 12).

Compelling evidence has been offered that both processes occurred via aldehyde–amine–alkyne coupling intermediates. In contrast to other well-known mechanisms for chalcone formation from aldehydes and alkynes, a replacement reaction pathway that involved propargyl amines as intermediates that did not undergo rearrangement was presented. The formation of indolizines or chalcones is driven by inductive and solvent effects, with a good array of both being reported. In both reactions, the nanoparticulate catalyst was superior to some commercially available Cu catalysts, and it could be recycled during chalcone synthesis.[96]

3.3 QUINOLIZINIUM SALTS

Ever since their first reported synthesis,[97] the quinolizinium salts **1** have occupied a prominent place within synthetic chemistry and medicine. The quinolizinium salts and their benzologs are classified as azonia-aromatic compounds where a bridgehead C is replaced by a quaternary N atom. This class of organic salts has been widely studied for their biological activities. Many alkaloids, such as berberine alkaloids,[98–101] palmatine,[102] columbamine,[103] jatrorrhizine, coptisine,[105] worenine,[106] dehydrocorydaline,[107] dehydrothialictrifoline,[108] simper-virine, coralyne, and flavopereurine[109–112] are known to possess a quinolizinium structure. Benzo[c]quinolizinium compounds are used for the treatment of diseases that are linked to smooth muscle fiber contractions, such as hypertension and asthma.[113] In addition, they act as activators of the CF transmembrane conductance regulator (CFTR).[114] Various berberine alkaloids exhibit antileukemic activity [115] and antitumor activity.[116,117] It will even be habituated to design DNA-targeting drugs for tumor treatment.[118]

The efficient synthesis of quinolizinium salts from 2-vinylpyridines and alkynes via Rhodium(III) or Rhodium(II)-catalyzed C–H activation and annulation reaction has been described. described. A possible mechanism that involved pyridine assisted vinylic ortho-C–H activation, alkyne insertion, and reductive elimination was proposed.[119]

A sealed tube that contained pentamethylcyclopentadienyl rhodium dichloride dimer ([Cp*RhCl$_2$]$_2$) (1.8 mg, 0.0028 mmoL) and copper(II) tetrafluoroborate hydrate (Cu(BF$_4$)$_2$.6H$_2$O) (49.0 mg, 0.14 mmoL) was evacuated and purged with O$_2$ three times. Then, 2-vinylpyridine **1** (0.28 mmoL) and alkyne **2** (0.34 mmoL) in MeOH (1.0 mL) were added to the system via syringe under an O$_2$ atmosphere and the reaction was stirred at 60°C for 18 h under O$_2$. When the reaction was completed, the mixture was diluted with CH$_2$Cl$_2$ (10 mL) and filtered through a celite pad and the celite pad was washed several times with CH$_2$Cl$_2$ (50 mL). The combined filtrate was

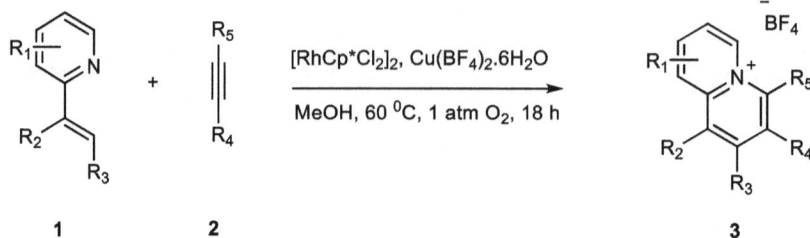

SCHEME 3.13 Synthesis of quinolizinium salts

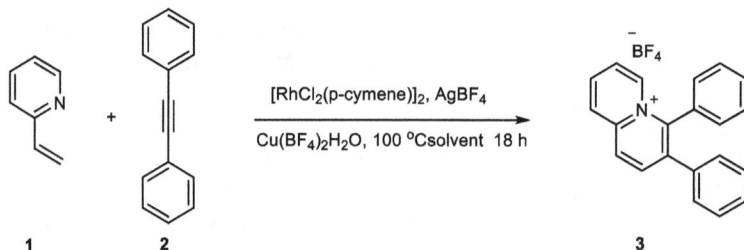

SCHEME 3.14 Synthesis of quinolizinium

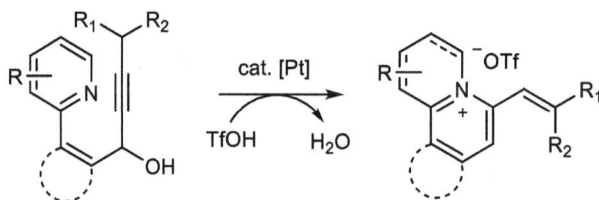

SCHEME 3.15 Synthesis of quinolizinium-type heteroaromatics by Pt(II)-catalyzed cyclization of 2-arylpyridine propargyl alcohol

concentrated in vacuo and the residue was purified by chromatography on a colloid column using DCM/MeOH (95:5) as eluent to select the specified pure product **3**. The synthesis of quinolizinium salts is shown in Scheme 3.13. The synthesis of quinolizinium is shown in Scheme 3.14.

The efficient synthesis of quinolizinium-type heteroaromatics by Pt(II)-catalyzed cyclization of 2-arylpyridine propargyl alcohol has been developed. The presence of a protic acid is crucial for the success of the reaction. Mechanistic studies disclosed that the reaction proceeds via a platinum–carbene intermediate. Additionally, the fluorescence properties of the synthesized heteroaromatics were investigated to provide perspectives for potential applications. The synthesis of quinolizinium-type heteroaromatics by Pt(II)-catalyzed cyclization of 2-arylpyridine propargyl alcohol is shown in Scheme 3.15.[120]

To a 50 mL-flask **1** (100 mg, 0.27 mmoL), Pd/C (6 mg, 0.027 mmoL), and MeOH (10 mL) were added. H_2 was bubbled through the suspension, then the mixture was stirred at 30°C for 16 h under one hydrogen gas atmosphere. After the reaction was completed, the mixture was filtered through a celite pad and the celite pad was washed several times with MeOH (30 mL). The combined filtrate was concentrated in vacuo and the mixture was separated by chromatography on a colloid column that used a mix of DCM/MeOH (95:5) as eluent to select the specified pure product **2**. The synthesis of Tetrahydroquinolizinium salt is shown in Scheme 3.16.

The association of heteroaromatic ligands with DNA might be a crucial and biologically relevant process, because it is has a strong influence on the function of the macromolecule. Therefore,

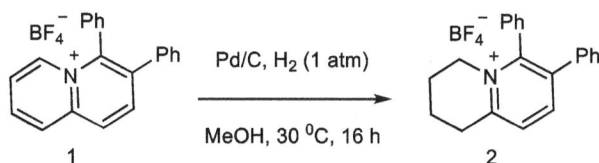

SCHEME 3.16 Synthesis of Tetrahydroquinolizinium salt

efficient and selective DNA-targeting ligands are considered promising lead structures for drugs. The quinolizinium ion was established as a versatile building block for the design of DNA-binding ligands, with the long-term goal to understand the structural parameters that govern the association of cationic hetarenes with DNA. During this, annelated quinolizinium derivatives were easily available and their structure and substitution pattern were highly variable. Of note, the availability of several derivatives of different sizes and shapes enabled the assessment of structure–property relationships for their DNA-binding properties. From the literature, the systematic variation in the ligand structure, in conjunction with analysis of the binding parameters, were often employed to research the structural requirements of a ligand to bind to different DNA forms, such as triplex, quadruplex, and a basic site-containing DNA.

3.4 CONCLUSION

Azidobenziodoxolone is the source of the azide radical. Other azide reagents, such as $TMSN_3$ and NaN_3 failed to produce the fused pyrrolines. This one-step synthesis of fused pyrrolines proceeded via the generation of the azide radical from azidobenziodoxolone with the aid of Cu^{2+} as a catalyst. Pyrroline and its derivatives are considered privileged structures, which is reflected by their presence in many bioactive compounds. The pyrroline showed antimicrobial, antihypertensive, anti-infective, antitumor, and anti-inflammatory activities.

Indolizine synthesis is an efficient and atom economical access that was developed by a Cu-catalyzed cyclization. Indolizine and its derivatives gave good to excellent yields under mild reaction conditions. Indolizine derivatives exhibit potential biological activities. Indolizine pharmacophore has become a crucial synthetic target for novel synthetic analogs with various pharmacological properties, such as CNS suppression, analgesic and anti-inflammatory, anticancer, antibacterial, antioxidant, larvicidal, and anti-HIV.

Quinolizinium salts have occupied a prominent place in synthetic chemistry and medicine. This class of organic salts has been widely studied because of their biological activities. They are known to act as activators of CFTR. Various berberine alkaloids exhibit antileukemic activity and antitumor activity. It cannot design the DNA-targeting drugs for tumor treatment. In addition, the fluorescent properties of the synthesized heteroaromatics were investigated to provide perspectives for potential applications.

REFERENCES

1. Clark VC, Raxworthy CJ, Rakotomalala V, Sierwald P, Fisher BL. Convergent evolution of chemical defense in poison frogs and arthropod prey between Madagascar and the Neotropics. *Proc Nat. Acad Sci USA*. 2005. 102:11617–22. doi.10.1073/pnas.0503502102
2. Rinehart KL, Kobayashi J, Harbour GC, Gilmore J, Mascal M, Holt TG. et al. Eudistomins A-Q, .beta.-carbolines from the antiviral Caribbean tunicate *Eudistoma olivaceum. J Am Chem Soc*. 1987. 109 3378–87. doi.10.1021/ja00245a031
3. Marti C, Carreira EM. Total Synthesis of (−)-Spirotryprostatin B: Synthesis and Related Studies. *J Am Chem Soc*. 2005. 127:11505–15. doi.10.1021/ja0518880
4. Tsukamoto D, Shibano M, Okamoto R, Kusano G. Studies on the constituents of Broussonetia species VIII. Four new pyrrolidine alkaloids, broussonetines R, S, T, and V and a new pyrroline alkaloid,

broussonetine U, from Broussonetia kazinoki Sieb. *Chem Pharm Bull*. 2001. 49:492–6. doi.10.1248/cpb.49.492

5. Adams A, Kimpe ND. Chemistry of 2-acetyl-1-pyrroline, 6-acetyl-1,2,3,4-tetrahydropyridine, 2-acetyl-2-thiazoline, and 5-acetyl-2,3-dihydro-4H-thiazine: Extraordinary Maillard flavor compounds. *Chem Rev*. 2006. 106:2299–319. doi.10.1021/cr040097y

6. Huang TC, Teng CS, Chang JL, Chuang HS, Ho CT, Wu ML. Biosynthetic Mechanism of 2-Acetyl-1-pyrroline and Its Relationship with Δ^1-Pyrroline-5-carboxylic Acid and Methylglyoxal in Aromatic Rice (*Oryza sativa* L.) Callus. *J Agric Food Chem*. 2008. 56:7399–404. doi.10.1021/jf8011739.

7. Cui B, Kakeya H, Osada H. Spirotryprostatin B, a Novel Mammalian Cell Cycle Inhibitor Produced by Aspergillus fumigatus. *J Antibiot*. 1996. 49:832–5. doi.10.7164/antibiotics.49.832.

8. Hurley LH, Petrusek R. Proposed structure of the anthramycin–DNA adduct. *Nature*. 1979. 282:529–31. doi.10.1038/282529a0

9. Ozawa M, Etoh T, Hayashi M, Komiyama K, Kishida A, Ohsaki A. Trail-enhancing activity of Erythrinan alkaloids from *Erythrina velutina*. *Bioorg Med Chem Lett*. 2009. 19:234–6. doi.10.1016/j.bmcl.2008.10.111

10. Kadish KM, Smith KM, Guilard R, Academic, San Diego (2002) The Porphyrin Handbook, ed. 354.

11. Tyroller S, Zwickenpflug W, Richter E. New sources of dietary myosmine uptake from cereals, fruits, vegetables, and milk. *J Agric Food Chem*. 2002. 50:4909–15. doi.10.1021/jf020281p

12. Bacos JJ, Basselier JP, Celerler C, Lange E, Marx G, Lhommet P. et al. Ant venom alkaloids from Monomorium species: natural insecticides. *Tetrahedron Lett*. 1988. 29:3061–4. doi.10.1016/0040-4039(88)85085-8

13. Castellano S, Fiji HDG, Kinderman SS, Watanabe M, de Leon P, Tamanoi F. et al. Small-Molecule Inhibitors of Protein Geranylgeranyltransferase Type I. *J Am Chem Soc*. 2007. 129:5843–5. doi.10.1021/ja070274n

14. Schann S, Bruban V, Pompermayer K, Feldman J, Pfeiffer B, Renard P. et al. Synthesis and biological evaluation of pyrolinic isosteres of rilmenidine. Discovery of cis-/trans-dicyclopropylmethyl-(4,5-dimethyl-4,5-dihydro-3H-pyrrol-2-yl)-amine (LNP 509), anI1 imidazoline receptor selective ligand with hypotensive activity. *J Med Chem*. 2001. 44:1588–93. doi.10.1021/jm001111b

15. Behr JB, Pearson MSM, Bello C, Vogel P, Plantier-Royon R. Synthesis and l-fucosidase inhibitory potency of a cyclic sugar imine and its pyrrolidine analogue. *Tetrahedron: Asymmetry*. 2008. 19:1829–32. doi.10.1016/j.tetasy.2008.06.019

16. Magedov V, Luchetti G, Evdokimov NM, Manpadi M, Steelant WFA, Van Slambrouck S. et al. Novel three-component synthesis and antiproliferative properties doi.10.1016/j.bmcl.2008.01.019

17. Mou QY, Chen J, Zhu YC, Zhou DH, Chi ZQ, Long YQ. 3-Pyrroline containing arylacetamides: a novel series of remarkably selective kappa-agonists. *Bioorg Med Chem Lett*. 2002. 12:2287–90. doi.10.1016/s0960-894x(02)00429-8.

18. Rondeau P, Gill M, Chan, Curry K, Lubell WD. Synthesis and pharmacology of new enantiopure Δ3-4-arylkainoids. *Bioorg Med Chem Lett*. 2000. 10:771–3. doi.10.1016/S0960-894X(00)00093-7

19. Cox CD, Coleman PJ, Breslin MJ, Whitman DB, Garbaccio RM, Fraley ME. Kinesin Spindle Protein (KSP) Inhibitors. 9. Discovery of (2S)-4-(2,5-Difluorophenyl)-N-[(3R,4S)-3-fluoro-1-methylpiperidin-4-yl]-2-(hydroxymethyl)-N-methyl-2-phenyl-2,5-dihydro-1H-pyrrole-1-carboxamide (MK-0731) for the Treatment of Taxane-Refractory Cancer. *J Med Chem*. 2008. 51:4239–52. doi.10.1021/jm800386y

20. Peddibhotla S, Tepe JJ. Stereoselective Synthesis of Highly Substituted Δ-Pyrrolines: exo-Selective 1,3-Dipolar Cycloaddition Reactions with Azlactones. *J Am Chem Soc*. 2004. 126:12776–7. doi.10.1021/ja046149i

21. Imbri NN, Kucukdisli M, Kammer LM, Jung P, Kretzschmann A, Opatz T. One-Pot Synthesis of Pyrrole-2-carboxylates and -carboxamides via an Electrocyclization/Oxidation Sequence. *J Org Chem*. 2014. 79:11750–8. doi.10.1021/jo5021823

22. Bai XF, Li L, Xu Z, Zheng ZJ, Xia CG, Cui YM. et al. Asymmetric Michael Addition of Aldimino Esters with Chalcones Catalyzed by Silver/Xing-Phos: Mechanism-Oriented Divergent Synthesis of Chiral Pyrrolines. *Chem Eur J*. 2016. 22:10399–404. doi.10.1002/chem.201601945

23. Majhail MK, Ylioja PM, Willis MC. Direct Synthesis of Highly Substituted Pyrroles and Dihydropyrroles Using Linear Selective Hydroacylation Reactions. *Chem Eur J*. 2016. 22:7879–84. doi.10.1002/chem.201600311

24. Dannhardt KW. 1-Pyrrolines (3,4-dihydro-2*H*-pyrroles) as a template for new drugs. *Arch Pharm.* 2001. 334:183–8. doi.10.1002/1521-4184(200106)334:6<183::aid-ardp183>3.0.co;2-u

25. Snider BB, Neubert BJ.Syntheses of ficuseptine, juliprosine, and juliprosopine by biomimetic intramolecular Chichibabin pyridine syntheses. *Org Lett.* 2005. 7:2715–18. doi.10.1021/ol0509311

26. Davis FA, Theddu N, Edupuganti R. Asymmetric total synthesis of (S)-(+)-cocaine and the first synthesis of cocaine C-1 analogs from N-sulfinyl β-amino ester ketals. *Org Lett.* 2010. 12:4118–21. doi.10.1021/ol1017118

27. Mei Z, Ma N, Weijun F, Chen X, Guanglong Z. Gold-Catalyzed Homocoupling Reaction of Terminal Alkynes to 1,3-Diynes. *Bull Korean Chem Soc.* 2012. 33(4), 1325–8. doi.10.5012/bkcs.2012.33.4.1325

28. Nebe MM, Kucukdisli M, Opatz T. 3,4-Dihydro-2H-pyrrole-2-carbonitriles: Useful Intermediates in the Synthesis of Fused Pyrroles and 2,2'-Bipyrroles. *J Org Chem.* 2016. 81:4112–21. doi.10.1021/acs.joc.6b00393

29. Humphrey JM, Liao Y, Ali A, Rein T, Wong YL, Chen HJ. et al. Enantioselective total syntheses of manzamine a and related alkaloids. *J Am Chem Soc.* 2002. 124:8584–92. doi.10.1021/ja0202964.

30. Martin R, Jager A, Bohl M, Richter S, Fedorov R, Manstein DJ. et al. Total Synthesis of Pentabromo- and Pentachloropseudilin, and Synthetic Analogues-Allosteric Inhibitors of Myosin ATPase. *Angew Chem Int Ed.* 2009. 48:8042–6. doi.10.1002/anie.200903743

31. Wegner J, Ley SV, Kirschning A, Hansen AL, Montenegro GJ, Baxendale IR. A total synthesis of millingtonine. *Org Lett.* 2012. 14:696–9. doi.10.1021/ol203158p

32. Zhang H, Curran DP. A short total synthesis of (±)-epimeloscine and (±)-meloscine enabled by a cascade radical annulation of a divinylcyclopropane. *J Am Chem Soc.* 2011. 133:10376–8. doi.10.1021/ja2042854

33. Ritthiwigrom T, Willis AC, Pyne SG. Total Synthesis of Uniflorine A, Casuarine, Australine, 3-epi-Australine, and 3,7-Di-epi-australine from a Common Precursor. *J Org Chem.* 2010. 75:815–24. doi.10.1021/jo902355p

34. Kaden S, Reissig HU. Efficient Approach to the Azaspirane Core of FR 901483. *Org Lett.* 2006. 8:4763–6. doi.10.1021/ol061538y.

35. Dhand V, Draper JA, Moore J, Britton R. A short, organocatalytic formal synthesis of (-)-swainsonine and related alkaloids. *Org Lett.* 2013. 15:1914–17. doi.10.1021/ol400566j

36. Garcia LL, Carpes MJS, de Oca ACBM, dos Santos MAG, Santana CC, Correia CRD. Synthesis of 4-Aryl-2-pyrrolidones and β-Aryl-γ-amino-butyric Acid (GABA) Analogues by Heck Arylation of 3-Pyrrolines with Arenediazonium Tetrafluoroborates. Synthesis of (±)-Rolipram on a Multigram Scale and Chromatographic Resolution by Semipreparative Chiral Simulated Moving Bed Chromatography. *J Org Chem.* 2005. 70:1050–3. doi.10.1021/jo0484880

37. Davies SG, Fletcher AM, Houlsby ITT, Roberts PM, Thomson JE. Asymmetric Synthesis of the Tetraponerine Alkaloids. *J Org Chem.* 2017. 82:6689–702. doi.10.1021/acs.joc.7b00837

38. Miyauchi R, Ono C, Ohnuki T, Shibad Y. Nectrisine Biosynthesis Genes in Thelonectria discophora SANK 18292: Identification and Functional Analysis. *Appl Environ Microbiol.* 2016. 82:6414–22. doi.10.1128/AEM.01709-16

39. Behr JB, Pearson MSM, Bello C, Vogel P, Plantier-Royon R. Synthesis and 1-fucosidase inhibitory potency of a cyclic sugar imine and its pyrrolidine analogue. *Tetrahedron: Asymmetry.* 2008. 19:1829–32. doi.10.1016/j.tetasy.2008.06.019

40. Tsujii E, Muroi M, Shiragami N, Takatsuki A. Nectrisine is a potent inhibitor of α-glucosidases, demonstrating activities similarly at enzyme and cellular levels. *Biochem Biophys Res Commun.* 1996. 220:459–66.

41. Schann S, Bruban V, Pompermayer K, Feldman J, Pfeiffer B, Renard P. et al. Synthesis and biological evaluation of pyrrolinic isosteres of rilmenidine. Discovery of cis-/transdicyclopropylmethyl-(4,5-dimethyl-4,5-dihydro-3H-pyrrol-2-yl)-amine (LNP 509), an I1 imidazoline receptor selective ligand with hypotensive activity. *J Med Chem.* 2001. 44:1588–93. doi.10.1021/jm001111b

42. Zhao MX, Zhu HK. Dai TL, Shi M. Cinchona alkaloid squaramide-catalyzed asymmetric Michael addition of α-aryl isocyanoacetates to β-trifluoromethylated enones and its application in the synthesis of chiral β-trifluoromethylated pyrrolines. *J Org Chem.* 2015. 80:11330–8. doi.10.1021/acs.joc.5b01829

43. Hagen TJ, Bergmanis AA, Kramer SW, Fok KF, Schmelzer AE, Pitzele BS. et al. 2-Iminopyrrolidines as Potent and Selective Inhibitors of Human Inducible Nitric Oxide Synthase. *J Med Chem.* 1998. 41:3675–83. doi.10.1021/jm970840x

44. Vaillancourt V, Sheehan SMK. Azetidine derivatives as antiparasitic agents. *PCT Int. Appl.* WO2013169622A1, 2013.

45. Aicher D, Wiehe A, Stark CBW, Albrechr V. Application of beta-functionalized dihydroxy-chlorins for pdt. United States patent application. US20130041307A1, 2013.

46. Aicher D, Albrecht V, Gitter B, Stark CBW, Wiehe A. Glyco-substituted dihydroxy-chlorins and b-functionalized chlorins for anti-microbial photodynamic therapy. *PCT Int. Appl.* WO201 3015774A1, 2013.

47. Aicher D, Grafe S, Stark, CBW, Wiehe A. Synthesis of β-functionalized Temoporfin derivatives for an application in photodynamic therapy. *Bioorg Med Chem Lett.* 2011. 21:5808–11. doi.10.1016/j.bmcl.2011.07.113

48. Aicher D, Wiehe A, Stark CBW, Albrecht V, Grafe S. Preparation of β-functionalized dihydroxy-chlorins for PDT. *PCT Int. Appl.* WO2012012809A2, 2012, 53.

49. Noelia S, Medran A, La-Venia SAT. Metal-mediated synthesis of pyrrolines. *RSC Adv.* 2019. 9:6804–44. doi.10.1039/C8RA10247C

50. Sanjaya S, Chua SH, Chiba S. Cu(II)-Mediated Aminooxygenation of Alkenylimines and Alkenylamidines with TEMPO. *Synlett.* 2012. 1657–61. doi.10.1055/s-0031-1291157

51. Debrouwer W, Heugebaert TSA, Van Hecke K, Stevens CV. Synthetic Entry into 1-Phosphono-3-azabicyclo[3.1.0]hexanes. *J Org Chem.* 2013. 78:8232–41. doi.10.1021/jo401185u

52. Ouyang XH, Song RJ, Liu Y, Hu M, Li JH. Copper-Catalyzed Radical [2 + 2 + 1] Annulation of Benzene-Linked 1,n-Enynes with Azide: Fused Pyrroline Compounds. *Org Lett.* 2015. 17:6038–41. doi.10.1021/acs.orglett.5b03040

53. Shanping C, Yunfeng L, Feng Z, Hongrui Q, Saiwen L, Guo-Jun, D. Palladium-Catalyzed Direct Arylation of Indoles with Cyclohexanones. *Org Lett.* 2014. 16(6):1618–21. doi.10.1021/ol500231c

54. Goutham K, Mangina N, Suresh S, Raghavaiah P, Karunakar GV. Gold-catalyzed Cyclization of N-Propargylic β-Enaminones to form 3-Methylene-1-pyrroline Derivatives. *Org Biomol Chem.* 2014. 12:2869–73. doi.10.1039/c3ob42513d.

55. Yang HB, Selander N. Divergent Iron-Catalyzed Coupling of O-Acyloximes with Silyl Enol Ethers. *Chem Eur J.* 2017. 23:1779–83. doi.10.1002/CHEM.201605636

56. Jackman MM, Cai Y, Castle SL. Recent advances in iminyl radical cyclizations. *Synthesis.* 2017. 49:1785–95. doi.10.1055/s-0036-1588707

57. Shimbayashi T, Okamoto K, Ohe K.Iron-Catalyzed Aminative Cyclization/Intermolecular Homolytic Aromatic Substitution Using Oxime Esters and Simple Arenes. *Chem Asian J.* 2018. 13:395–9. doi.10.1002/asia.201701634

58. Huang W, Zuo T, Jin H, Liu Z, Yang Z, Yu X. Design, synthesis and biological evaluation of indolizine derivatives as HIV-1 VIF-ElonginC interaction inhibitors. Mol Diversity. 2013. 17:221–43. doi.10.1007/s11030-013-9424-3

59. Dinica RM, Furdui B, Ghinea IO, Bahrim G, Bonte S, Demeunynck M. Novel One-Pot Green Synthesis of Indolizines Biocatalysed by *Candida antarctica* Lipases. *Marine Drugs.* 2013. 11:431–9. doi.10.3390/md11020431

60. Wan J, Zheng CJ, Fung MK, Liu ZK, Lee CS, Zhang XH. Multifunctional electron-transporting indolizine derivatives for highly efficient blue fluorescence, orange phosphorescence host and two-color based white OLEDs. *J Mater Chem.* 2012. 22:4502–10. doi.10.1039/C2JM14904D

61. Dumitrascu F, Vasilescu M, Draghici C, Caproiu M, Teodor B, Loredana DDG. New fluorescent indolizines and bisindolizinylethylenes. *Arkivoc.* 2011 (x): 338–350. www.researchgate.net/publication/267943963_New_fluorescent_indolizines_and_bisindolizinylethylenes

62. Becuwe M, Landy, D Delattre F, Cazier F, Foumentin S. Fluorescent Indolizine-b-Cyclodextrin Derivatives for the Detection of Volatile Organic Compounds. *Sensors.* 2008. 8:3689–705. doi.10.3390/s8063689

63. Sharma V, Kumar V. Indolizine: a biologically active moiety. *Med Chem Res.* 2014. 23:3593–606. doi.10.1007/s00044-014-0940-1

64. Singh GS, Mmatli EE. Recent progress in synthesis and bioactivity studies of indolizines. *Eur J Med Chem.* 2011. 46 5237–57. doi.10.1016/j.ejmech.2011.08.042.

65. Lazzaroni R, Settambolo R, Rocchiccioli S, Guazzelli G. From chiral and prochiral N-allylpyrroles to stereodefined pyrrole fused architectures: A particular application of the rhodium-catalyzed hydroformylation. *J Organometal Chem.* 2007. 692:1812–16. doi.10.1016/j.jorganchem.2006.11.020

66. Nishiwaki N, Furuta K, Komatsu M, Ohshiro YJ. Functionalized indolizines from 2-ethynylpyridines. *Chem Soc Chem Commun.* 1990. 1151–2.
67. Singh GS, Mmatli EE. Recent progress in synthesis and bioactivity studies of indolizines. *Eur J Med Chem.* 2011. 46:5237–57.
68. Xue YJ, Tang X, Ma Q, Li B, Xie Y, Hao H. et al. Synthesis and biological activities of indolizine derivatives as alpha-7 nAChR agonists. *Eur J Med Chem.* 2016. 115:94–108. doi.10.1016/j.ejmech.2016.03.016.
69. Elattar KM, Youssef I, Fadda AA. Reactivity of indolizines in organic synthesis. *Synth Commun.* 2016. 46:719–44. doi.10.1080/00397911.2016.1166252
70. Park S, Kim I. Electron-withdrawing group effect in aryl group of allyl bromides for the successful synthesis of indolizines via a novel [3+3] annulation approach. *Tetrahedron.* 2015. 71:1982–91. doi.10.1016/j.tet.2015.02.013
71. Jung Y, Kim I. Deformylative Intramolecular Hydroarylation: Synthesis of Benzo[e]pyrido[1,2-a] indoles. *Org Lett.* 2015. 17:4600–3. doi.10.1021/acs.orglett.5b02331.
72. Kim M, Jung Y, Kim I. Domino Knoevenagel condensation/intramolecular aldol cyclization route to diverse indolizines with densely functionalized pyridine units. *J Org Chem.* 2013. 78:10395–404. doi.10.1021/jo401801j
73. Liu R, Cai Z, Lu C, Ye S, Bin X, Jianrong G. et al. Indolizine synthesis via Cu-catalyzed cyclization of 2-(2-enynyl)pyridines with nucleophiles. *Org Chem Front.* 2015. 2:226–230. doi.10.1039/C4QO00336E
74. Robarge KD, Brunton SA, Castanedo GM. GDC-0449—A potent inhibitor of the hedgehog pathway. *Bioorg Med Chem Lett.* 2009. 19:5579–81. doi.10.1016/j.bmcl.2009.08.049
75. Kim ND, Park ES, Kim YH. Structure-based virtual screening of novel tubulin inhibitors and their characterization as anti-mitotic agents. *Bioorg Med Chem.* 2010. 18:7092–100. doi.101021/jo960438a
76. Shen YM, Cheng LP, Chen W. Synthesis and antiproliferative activity of indolizine derivatives incorporating a cyclopropylcarbonyl group against Hep-G2 cancer cell line. *Eur J Med Chem.* 2010. 45:3184–90. doi.10.1016/j.ejmech.2010.02.056
77. Dumea C, Belei D, Ghinet A. Novel indolizine derivatives with unprecedented inhibitory activity on human farnesyl transferase. *Bioorg Med Chem Lett.* 2014. 24:5777–81. doi.10.1016/j.bmcl.2014.10.044
78. Abuhaie CM, Bicu E, Rigo B. Synthesis and anticancer activity of analogues of phenstatin, with a phenothiazine A-ring, as a new class of microtubule-targeting agents. *Bioorg Med Chem Lett.* 2013. 23:147–52. doi.10.1016/j.bmcl.2012.10.135.
79. Boot A, Brito A, Wezell TV. Anticancer Activity of Novel pyrido[2,3-b]indolizineDerivatives: The Relevance of Phenolic Substituents. *Anticancer Res.* 2014. 34:1673–8.
80. Huang W, Zuo T, Luo X. Indolizine Derivatives as HIV-1 VIF–Elongin C Interaction Inhibitors. Chem *Biol Drug Des.* 2013. 81:730–41. doi.10.1111/cbdd.12119.
81. Sinha C, Nischal A, Bandaru S. An in silico approach for identification of novel inhibitors as a potential therapeutics targeting HIV-1 viral infectivity factor. *Curr Top Med Chem.* 2015. 15:65–72. doi.10.2174/1568026615666150112114337.
82. Huang W, Zuo T, Jin H. Design, synthesis and biological evaluation of indolizine derivatives as HIV-1 VIF–Elongin C interaction inhibitors. *Mol Divers.* 2013. 17: 21–243. doi.10.1007/s11030-013-9424-3.
83. Zuo T, Liu D, Lv W. Small-molecule inhibition of human immunodeficiency virus type 1 replication by targeting the interaction between Vif and Elongin C. *J Virol.* 2012. 86: 5497–507. doi.10.1128/JVI.06957-11.
84. Lee WG, Frey KM, Gallardo-Macias R. Discovery and crystallography of bicyclic arylaminoazines as potent inhibitors of HIV-1 reverse transcriptase. *Bioorg Med Chem Lett.* 2015. 25:4824–7. doi.10.1016/j.bmcl.2015.06.074
85. Zhang L, Yu X, Huang W. Preparation of indolizine derivatives as antiviral agents. Faming Zh Shenqing. (2013) CN103087061A 20130508.
86. Bosanac T, De LS, Lo HY. Preparation of indolizine inhibitors of leukotriene production. *PCT Int. Appl.* (2010) WO2010027762A1 20100311.
87. Cao CQ, Wei Y, Zou K. Synthesis and interleukin-6 inhibitory activities of 3-alkyloxylindolizine derivatives. *Adv Mat Res.* 2013. 781: 1089–92. doi.10.4028/www.scientific.net/AMR.781-784

88. Wei1 Y, Cao CQ, Lu XF. Facile Synthesis, Characterization and Anti-inflammatory Effect of 3-Aminoindolizine Derivatives. *Adv Mat Res*. 2014. 881:446–9. doi.10.4028/www.scientific.net/AMR.881-883

89. Hazra A, Mondal, S, Maity A.Amberlite-IRA-402 (OH) ion exchange resin mediated synthesis of indolizines, pyrrolo [1,2-a] quinolines and isoquinolines: Antibacterial and antifungal evaluation of the products. *Eur J Med Chem*. 2011. 46:2132–40. doi.10.1016/j.ejmech.2011.02.066

90. Gomha SM, Dawood, KM. Synthesis of novel indolizine, pyrrolo[1,2-a] quinoline, and 4,5-dihydrothiophene derivatives via nitrogen ylides and their antimicrobial evaluation. *J Chem Res*. 2014. 38:515–19. doi.10.3184/174751914x14067338307126

91. Faghih-Mirzaei E, Seifi M, Abaszadeh M. Design, Synthesis, Biological Evaluation and Molecular Modeling Study of Novel Indolizine-1-Carbonitrile Derivatives as Potential Anti-Microbial Agents. *Iran J Pharm Res*. 2018. 17(3):883–95.

92. Olejnikova P, Birosova L, Svorc L. Newly synthesized indolizine derivative antimicrobial and antimutagenic properties. *Chem Pap*. 2015. 69:983–2. doi.10.1515/chempap-2015-0093

93. Muthusaravanan S, Perumal S, Yogeeswari P, Sriram D. Facile three-component domino reactions in the regioselective synthesis and antimycobacterial evaluation of novel indolizines and pyrrolo[2,1-a] isoquinolines. *Tetrahedron Lett*. 2010. 51:6439–43. doi.10.1016/j.tetlet.2010.09.128

94. Danac R. Mangalagiu II. Antimycobacterial activity of nitrogen heterocycles derivatives: Bipyridine derivatives. Part III. *Eur J Med Chem*. 2014. 74:664–70. doi.10.1016/j.ejmech.2013.09.061

95. Matviiuk T, Mori DG, Lherbet L. Synthesis of 3-heteryl substituted pyrrolidine-2,5-diones via catalytic Michael reaction and evaluation of their inhibitory activity against InhA and Mycobacterium tuberculosis. *Eur J Med Chem*. 2014. 71:46–52. doi.10.1016/j.ejmech.2013.10.069

96. Albaladejo MJ, Alonso F, Gonzalez-Soria MJ. Synthetic and Mechanistic Studies on the Solvent-Dependent Copper-Catalyzed Formation of Indolizines and Chalcones. *ACS Catal*. 2015. 5(6):3446–56. doi.10.1021/acscatal.5b00417

97. Boekelheide V, Gall WG. Syntheses in the Thioctic Acid Series. *J Am Chem Soc*. 1954. 76:1832–6.

98. Perkin Jr. WH, Ray JH. CIII.—A synthesis of oxyberberine. *J Am Chem Soc*. 1925. 127:740–4. doi.10.1039/CT9252700740

99. Haworth RD, Perkin Jr. WH, Raukin J. CCXIX.—ψ-Berberine. *J Chem Soc*. 1924. 125:1686–701 doi.10.1039/CT9242500032

100. Perkin Jr. WH, Ray JH. XLII.-epiBerberine. *J Chem Soc Trans*. 1918. 113:492–522.

101. Buck JS, Perkin Jr. WH. CCXIX.—ψ-Berberine. *J Chem Soc*. 1924. 125:1675–86.

102. Haworth RD, Koepfli WH, Perkin Jr. WH. LXXXII.—A new synthesis of oxyberberine and a synthesis of palmatine. *J Chem Soc*. 1927. 548–54.

103. Spath E, Mosettig E. (1927) *Ber*. 60: 383.

104. Spath E, Mosettig E (1925) *Ber*, 58: 2133.

105. Spath E, Mosettig E. Posega K. (1929) *Ber*, 62: 1029.

106. Henry TA. The Plant Alkaloid. 4th ed. Philadelphia: Blakiston Co.; 1949. 344 p.

107. Kopfl J, Perkin Jr. WH. *J Chem Soc*. 1928. 2989.

108. Manske RF. *J Research*. 1943. 21B: 111.

109. Thyagrajan BS. *Adv Heterocycl Chem*. 1965. 5: 291.

110. Jones G. Adv Heterocycl Chem. 1982. 31: 1.

111. Bradshe CK in Comprehensive Heterocyclic Chemistry,Vol. 2, edited by A R Katritzsky & C W Rees (PergamonPress, Oxford), 1984. 525.

112. Arai S, Hida M. Polycyclic Aromatic Nitrogen Cations. *Adv Heterocycl Chem*. 1992. 55:261–358.

113. Becq F, Robert R, Pignoux L, Rogier C, Mettey Y, Vierfond JM. et al. Marivingt-Mounir C. US Patent 7 897 610, 2011.

114. Marivingt-Mounir C, Rand R, Bulteu-Pignoux L, Nguyen-Huy D, Viosat B, Margant G. et al. Synthesis, SAR, Crystal Structure, and Biological Evaluation of Benzoquinoliziniums as Activators of Wild-Type and Mutant Cystic Fibrosis Transmembrane Conductance Regulator Channels. *J Med Chem*. 2004. 47:962–72. doi.10.1021/jm0308848

115. Philips SD, Castle RN. A review of the chemistry of the antitumor benzo[c]phenanthridine alkaloids nitidine and fagaronine and of the related antitumor alkaloid coralyne. *J Heterocycl Chem*. 1988. 18:223–32.

116. Gupta RS, Murray W, Gupta R. Cross resistance pattern towards anticancer drugs of a human carcinoma multidrug-resistant cell line. *Br J Cancer*. 1988. 58:441–7.

117. Gatto B, Sanders MM, Yu C, Yu HY, Makhey D, Lavoie EJ, Liu LF. Identification of topoisomerase I as the cytotoxic target of the protoberberine alkaloid coralyne. *Cancer Res*. 1996. 56:2795–800.

118. Ihmels H, Faulhaber K, Vedaldi D, Dall'Acqua F, Viola G. Intercalation of organic dye molecules into double-stranded DNA. Part 2: the annelated quinolizinium ion as a structural motif in DNA intercalators. *Photochem Photobiol*. 2005. 81:1107–15. doi./10.1562/2005-01-25-IR-427

119. Ching-Zong L, Parthasarathy G, Chien–Hong C. A convenient synthesis of quinolizinium salts through Rh(iii) or Ru(ii)-catalyzed C–H bond activation of 2-alkenylpyridines. *Chem Commun*. 2013. 49:8528–30. doi.10.1039/C3CC45004J

120. Feng L, Jihee C, Shenpeng T, Kim S.Synthesis of Quinolizinium-Type Heteroaromatics via a Carbene Intermediate. *Org Lett*. 2018. 20(3):824–7. doi.10.1021/acs.orglett.7b03964.

4 Nanocatalyzed Synthesis of Bioactive Pyrrole, Indole, Furan, and Benzofuran Derived Heterocycles

S. U. Deshmukh,[1] Ajit K. Dhas,[1] Vidya D. Dofe,[1]
Satish A. Dake,[2] Jaiprakash N. Sangshetti,[3]
Keshav Lalit Ameta,[4] and R. P. Pawar[5]

[1] Department of Chemistry, Deogiri College, Aurangabad, India
[2] Department of Chemistry, Sunderrao Solanke Mahavidyalaya, Majalgaon, Maharashtra, India
[3] Department of Chemistry, Y. B. Chavan College of Pharmacy, Aurangabad, Maharashtra, India
[4] Department of Chemistry, School of Liberal Arts and Sciences, Mody University of Science and Technology, Lakshmangarh, Rajasthan, India
[5] Department of Chemistry, Shiv Chattrapati College, Aurangabad, Maharashtra, India

4.1 INTRODUCTION

This chapter describes nanocatalyst and their application in the organic transformation of biological activated heterocyclic compounds, such as pyrrole, indole, furan, and benzofuran derivatives. Recently, nanotechnology is a branch of science and engineering that is growing into one of the most attractive research areas. The catalytic action of nanoparticles (NPs) is due to very high surface-to-volume ratios.

Today, nanocatalysts have a vital role in green chemistry. The advantages of nanocatalysts are the required small quantity, decreased size of the nanocatalyst, more surface area, exposure to the reactant, and non-toxic. Using a nanocatalyst, a minimum time is required for the formation of the desired product. Researchers in the pharmaceutical industry are continually searching for highly efficient, active, and stable catalysts.

This chapter will compile a literature survey on nanocatalyst and their applications in the organic synthesis of bioactive heterocyclics, such as pyrrole, indole, furan, and benzofuran. A recently updated literature survey is very significant for researchers, chemists, and scientists that work in this field to reveal important information about the synthesis of bioactive heterocyclic compounds that use various nanocatalysts.

4.1.1 INTRODUCTION OF PYRROLES

Pyrroles **1** moiety is present in several natural and synthetic pharmaceutically active compounds.[1,2] The chemistry of pyrroles heterocyclic compounds are more reactive at the second carbon (C) atom.

DOI: 10.1201/9781003141488-4

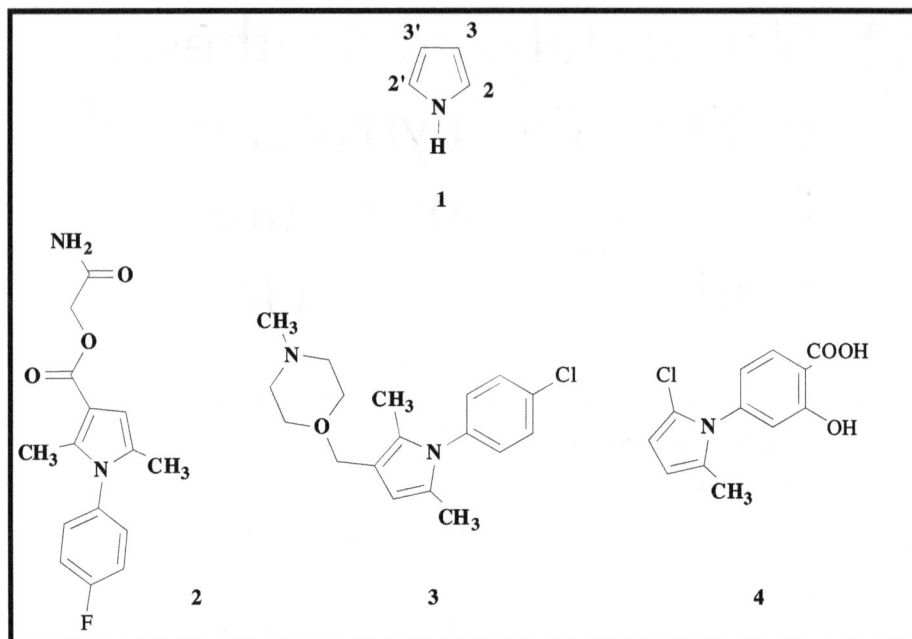

FIGURE 4.1 Some bioactive pyrrole systems

The pyrrole derivatives have new structures and exhibit a broad range of biological activities. Pyrroles show potential antimalarial **2**,[3] antibacterial **3**,[4] antiviral **4**,[5] (Figure 4.1) and HIV fusion inhibitors.[6] Among many others, pyrroles that contain an important class of heterocyclic are drugs. Some of the top-selling drugs worldwide are valuable building blocks for the non-steroidal anti-inflammatory moiety tolmetin **5,** the cholesterol-lowering compound atorvastatin **6,** and the anticancer drug candidate tallimustine **7** (Figure 4.2).

4.1.2 SYNTHESIS OF PYRROLE DERIVATIVES USING NANOCATALYST

Saeidian et al. reported an efficient synthetic method for substituted pyrrole derivatives that used β-ketoester, an aryl aldehyde, amine, and nitromethane in the presence of copper oxide (CuO) NPs under reflux conditions (Scheme 4.1).[7]

Moghaddam et al. investigated the use of $NiFe_2O_4$ NPs for the synthesis of tetrasubstituted pyrroles from aryl aldehyde, 1,3-dicarbonyl compound, amine, and nitromethane by stirring at 100°C (Scheme 4.2).[8]

Mukherjee et al. studied the reaction of an environmentally benign one-pot synthesis for biologically significant chromeno[4,3-b] pyrrol-4(1H)-one derivative. A three-component domino condensation of arylglyoxal monohydrates, arylamines, and 4-amino-coumrins, produced functionalized chromeno[4,3-b] pyrrol-4(1H)-ones in the presence of $Fe_3O_4@SiO_2-SO_3H$ NPs as a solid acid catalyst under room temperature (Scheme 4.3).[9]

Veisi et al. prepared sulfonic acid group-loaded amino-functionalized iron (III) oxide (Fe_3O_4) NPs as an active and stable magnetically separable acidic nanocatalyst and used them for the synthesis of one-pot two-component condensation of γ-diketones and 1^0 amines under water:ethanol (H_2O:EtOH) (1:1) at room temperature (RT) to yield the product N-substituted pyrroles (Scheme 4.4).[10]

Hemmati et al. prepared an active and stable magnetically separable acidic nanocatalyst that contained carboxylic acid group-loaded amino-functionalized Fe_3O_4 nanoparticles diethylenetriamine

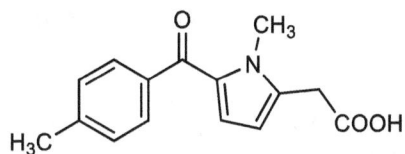

5, Tolmetin

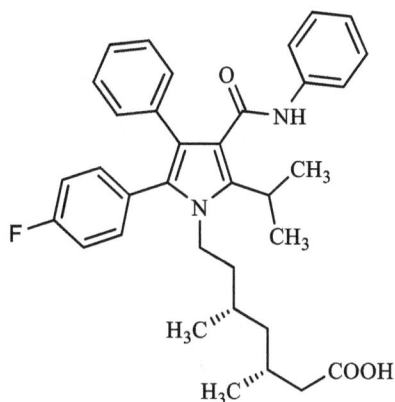

6, Atorvastain

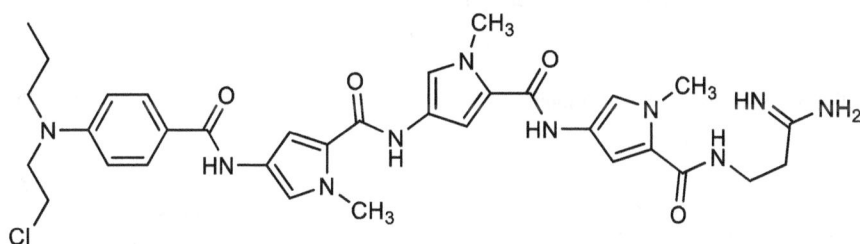

7 , Tallimustine

FIGURE 4.2　Pyrrole that contains active drugs

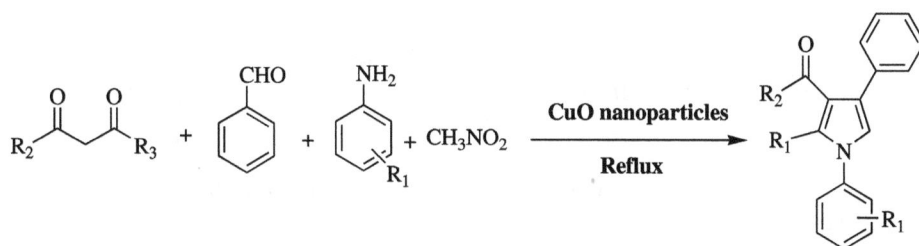

SCHEME 4.1　Synthesis of pyrrole derivatives by CuO NPs

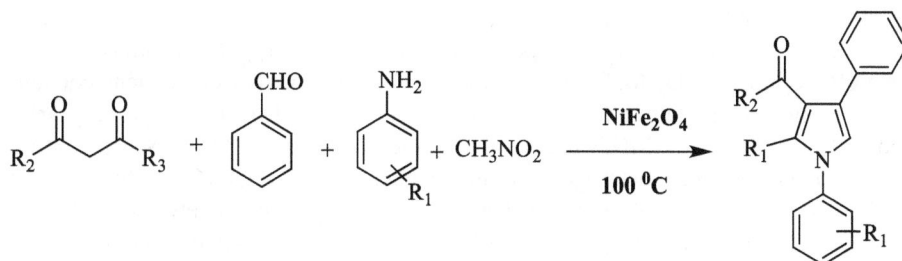

SCHEME 4.2　Synthesis of tetrasubstituted pyrrole using $NiFe_2O_4$ NPs

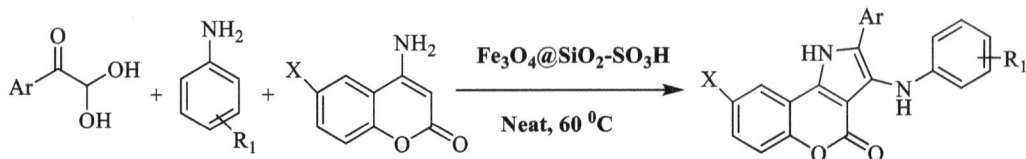

SCHEME 4.3   Synthesis of chromeno[4,3-b]pyrrol-4(1H)-one derivative using Fe$_3$O4@SiO2-SO$_3$H NPs

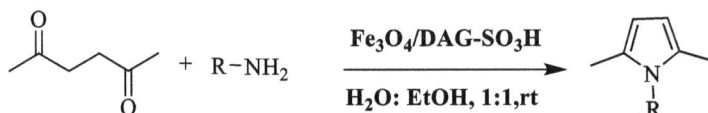

SCHEME 4.4   Synthesis of γ-diketones and 1⁰ amines using Fe$_3$O$_4$/DAG-SO$_3$H

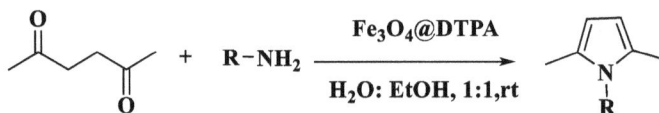

SCHEME 4.5   Synthesis of N-substituted pyrroles was carried out at RT catalyzed by Fe$_3$O$_4$@DTPA11

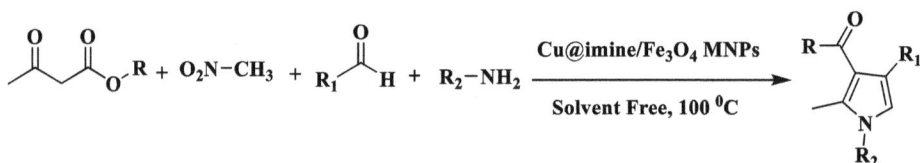

SCHEME 4.6   Polysubstituted pyrroles synthesis using Cu@imine/ Fe$_3$O$_4$ MNPs as a catalyst

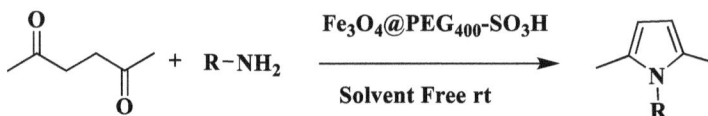

SCHEME 4.7   Synthesized pyrrole a heterogeneous and magnetically recyclable core/shell nanostructure Fe$_3$O$_4$@PEG40-SO$_3$H nanocatalyst

penta acetic acid (MNPs/DTPA) catalyst. The synthesis of N-substituted pyrroles was carried out by a one-pot two-component condensation of γ-diketones and 1° amines under an aqueous phase at RT and catalyzed using Fe$_3$O$_4$@DTPA (Scheme 4.5).[11]

Thwin et al. developed an effective, rapid, and green process for polysubstituted pyrroles synthesis using Cu@imine/Fe$_3$O$_4$ MNPs as a catalyst. The one-pot four-component condensations of ethyl or methyl acetoacetate, nitromethane, substituted benzaldehyde, and primary amine was catalyzed by Cu@imine/Fe$_3$O$_4$ MNPs under solvent-free conditions at 100°C (Scheme 4.6).[12]

Bonyasi et al. synthesized a heterogeneous and magnetically recyclable core/shell nanostructure Fe$_3$O$_4$@PEG400-SO$_3$H nanocatalyst. A Paal-Knorr condensation reaction between γ-diketones with amines was catalyzed by Fe$_3$O$_4$@PEG400-SO$_3$H at RT under solvent-free conditions to yield N-substituted pyrroles (Scheme 4.7).[13]

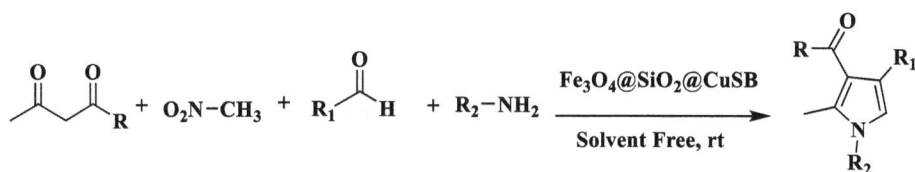

SCHEME 4.8   Synthesized pyrrole using $Fe_3O_4@SiO_2@CuSB$ nanocatalyst

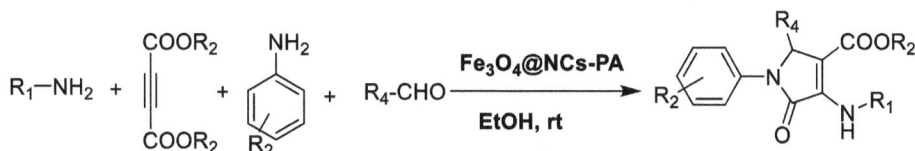

SCHEME 4.9   Catalyzed using $Fe_3O_4@$nano-cellulose-OPO_3H as a novel biobased magnetic nanocatalyst

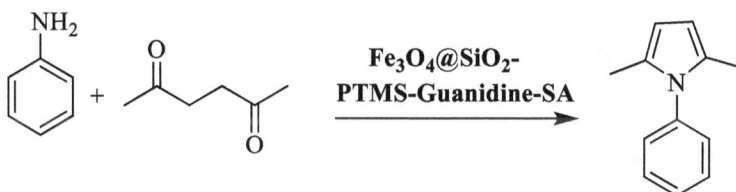

SCHEME 4.10   Synthesis of pyrrole using acidic nanocatalyst $Fe_3O_4@SiO_2$-PTMS-Guanidine-SA

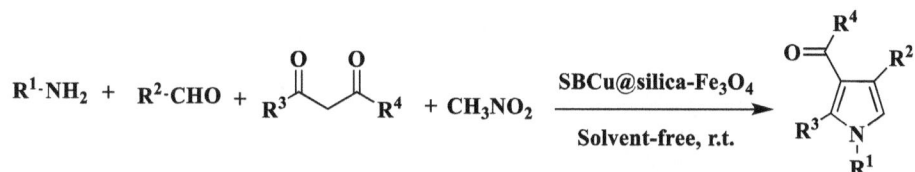

SCHEME 4.11   Synthesis of substituted pyrrole derivatives using catalyst SBCu@silica-Fe_3O_4

Rakhtshah et al. synthesized a $Fe_3O_4@SiO_2@CuSB$ nanocatalyst by immobilizing Cu Schiff base complex on silica-coated Fe_3O_4 NPs, which was an efficient catalyst for polysubstituted pyrrole derivative synthesis using ethyl acetoacetate, nitromethane, aldehyde, and amine at RT under solvent-free conditions (Scheme 4.8).[14]

Salehin et al. developed a green and environmentally benign approach for dihydro-2-oxopyrrole derivatives synthesis via a one-pot four-component condensation reaction of amines, dialkylacetylenedicarboxylate, other amines, and aldehyde catalyzed using $Fe_3O_4@$nano-cellulose-$OPO3H$ as a novel biobased magnetic nanocatalyst in ethanol at RT (Scheme 4.9).[15]

Rostami et al. developed a new method for the synthesis of N-substituted pyrroles using an amine derivative and γ-diketone under neat conditions, which was stirred for 3 h at RT in an acidic nanocatalyst $Fe_3O_4@SiO_2$-PTMS-Guanidine-SA to give the final product (Scheme 4.10).[16]

Hamrahian et al. studied the synthesis of substituted pyrrole derivatives using the catalyst copper Schiff base complex immobilized on silica-coated Fe_3O_4 nanoparticles (SBCu@silica-Fe_3O_4) by treating amine, aryl aldehyde, a 1,3-dicarbonyl compound, and nitromethane at RT under solvent-free conditions (Scheme 4.11).[17]

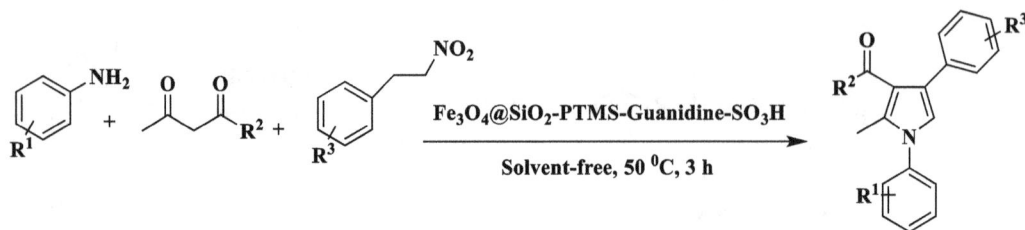

SCHEME 4.12   Synthesis of pyrole by reusable magnetic nanocatalyst Fe_3O_4H SiO-CPTMS-guanidine-SO_3H

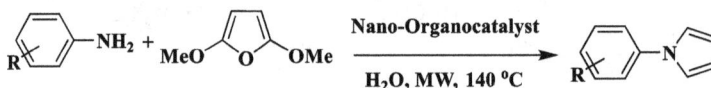

SCHEME 4.13   Synthesis of pyrrole using nano-organo catalysts

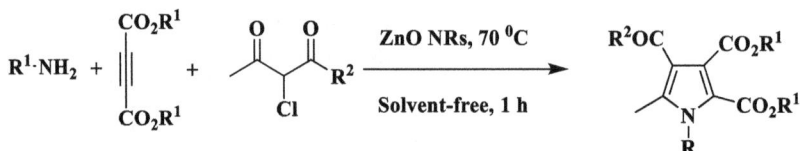

SCHEME 4.14   ZnO nanorods catalyzed for the synthesis of pyrrole derivatives

Rostami et al. described a synthetic method of polysubstituted pyrrole derivatives that used anilines, β-diketones or β-ketoesters, and β-nitrostyrene derivatives under solvent-free conditions in the presence of a reusable magnetic nanocatalyst Fe_3O_4@SiO_2-CPTMS-guanidine-SO_3H at 50°C (Scheme 4.12). [18]

Polshettiwar et al. developed a unique and high selectivity of nano-organocatalysts for a microwave-assisted Paal-Knorr reaction, aza-Michael addition, and pyrazole synthesis that used aromatic amines and 2,5-dimethoxyfuran (Scheme 4.13). [19]

Sabbaghan et al. described zinc oxide (ZnO) nanorods that were catalyzed for the synthesis of pyrrole derivatives that used primary alkylamines, dialkylacetylenedicarboxylates, and 2-chloro-1,3-dicarbonyl compounds at 70°C under solvent-free conditions (Scheme 4.14). [20]

4.2   INTRODUCTION TO INDOLE

Indole is non-basic nitrogen (N) containing compound in which a benzene ring and a pyrrole nucleus are fused in 2, 3 positions. The indole **8** moiety is present in many natural products. The chemistry of indole heterocyclic compounds was more reactive at the third position C atom. Bisindolylmethanes (BIMs) have new structures and exhibit a wide range of biological activities. BIMs show potential growth inhibitory activity on lung cancer cells **9**. [21] BIM derivatives possess different biological activities, for instance, streptindole **10** has gene toxic and DNA damaging activities. [22] A patent [23,24] disclosed the methodology for chromomeric 3,3′-bisindolyl-4-azaphthalides **11** and their purpose as color formers in a pressure and heat interested recording resource. [25] Newer patents explain the synthesis of BIM forming complexes **12** with radioactive metal ions gadolinium (Gd^{3+}), to assist different agents for radioimaging and visualization of various tissues and organs. [26]

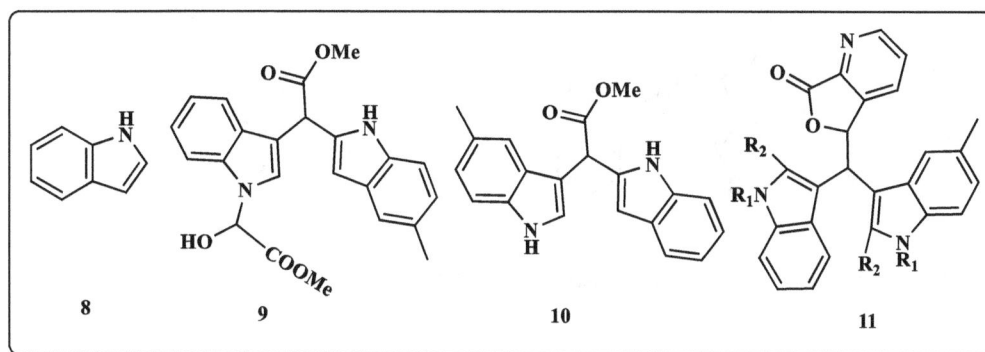

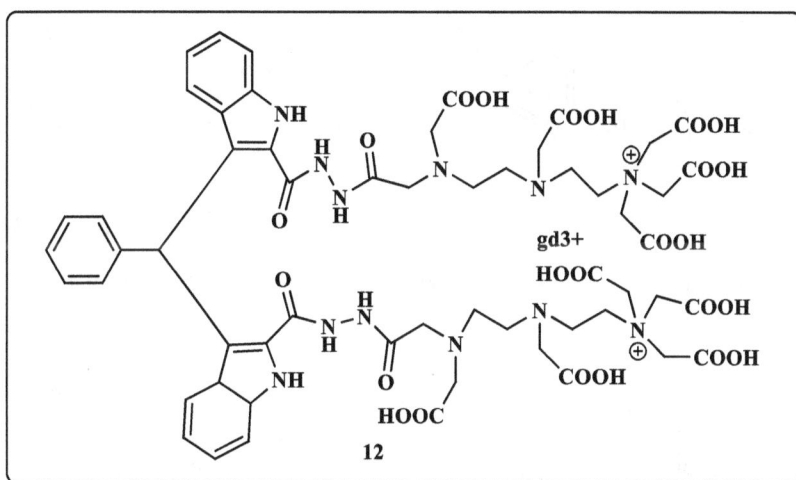

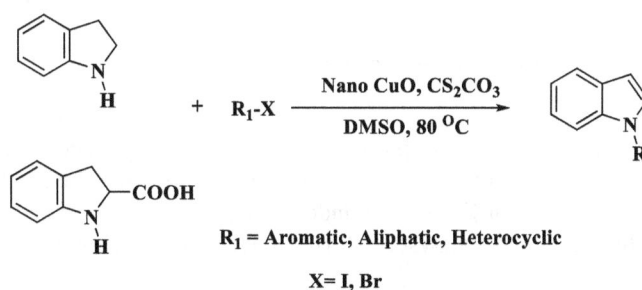

SCHEME 4.15   Synthesis of substituted indoles using nano CuO as a catalyst

4.2.1 SYNTHESIS OF INDOLE DERIVATIVES USING NANOCATALYSTS

Reddy et al. reported the synthesis of substituted indoles using nano CuO as a catalyst and cesium carbonate (Cs_2CO_3) as a base in dimethyl sulfoxide (DMSO) at 80°C. Using nano CuO as a recyclable catalyst followed by a C–N cross-coupling reaction aromatization of indoline and indoline carboxylic acid, and different aryl halides (Scheme 4.15).[27]

Dastmard et al. described a protocol for the synthesis of polyfunctional indole pyrido[2,3-d] pyrimidine hybrids that used a nickel-incorporated fluorapatite encapsulated iron oxide (Fe_3O_4@

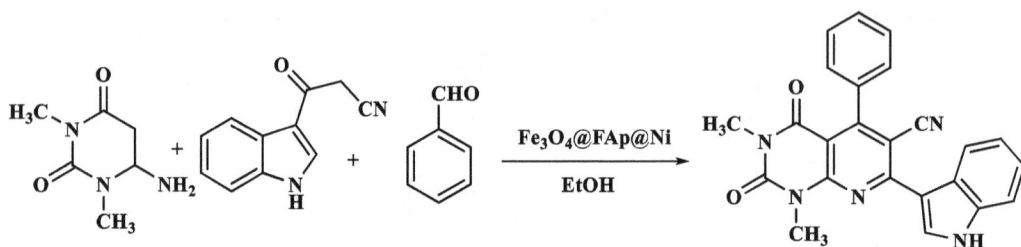

SCHEME 4.16   Synthesis of polyfunctional indole pyrido[2,3-d] pyrimidine using Fe$_3$O$_4$@FAp@Ni catalyst

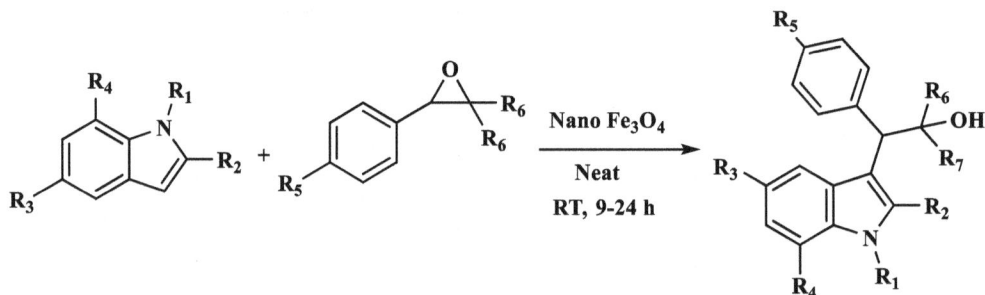

SCHEME 4.17   Synthesis of C-alkylated indole compounds by magnetic nano Fe$_3$O$_4$ catalyst

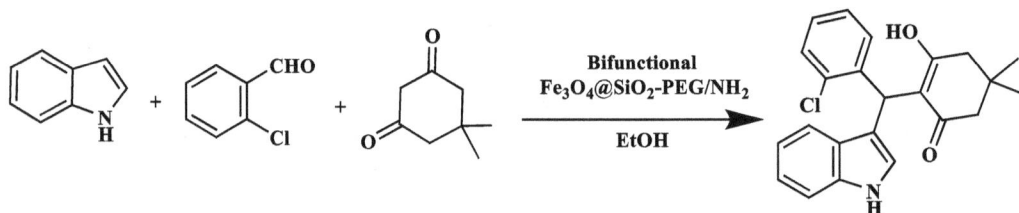

SCHEME 4.18   Synthesis of active 3-alkylated indoles using recyclable bifunctional Fe$_3$O$_4$@SiO$_2$-PEG/NH$_2$

FAp@Ni) magnetic nanocatalyst in the presence of EtOH from 6-amino-N, N-dimethyl uracil, 3-cyanoacetylindole and aryl aldehydes at 60°C to manufacture product (Scheme 4.16).[28]

Parella et al. derived a series of C-alkylated indole compounds from indole styrene oxide in the presence of a magnetic nano Fe$_3$O$_4$ catalyst by stirring at RT under neat conditions for 24 h (Scheme 4.17).[29]

Kardooni et al. described a one-pot synthesis for active 3-alkylated indoles that used indole, aldehydes, and dimedone in EtOH and the presence of green and recyclable bifunctional PEG/NH2 silica-coated magnetic nanocomposite (Fe$_3$O$_4$@SiO$_2$-PEG/NH$_2$) and the reaction mixture was stirred at 80°C (Scheme 4.18).[30]

Bahuguna et al. reported the synthesis of 3-C functionalized indole derivatives. Initially, the reaction with indole and nitroalkenes was catalyzed by a nanocomposite of MoS2-graphitic carbon nitride (MoS$_2$-GCN) catalyst in an aqueous medium at 55°C, gives product. Further reactions with indole and isatin in the presence of a nanocomposite gave the final product of 3-C functionalized indole derivatives and synthesized the precursor of substituted tryptamine using 5-hydroxyindole and of β-nitrostyrene (Scheme 4.19).[31]

Shaikh et al. developed indole based heterocyclic motifs that were catalyzed by polymer grafted ZnO (PLA/ZnO) nanoparticles. The synthesis of 3-substituted indoles under ultrasonication in

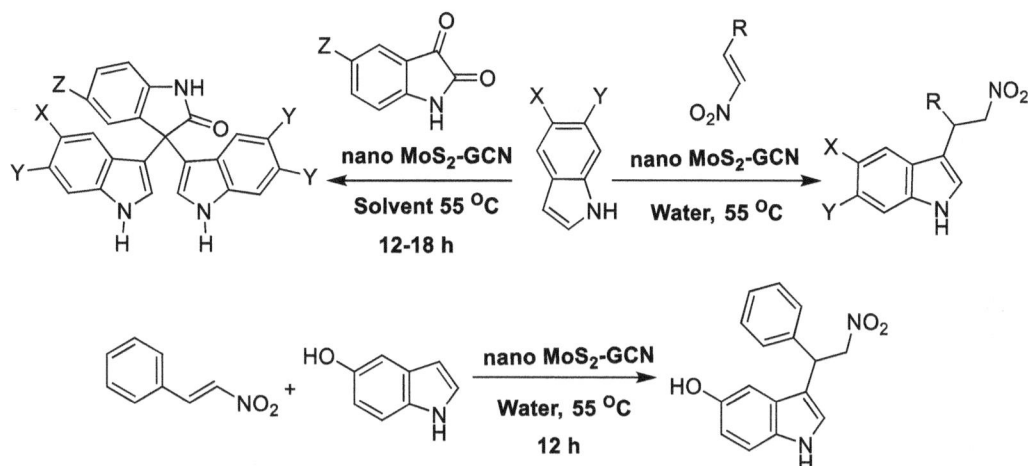

SCHEME 4.19 Synthesis of 3-C-functionalized indole derivatives catalyzed by nano MoS$_2$-GCN catalyst

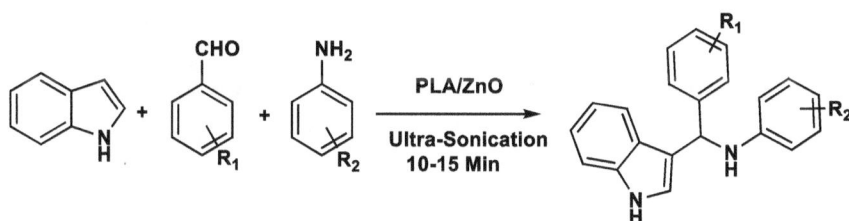

SCHEME 4.20 Synthesis of 3-substituted indole catalyzed by PLA/ZnO NPs

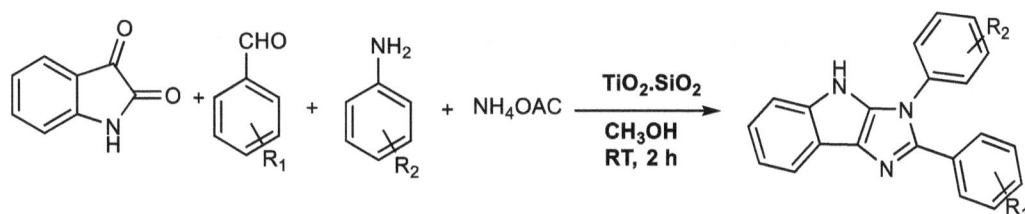

SCHEME 4.21 Synthesis of motifs 2,3-diaryl- 3,4-dihydroimidazo[4,5-b] indole derivatives TiO$_2$ SiO$_2$ NPs

aqueous media from indole substituted aldehydes and different substituted amines were reported (Scheme 4.20).[32]

Geedkar *et al.* synthesized a series of biological potent motifs 2,3-diaryl- 3,4-dihydroimidazo[4,5-b] indole derivatives from a mixture of isatin, substituted aniline derivative aryl aldehyde, ammonium acetate, and TiO$_2$.SiO$_2$ NPs followed by the addition of methanol as solvent at RT (Scheme 4.21).[33]

Garkoti et al. prepared a series of a biologically important class of 3-amino alkylated indoles using a Mannich reaction. The synthesis of 3-amino alkylated indoles motifs from indole, benzaldehyde, pyrrolidine, and added an amine-terminated ionic liquid modified magnetic graphene oxide (MGO-IL-NH$_2$) as a catalyst was reported (Scheme 4.22).[34]

Pradhan et al. extended the NPs scope for the general synthesis of 3-substituted indoles using heterogeneous phosphate grafted SnO$_2$-ZrO$_2$ nanocomposite oxides. The synthesis of pharmaceutically

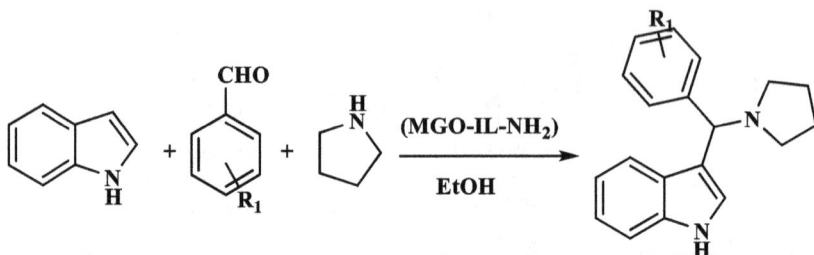

SCHEME 4.22 Synthesis of 3-amino alkylated indoles using ionic liquid modified magnetic graphene oxide (MGO-IL-NH$_2$)

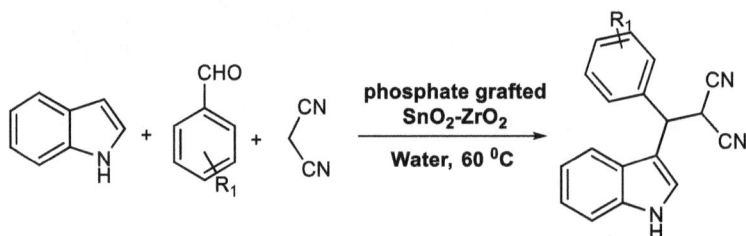

SCHEME 4.23 Synthesis of 3- substituted indoles using heterogeneous phosphate grafted SnO$_2$-ZrO$_2$ nanocomposite oxides

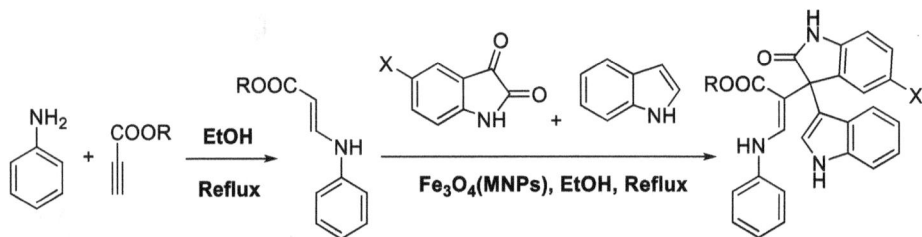

SCHEME 4.24 Synthesis of indoles by Fe$_3$O$_4$ MNPs

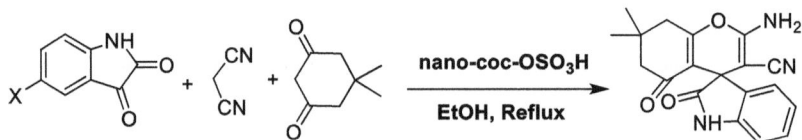

SCHEME 4.25 Synthesis of spirooxinole derivatives using nano-coc-OSO$_3$H

potent 3-substituted indoles occurred via the multicomponent one-pot condensation of indole, aryl aldehydes, and malononitrile (Scheme 4.23).[35]

Hajighasemi et al. established the application of magnetic Fe$_3$O$_4$ NPs (Fe$_3$O$_4$ MNPs) as an easily available, highly proficient, and ecofriendly catalyst. The reaction between aryl amine and alkyl propionate in EtOH obtained the desired products. A mixture of motifs isatin, indolein, and EtOH was heated at reflux in the presence of a Fe$_3$O$_4$ MNPs catalyst to give the final product (Scheme 4.24).[36]

Sadeghi et al. employed spirooxinoles using isatin derivatives, malononitrile, and dimedone in EtOH at reflux condition and chlorosulfonic acid supported on coconut shell (nano-coc-OSO$_3$H) was used as a catalyst to give spirooxinole derivatives (Scheme 4.25).[37]

4.3   INTRODUCTION TO FURAN

Nanotechnology is an attractive field for research. NPs have very high surface-to-volume ratios due to their catalytic activity. The high catalytic potential of nanocatalysts is recovery, and the recycling of expensive nanocatalysts is an important process in modern nanocatalysts. Reusability could provide significant subsidies for the economic viability and sustainable development of nanocatalysis.[38] Furan is a significant heterocyclic compound that exhibits outstanding biological activities during the synthesis of natural products.[39] Derivatives of these compounds possess important pharmaceutical,[40]antifunga,l[41] and antitumor[42]properties. Recently, nanocatalysts have been used as heterogeneous catalysts in several organic transformations.[43] Nanocatalysts have gained significant attention due to their high reactivity, low cost, and they are non-toxic and can be applied in coupling reactions.[44] The one-pot synthesis of benzo[b] furans via the three-component coupling of aldehydes, amines, and alkyne by a copper iodide nanoparticle (CuI-NP) catalyst. Some examples of furan **13** containing biological active drug molecules, such as furazolidone **14**, nitrofural **15**, ranitidine **16**, and nitrofurantoin **17** follow.

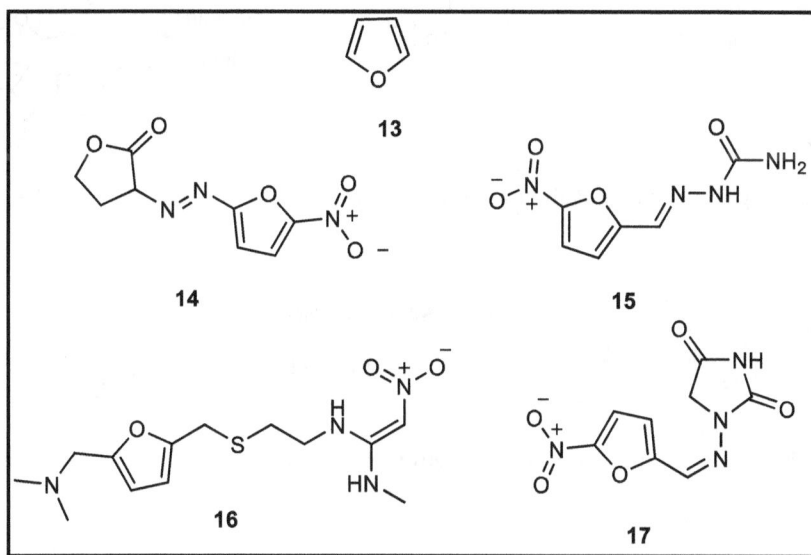

4.3.1   SYNTHESIS OF FURAN DERIVATIVES USING NANOCATALYSTS

Baharfar et al. reported magnesium oxide (MgO) NPs supported ionic liquid-based periodic mesoporous organosilica (MgO@PMO-IL) as a reusable nanocatalyst for the synthesis of a novel spirooxindole–furan derivative in EtOH at 50°C (Scheme 4.26).[45]

Vatanchian et al. synthesized a series of dihydroindeno[1,2-b] furan derivatives using 1,3-indanedione, aryl glyoxal, and pyridinium ylide that used a nano γ-Fe_2O_3-quinuclidine-based catalyst in water (Scheme 4.27).[46]

Khodaei et al. manufactured 4-carboxybenzyl sulfamic acid functionalized Fe_3O_4 NPs as a novel catalyst and used t to synthesize furan-2(5H)-one derivative from aryl aldehydes, anilines, and dimethyl acetylenedicarboxylate in EtOH at 70°C (Scheme 4.28).[47]

Payra et al. reported CuO NPs catalyzed synthesis of furan derivatives using α, β-unsaturated carbonyl compounds, and 1,3-dicarbonyl compounds in an EtOH: water (1:1) solvent system (Scheme 4.29).[48]

Shirzaei et al. reported furan derivatives by reacting aromatic aldehydes and aromatic amines and dialkylacetylenedicarboxylate in the presence of $Fe_3O_4.SiO_2$ NPs as a catalyst (Scheme 4.30).[49]

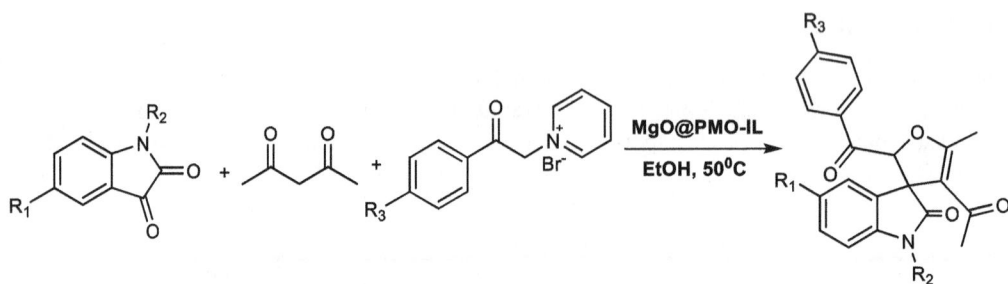

SCHEME 4.26   Synthesis of novel spiro oxindole furan derivatives using organosilica (MgO@PMO-IL)

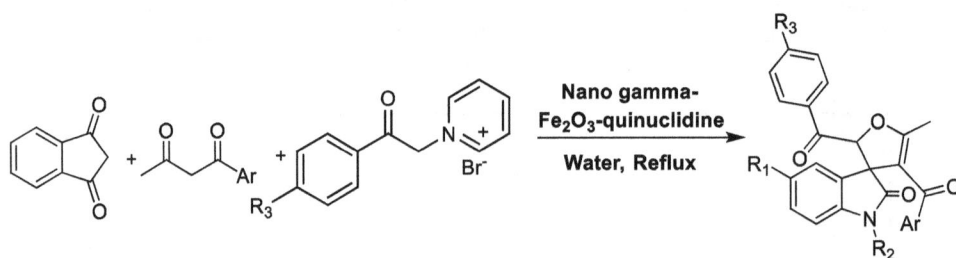

SCHEME 4.27   Synthesis of furan derivatives by using nano γ-Fe₂O₃-quinuclidine-based catalyst

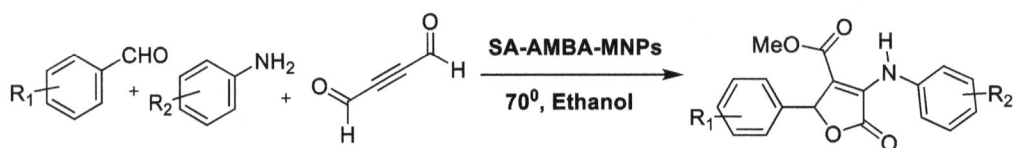

SCHEME 4.28   Synthesize furan-2(5H)-one derivative using 4-carboxybenzyl sulfamic acid functionalized Fe₃O₄ NPs

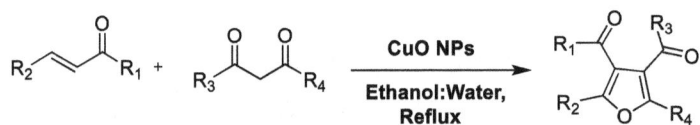

SCHEME 4.29   Synthesis of furan derivatives catalyzed CuO NPs

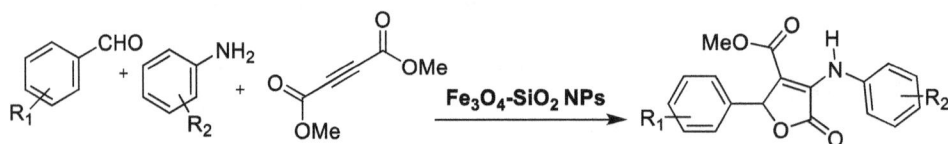

SCHEME 4.30   Synthesis of furan derivatives by Fe₃O₄ SiO₂ NPs

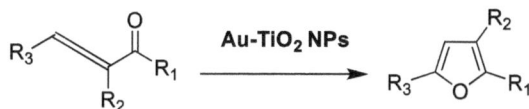

SCHEME 4.31   Synthesis furans catalyzed by Au NPs

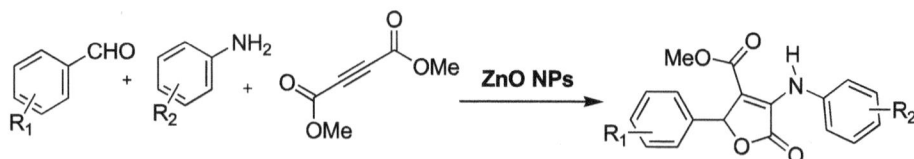

SCHEME 4.32   Synthesis furans catalyzed by ZnO NPs

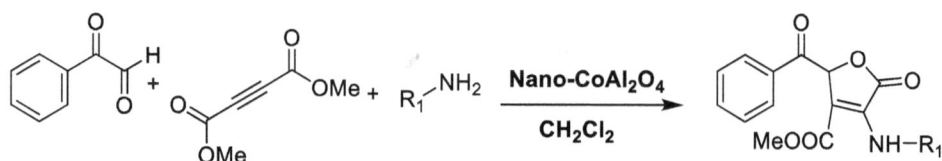

SCHEME 4.33   Synthesis of furan by nano CoAl $_2$O$_4$ catalyst

Zorba et al. reported the cycloisomerization of conjugated allenones into furans catalyzed by Au NPs supported on TiO$_2$ (1 mol %) under mild conditions (Scheme 4.31).[50]

Banerjee reported ZnO NP catalyzed synthesis of 3,4,5-trisubstituted furan-2(5H)-ones using a multicomponent approach (Scheme 4.32).[51]

Seyyed et al. reported the synthesis of 5-oxo-2,5-dihydro-3 furancarboxylates by treating phenylglyoxal, dimethyl acetylenedicarboxylate, and primary amines in the presence of a nano CoAl$_2$O$_4$ catalyst. The best results were obtained in the presence of 4 mg of nano CoAl$_2$O$_4$ in CH$_2$Cl$_2$ at RT (Scheme 4.33).[52]

4.4   INTRODUCTION TO BENZOFURAN

Benzofuran **18** is six-membered ring benzene and five-member ring fused aromatic compound. The structure of benzofuran is shown here:

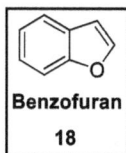

Benzofuran is a significant heterocyclic scaffold found in diverse pharmaceuticals and natural products with promising biological activities,[53–60] such as anti-estrogen breast cancer agent **19**, antifungal **20**, antimicrobial **21**, antimycobacterial **2, 2**and antitumor agent **23**.

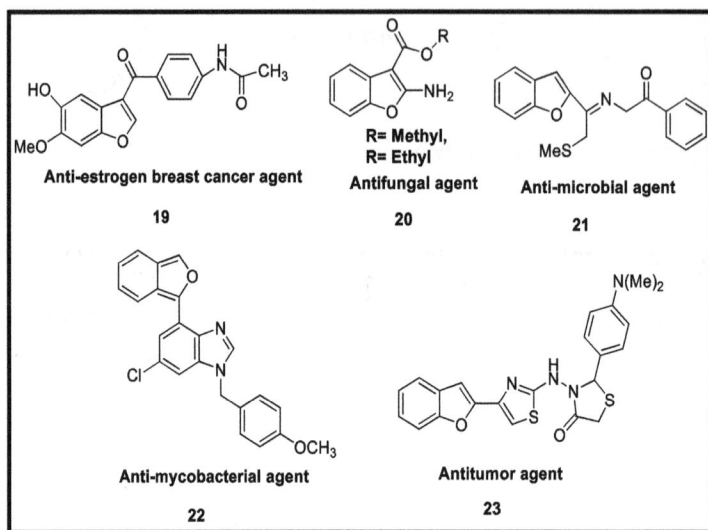

4.4.1 Synthesis of Benzofuran using Nanocatalysts

Purohit et al. reported an efficient process for the synthesis of benzofuranamine A and dihydro-benzofuranamine B that was catalyzed by an arranged porous sphere-like copper oxide (HS-CuO) NPs. Compounds A and B are synthesized from the annulated coupling of salicylaldehyde, secondary amines, and phenylacetylenes in the presence of HS-CuO NPs catalyst at 110°C under neat conditions (Scheme 4.34).[61]

Safaei-Ghomi et al. developed a method for the synthesis of 2,3-disubstituted benzo[b]furan derivatives by reacting aldehydes, secondary amines, and alkynes in equimolar concentrations of EtOH: water system in the presence of ZnO NPs catalyst (Scheme 4.35).[62]

Bruneau et al. reported the synthesis of benzofuran using o-iodophenols with acetylenes to give 2-substituted benzofurans in the presence of heterogeneous catalysts, consisting of Pd nanoparticles supported on a siliceous mesocellular foam (Pd0-AmP-MCF) at 70°C (Scheme 4.36).[63]

Sajjadi-Ghotbabadi et al. synthesized a series of 2-oxochromene and benzofuran derivatives from the addition or intramolecular cyclization reactions of 1-(6-hydroxy- 2-isopropenyl-1-benzofuran-5-yl)-1-ethanone, activated acetylenic compounds and triphenylphosphine in the

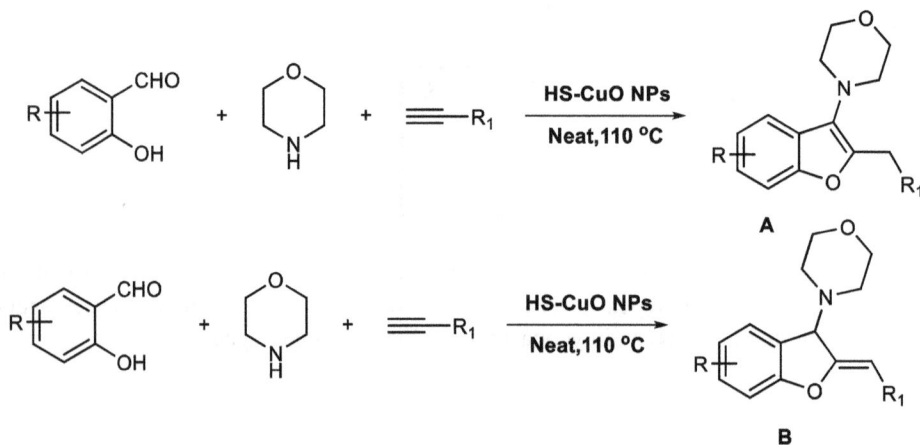

SCHEME 4.34 Synthesis of benzofuran amine dihydro-benzofuran amine catalyzed by HS-CuO NPs

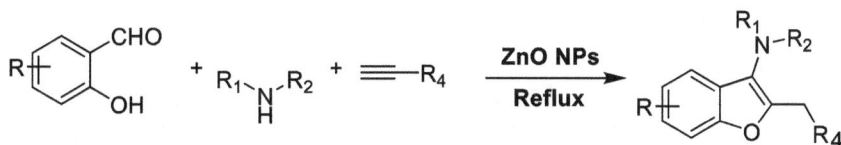

SCHEME 4.35   Synthesis of 2,3-disubstituted benzo[b]furan derivatives by of ZnO NPs

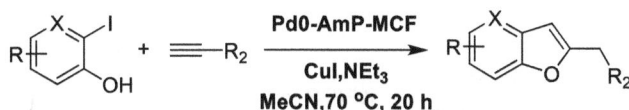

SCHEME 4.36   Synthesis of benzofuran by heterogeneous catalyst Pd0-AmP-MCF

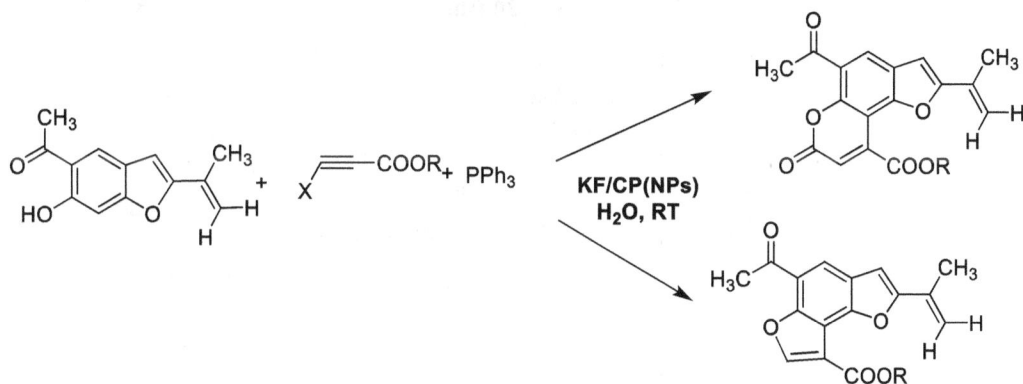

SCHEME 4.37   Synthesized benzofuran derivatives using KF impregnated clinoptilolite NPs

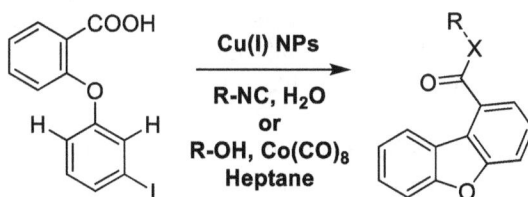

SCHEME 4.38   Synthesis of dibenzofuran using Cu(I) as a catalyst

presence of potassium fluoride (KF) impregnated clinoptilolite nanocatalyst in aqueous medium at RT (Scheme 4.37).[64]

Pal et al. reported the synthesis of new green one-step carbonyl dibenzofurans derivatives. This protocol has regio-selective decarboxylative C–H arylation and carbonylative aryl halide with isocyanides or alcohol in the presence of CuI as a catalyst in an aqueous solution and gives carbonyl dibenzofurans (Scheme 4.38).[65]

Woo et al. developed the synthesis of 2-phenyl benzofuran from 2-iodophenol with phenyl propionic acids in the presence of a Cu-doped Pd-Fe$_3$O$_4$ catalyst at 130°C for 1 h. The use of more catalysts influenced the base conversion achieved with sodium acetate (NaOAc) (90%) (Scheme 4.39).[66]

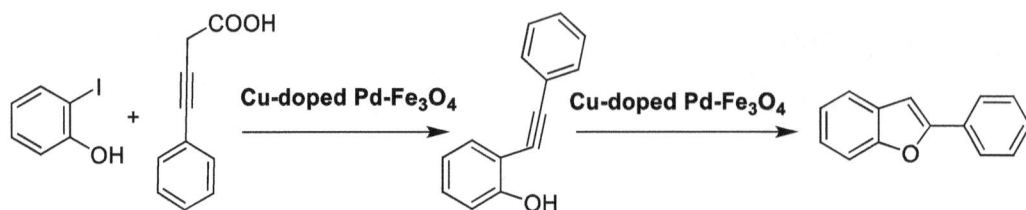

SCHEME 4.39 Synthesis of 2-phenyl benzofuran by Cu-doped Pd- Fe_3O_4 catalyst

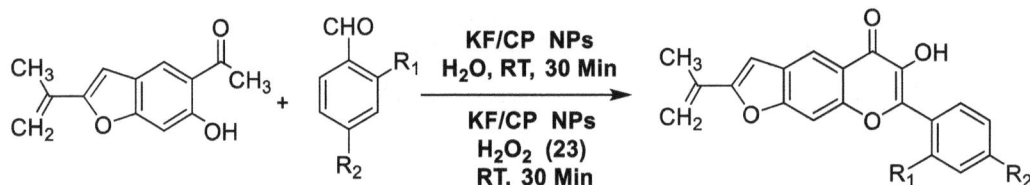

SCHEME 4.40 Synthesis of by KF/CP nanocatalyst

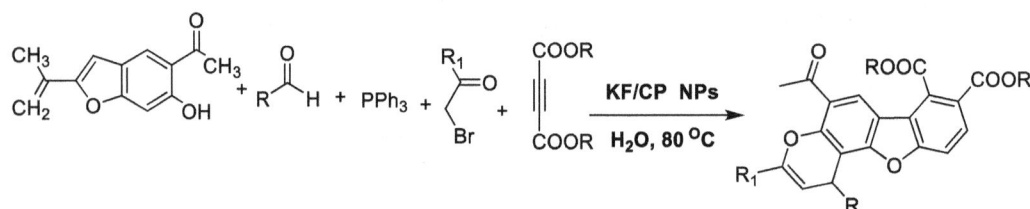

SCHEME 4.41 Synthesis of benzochromene derivatives by using heterogeneous nanocatalyst KF/CP NPs

Sajjadi-Ghotbabadi et al. described the synthesis of newer 3-hydroxy flavones by a three-component, one-pot aldol condensation and intramolecular cyclization reaction of 1-[6-hydroxy-2-(prop-1-en-2-yl)-1-benzofuran-5-yl] ethanone, substituted benzaldehyde, and hydrogen peroxide in the presence of a potassium fluoride/clinoptilolite nanocatalyst (KF/CP) in an aqueous medium at RT (Scheme 4.40).[67]

Ezzatzadeh et al. developed the synthesis of benzochromene derivatives by treating 1-(6-hydroxy-2-isopropenyl-1-benzofuranyl)-1-ethanone, aldehydes, alkyl bromides, dialkylacetylenedicarboxylate, and triphenylphosphine using heterogeneous nanocatalyst nano-potassium fluoride/clinoptilolite (KF/CP) NPs as basic catalyst in an aqueous medium at 80°C (Scheme 4.41).[68]

4.5 CONCLUSION

This chapter focused on the study of nanocatalysts and their applications in the synthesis of bio-active pyrrole, indole, furan, and benzofuran heterocyclic derivatives. Today, nanotechnology is a growing area of research. Therefore, this chapter could be helpful for researchers in chemistry and nanotechnology. The following are the advantages of nanocatalyst in the synthesis of biologically active heterocyclic compounds:

1. Environment-friendly approach.
2. Short reaction time.

3. Easy workup procedure.
4. High yield of product.
5. Non-toxic.
6. Maximize atom economy.

REFERENCES

1. Zhang M, Neumann H, Beller M. Selective Ruthenium-Catalyzed Three-Component Synthesis of Pyrroles. Angew Chem Int Ed. 2012. 52(2):597–601. Doi:10.1002/anie.201206082.
2. St Cyr DJ, Arndtsen BA. A New Use of Wittig-Type Reagents as 1,3-Dipolar Cycloaddition Precursors and in Pyrrole Synthesis. J Am Chem Soc. 2007. 129(41):12366–7. Doi:10.1021/ja074330w.
3. Calderon F, Barros D, Bueno JM, Coteron J M, Fernandez E, Gamo FJ. et al. An Invitation to Open Innovation in Malaria Drug Discovery: 47 Quality Starting Points from the TCAMS. ACS Med Chem Lett. 2011. 2(10):741–6. Doi:10.1021/ml200135p.
4. Biava M, Porretta GC, Poce G, De Logu A, Meleddu R, De Rossi E. et al. 1,5-Diaryl-2-ethyl pyrrole derivatives as antimycobacterial agents: Design, synthesis, and microbiological evaluation. Eur J Med Chem. 2009 44(11): 4734–8. Doi: 10.1016/j.ejmech.2009.06.005.
5. Jiang S, Lu H, Liu S, Zhao Q, He Y, Debnath AK. N-Substituted Pyrrole Derivatives as Novel Human Immunodeficiency Virus Type 1 Entry Inhibitors That Interfere with the gp41 Six-Helix Bundle Formation and Block Virus Fusion. Antimicrob Agents Chemother. 2004. 48(11):4349–59. Doi:10.1128/aac.48.11.4349-4359.2004
6. Teixeira C, Barbault F, Rebehmed J, Liu K, Xie L, Lu H. et al. Molecular modeling studies of N-substituted pyrrole derivatives-Potential HIV-1 gp41 inhibitors. Bioorganic & Medicinal Chemistry. 2008. 16(6):3039–048. doi:10.1016/j.bmc.2007.12.034.
7. Saeidian H, Abdoli M, Salimi R. One-pot synthesis of highly substituted pyrroles using nano copper oxide as an effective heterogeneous nanocatalyst. C R Chim. 2013. 16(11):1063–70. doi:10.1016/j.crci.2013.02.008.
8. Moghaddam F M, Koushki Foroushani B, Rezvani HR. Nickel ferrite nanoparticles: an efficient and reusable nanocatalyst for a neat, one-pot and four-component synthesis of pyrroles. RSC Adv. 2015. 5(23):18092–6.doi:10.1039/c4ra09348h.
9. Mukherjee S, Sarkar S, Pramanik A. A Sustainable Synthesis of Functionalized Pyrrole Fused Coumarins under Solvent-Free Conditions Using Magnetic Nanocatalyst and a New Route to Polyaromatic Indolocoumarins. ChemistrySelect. 2018. 3(5):1537–44. doi:10.1002/slct.201703146.
10. Veisi H, Mohammadi P, Gholami J. Sulfamic acid heterogenized on functionalized magnetic Fe_3O_4 nanoparticles with diaminoglyoxime as a green, efficient and reusable catalyst for one-pot synthesis of substituted pyrroles in aqueous phase. Appl Organomet Chem. 2014. 28(12): 868–73. doi:10.1002/aoc.3228.
11. Hemmati S, Mohammadi P, Sedrpoushan A, Maleki B. Synthesis of 2,5-Dimethyl-N-substituted Pyrroles Catalyzed by Diethylenetriaminepentaacetic Acid Supported on Fe_3O_4 Nanoparticles. Org Prep Proc Int. 2018. 50(5):465–81. doi:10.1080/00304948.2018.1525668.
12. Thwin M, Mahmoudi B, Ivaschuk OA, Yousif QA. An efficient and recyclable nanocatalyst for the green and rapid synthesis of biologically active polysubstituted pyrroles and 1,2,4,5-tetrasubstituted imidazole derivatives. RSC Adv.2019. 9(28):15966–75. doi:10.1039/c9ra02325a.
13. Bonyasi F, Hekmati M, Veisi H. Preparation of core/shell nanostructure Fe_3O_4@PEG400-SO_3H as heterogeneous and magnetically recyclable nanocatalyst for one-pot synthesis of substituted pyrroles by Paal-Knorr reaction at room temperature. Journal of Colloid and Interface Science, 2017. 496:177–87. doi:10.1016/j.jcis.2017.02.023.
14. Rakhtshah J, Shaabani B, Salehzadeh S, Hosseinpour, Moghadam N. The solvent-free synthesis of polysubstituted pyrroles by a reusable copper Schiff base complex immobilized on silica coated Fe_3O_4, and DNA binding study of one resulting derivative as a potential anticancer drug. Appl Organometal Chem. 2018. e4754: 1–15. doi:10.1002/aoc.4754.
15. Salehi N, FatamehMirjalili BB. Synthesis of highly substituted dihydro-2-oxopyrroles using Fe_3O_4@nano-cellulose-OPO_3H as a novel bio-based magnetic nanocatalyst. RSC Adv. 2017. 7(48):30303–9. doi:10.1039/c7ra04101b.

16. Rostami H, Shiri L. Fe$_3$O$_4$@SiO$_2$-PTMS-Guanidine-SA nanoparticles as an effective and reusable catalyst for the synthesis of *N*-substituted pyrroles. J Iranian Chem Soc. 2020. 17:1329–35.doi.10.1007/s13738-020-01857-7.
17. Hamrahian SA, Rakhtshah J, MousaviDavijani SM, Salehzadeh S. Copper Schiff base complex immobilized on silica coated Fe$_3$O$_4$ nanoparticles: a recoverable and efficient catalyst for synthesis of polysubstituted pyrroles. Appl Organometal Chem. 2018. e4501: doi.10.1002/aoc.4501.
18. Rostami H, Shiri L. Fe$_3$O$_4$@SiO$_2$-CPTMS-Guanidine-SO$_3$H-catalyzed One-Pot Multicomponent Synthesis of Polysubstituted Pyrrole Derivatives under Solvent-Free Conditions. Russian J Org Chem. 2019. 55(8):1204–11. doi.10.1134/S1070428019080207.
19. Polshettiwar V, Varma RS. Nano-organocatalyst: magnetically retrievable ferrite-anchored glutathione for microwave-assisted Paal-Knorr reaction, aza-Michael addition, and pyrazole synthesis. Tetrahedron. 2010. 66:1091–7. doi.10.1016/j.tet.2009.11.015
20. Sabbaghan M, Sanaeishoar H, Ghalaei A, Sofalgar, P. Solvent-free synthesis of polysubstituted pyrroles catalyzed by ZnO nanorods. J Iran Chem Soc. 2015. 12:2199–204 doi.10.1007/s13738-015-0697-6.
21. Chite N, Chougule MB, Jackson T, Fulzele SV, Safe S, Singh M. Enhancement of Docetaxel Anticancer Activity by a Novel Diindolylmethane Compound in Human Non-Small Cell Lung Cancer. Clin Cancer Res. 2009.15: 543–52.doi:10.1158/1078-0432.
22. Sarma P, Ramaiah M J, Kamal A, Bhadra U, Bhadra MP. A novel bisindole-PBD conjugate causes DNA damage induced apoptosis via inhibition of DNA repair pathway. Cancer Biology & Therapy. 2014. 15(10):1320–2. doi.10.4161/cbt.29705.
23. Bedekovic D, Fletcher IJ. (1986), *U.S. patent*, 4, 587, 343.
24. Bedekovic D, Fletcher IJ. (1987), *U.S. patent*, 4, 705, 776.
25. Fletcher IJ, Rudolf Z. Chemistry and Applications of Leuco Dyes. New York: Plenum Press; 1997.
26. Gresens E, Adriaens NY, Verbruggen PA, Marchal G. (200) *U.S. patent* 0053911A1.
27. Reddy KHV, Satish G, Ramesh K, Karnakar K, Nageswar YVD. An efficient synthesis of N-substituted indoles from indoline/indoline carboxylic acid via aromatization followed by C–N cross-coupling reaction by using nano copper oxide as a recyclable catalyst. Tetrahedron Lett. 2012. 53(24):3061–5. doi:10.1016/j.tetlet.2012.04.012.
28. Dastmard S, Mamaghani M, Farahnak L, Rassa M. Facile Synthesis of Polyfunctional Indole-Pyrido[2,3-d] Pyrimidine Hybrids Using Nickel-Incorporated Fluorapatite Encapsulated Iron Oxide Nanocatalyst and Study of Their Antibacterial Activities. Polycyclic Aromatic Compounds. 2020.1–14. doi10.1080/10406638.2020.1804413.
29. Parella R, Naveen, Babu SA. Magnetic nano Fe$_3$O$_4$ and CuFe$_2$O$_4$ as heterogeneous catalysts: A green method for the stereo- and regioselective reactions of epoxides with indoles/pyrroles. Catal Comms. 2012. 29: 118–21. doi:10.1016/j.catcom.2012.09.030.
30. Kardooni R, Kiasat AR. Bifunctional PEG/NH$_2$ silica-coated magnetic nanocomposite: An efficient and recoverable core–shell-structured catalyst for one pot multicomponent synthesis of 3-alkylated indoles *via* Yonemitsu-type condensation. J Taiwan Inst Chem Engineers. 2018. 87: 241–51. doi:10.1016/j.jtice.2018.03.029.
31. Bahuguna A, Kumar A, Kumar S, Chhabra T, Krishnan V.2D-2D Nanocomposite of MoS$_2$ -Graphitic Carbon Nitride as Multifunctional Catalyst for Sustainable Synthesis of C3-Functionalized Indoles. ChemCatChem. 2018. 10(14):3121–32. doi:10.1002/cctc.201800369.
32. Shaikh T, Sharma A, Kaur H. Ultrasonication-Assisted Synthesis of 3-Substituted Indoles in Water Using Polymer Grafted ZnO Nanoparticles as Eco-Friendly Catalyst. ChemistrySelect. 2019. 4(1): 245–49. doi:10.1002/slct.20180270.
33. Geedkar D, Kumar A, Reen GK, Sharma P. Titania-silica nanoparticles ensembles assisted heterogeneous catalytic strategy for the synthesis of pharmacologically significant 2,3-diaryl-3,4-dihydroimidazo[4,5-b] indole scaffolds. *J Heterocyclic Chem.* 2020. 57(4):1–11.doi:10.1002/jhet.3925.
34. Garkoti C, Shabir J, Mozumdar S. Amine-Terminated Ionic Liquid Modified Magnetic Graphene Oxide (MGO-IL-NH 2): A Highly Efficient and Reusable Nanocatalyst for the Synthesis of 3-Amino Alkylated Indoles. ChemistrySelect. 2020. 5(14):4337–46. doi:10.1002/slct.20200033.
35. Pradhan S, Jagannath SBG. Mishra morphology controlled phosphate grafted SnO$_2$-ZrO$_2$ nanocomposite oxides prepared by a urea hydrolysis method as efficient heterogeneous catalysts towards the synthesis of 3-substituted indoles. New J Chem. 2017. 14:6616–29.doi.org/10.1039/C7NJ00249A.

36. Hajighasemi H, Yazdani-Elah-Abadi A, Shams N. An Efficient and Green Stereoselective Synthesis of Functionalized 3-Indol-3-yl-oxoindolin-3-yl-3-acrylates *via* Nano-Fe$_3$O$_4$-Promoted One-Pot Four-Component Domino Reactions. Polycyclic Aromatic Compounds. 2017. 1–12. doi:10.1080/10406638.2017.1355326

37. Sadeghi B, Mousavi, SA. Preparation and Characterization of Nano-coc-OSO$_3$H as a Novel Nanocatalyst for the One-Pot Synthesis of Spirooxindoles. Polycyclic Aromatic Compounds. 2020. 1–13. 424–36. doi:10.1080/10406638.2020.1737828.

38. Xiang F, Wangqing K, Xin C, Xuejiao J, Zhengzhong S, Jim-Yang L. A Recycling-Free Nanocatalyst System: The Stabilization of In Situ-Reduced Noble Metal Nanoparticles on Silicone Nanofilaments via a Mussel-Inspired Approach. ACS Catal. 2017. 7:(4)2412–18.doi.org/10.1021/acscatal.6b03185

39. Safaei-Ghomi J, Ghasemzadeh M A, Kakavand-Qalenoei A. CuI-Nanoparticles-Catalyzed One-Pot Synthesis of Benzo[b]Furans *via* Three-Component Coupling of Aldehydes, Amines and Alkyne. J Saudi Chem Soc. 2016. 20(5):502–9. doi.org/10.1016/j.jscs.2012.07.010.

40. Shridhar DR, Sastry CV, Moorty SR, Vaidya NK, Reddy PG, Reddi GS. et al. Synthesis and Biological Activity of Some New Furan Quaternary Salts. J Med Chem. 1977. 20(1):149–54. doi.org/10.1021/jm00211a032.

41. Ahmed W, Yan X, Hu D, Adnan M, Tang RY, Cui ZN. Synthesis and Fungicidal Activity of Novel Pyrazole Derivatives Containing 5-Phenyl-2-Furan. Bioorg Med Chem. 2019. 27(19):115048. doi.org/10.1016/j.bmc.2019.115048.

42. Lu D, Zhou Y, Li Q, Luo J, Jiang Q, He B. et al. Synthesis, *In Vitro* Antitumor Activity and Molecular Mechanism of Novel Furan Derivatives and Their Precursors. Anticancer Agents Med Chem. 2020. 20(12):1475–86. doi.org/10.2174/1871520620666200424130204.

43. Prinsen P, Luque R. Introduction to Nano catalysts. Nanoparticle Design and Characterization for Catalytic Applications in Sustainable Chemistry. (2019). 1–36. doi.org/10.1039/9781788016292-00001. eISBN: 978-1-78801-629-2

44. Sharma RK, Dutta S, Sharma S, Zboril R, Varma RS, Gawande MB. Fe$_3$O$_4$ (Iron Oxide)-Supported Nano-catalysts: Synthesis, Characterization and Applications in Coupling Reactions. Green Chem. 2016. 18(11):3184–209. doi.org/10.1039/C6GC00864J.

45. Baharfar R, Zareyee D, Allahgholipour SL. Synthesis and Characterization of MgO Nanoparticles Supported on Ionic Liquid based Periodic Mesoporous Organosilica (MgO@PMO-IL) as a Highly Efficient and Reusable Nanocatalyst for the Synthesis of Novel Spirooxindole furan Derivatives. Appl Organomet Chem.2019. 33(4): e-4923. doi.10.1002/AOC.4805.

46. Vatanchian R, Mosslemin, MH, Tabatabaee M, Sheibani A. Synthesis of Trans-Dihydroindeno[1,2-b] Furans *via* Nano γ-Fe$_2$O$_3$-Quinuclidine-Based Catalyst in an Aqueous Medium. J Chem Res. 2018. 42(12):598–600. doi.org/10.3184/174751918X15411641337056.

47. Khodaei MM, Alizadeh A, Haghipour M. Supported 4-Carboxybenzyl Sulfamic Acid on Magnetic Nanoparticles as a Recoverable and Recyclable Catalyst for Synthesis of 3,4,5-Trisubstituted Furan-2(5H)-One Derivatives. J Organometal Chem. 2018. 870:58–67. doi.org/10.1016/j.jorganchem.2018.06.012.

48. Payra S, Saha A, Guchhait S, Banerjee S. Direct CuO nanoparticle-catalyzed synthesis of poly-substituted furans *via* oxidative C–H/C–H functionalization in aqueous medium. RSC Adv. 2016. 6(40):33462–7. doi:10.1039/c6ra04181g.

49. Shirzaei M, Mollashahi E, Taher Maghsoodlou M, Lashkari M. Novel Synthesis of Silica-Coated Magnetic Nano-Particles Based on Acidic Ionic Liquid, as a Highly Efficient Catalyst for Three Component System Leads to Furans Derivatives. J Saudi Chem Soc. 2020. 24(2):216–22. doi.org/10.1016/j.jscs. 2020.01.001.

50. Zorba L, Kidonakis M, Saridakis I, Stratakis M. Cycloisomerization of Conjugated Allenones into Furans under Mild Conditions Catalyzed by Ligandless Au Nanoparticles. Organic Lett. 2019. 21(14):5552–5.doi.org/10.1021/acs.orglet t.9b01869.

51. Banerjee B. Recent Developments on Nano-ZnO Catalyzed Synthesis of Bioactive Heterocycles. J Nano Struct Chem. 2017. 7(4):389–413. doi.org/10.1007 /s40097-017-0247-0.

52. Seyyed ME, Ali KA, Shahbazi-Alavi H, Safaei-Ghomi J. Synthesis of2,5-dihydro-3-furans using nano-CoAl$_2$O$_4$ Res Chem Intermed. 2021. 230. doi.org/10.1007/s11164-021-04463-1.

53. Boto A, Alvarez L. Furan and Its Derivatives. In: Heterocycles in Natural Product Synthesis; Berlin: Wiley-VCH: 2011. p. 97–152.

54. Rao MLN, Murty VN. Rapid Access to Benzofuran-Based Natural Products through a Concise Synthetic Strategy. Eur J Org Chem. 2016. 12: 2177–86. doi.org/10.1002/ejoc.201600154.

55. Li XY, He BF, Luo HJ, Huang NY, Deng WQ. 3-Acyl-5-hydroxybenzofuran derivatives as potential anti-estrogen breast cancer agents: A combined experimental and theoretical investigation. Bioorg Med Chem Lett. 2013. 15;23(16):4617–21. doi: 10.1016/j.bmcl.2013.06.022.

56. Ryu CK, Song AL, Lee JY, Hong JA, Yoon JH, Kim A. Synthesis and antifungal activity of benzofuran-5-ols. Bioorg Med Chem Lett. 2010.15;20(22):6777–80. doi: 10.1016/j.bmcl.2010.08.129.

57. Kirilmis C, Ahmedzade M, Servi S, Koca M, Kizirgil A, Kazaz C. Synthesis and antimicrobial activity of some novel derivatives of benzofuran: Part 2. The synthesis and antimicrobial activity of some novel 1-(1-benzofuran-2-yl)-2-mesitylethanone derivatives. Eur J Med Chem. 200843: 300–8. doi.10.1016/j.ejmech.2007.03.023.

58. Brndvang M, Bakken V, Gundersen LL. Synthesis, structure, and antimycobacterial activity of 6-[1(3H)-isobenzofuranylidenemethyl]purines and analogs. Bioorg Med Chem. 2009. 15;17(18):6512–6. Doi.10.1016/j.bmc.2009.08.012.

59. Othman Dina I, Abdelal Ali MM, El-Sayed Magda A, El Bialy, Serry AA. Novel benzofuran derivatives: synthesis and antitumor activity. Heterocyclic Comm. 2013. 19(1):29–35. doi.10.1515/hc-2012–0119.

60. Khodarahmi G, Asadi P, Hassanzadeh F, Khodarahmi E. Benzofuran as A Promising Scaffold for the Synthesis of Antimicrobial and Anti breast Cancer Agents: A review. J Res Med Sci. 2015. 20:1094–104. doi.10.4103/1735-1995.172835.

61. Purohit GU Chinna R, Rawat DS. Hierarchically Porous Sphere-Like Copper Oxide (HS-CuO) Nanocatalyzed Synthesis of Benzofuran Isomers with Anomalous Selectivity and Their Ideal Green Chemistry Metrics. ACS Sustain Chem Eng. 2017. 5(8):6466–77.doi.10.1021/acssuschemeng.7b00500.

62. Safaei-Ghomi J, Ghasemzadeh, MA. Zinc oxide nanoparticle promoted highly efficient one pot three-component synthesis of 2,3-disubstituted benzofurans. Arabian J Chem. 2017. 10:(2)S1774–80. doi.org/10.1016/j.arabjc.2013.06.030.

63. Bruneau A, Gustafson KPJ, Yuan N, Cheuk-Wai T, Persson I, Zou X. et al. Synthesis of Benzofurans and Indoles from Terminal Alkynes and Iodoaromatics Catalyzed by Recyclable Palladium Nanoparticles Immobilized on Siliceous Mesocellular Foam. Chem A Eur J. 2017. 23(52):12886–91.doi.10.1002/chem.201702614.

64. Sajjadi-Ghotbabadi H, Javanhir S, Rostami-Charati F. Synthesis, Characterization, and Antioxidant Evaluations of New 2-Oxochromene and Benzofuran Derivatives Catalyzed by KF/CP: Synthesis, Characterization, and Antioxidant Evaluations of New 2-Oxochromene and Benzofuran Derivatives. J Heterocyclic Chem. 2016. 54(2): doi:10.1002/jhet.2662.

65. Pal R, Chatterjee N, Roy M, Sarkar S, Sen AK. Cubic nano-copper(I) oxides as reusable catalyst in consecutive decarboxylative C-H arylation and carbonylation: rapid synthesis of carbonyl dibenzofurans. Tetrahedron Lett. 2016. 57(45): 4956–60. doi.10.1016/j.tetlet.2016.09.074.

66. Woo H, Kim D, Park JC, Kim JW, Park S, Lee JM, Park KH. A new hybrid nanocatalyst based on Cu-doped Pd-Fe$_3$O$_4$ for tandem synthesis of 2-phenylbenzofurans. J Mater Chem A 2015. 3:20992–8 doi.10.1039/C5TA05111H.

67. Sajjadi-Ghotbabadi H, Javanshir S, Rostami-Charati F, Sayyed-Alangi SZ. Eco-compatible synthesis of novel 3-hydroxyflavones catalyzed by KF-impregnated mesoporous natural zeolite clinoptilolite. Chem Heterocyclic Comp. 2018. 54(5):508–13.doi.10.1007/s10593-018-2297-8.

68. Ezzatzadeh E, Hossaini Z. Four-component green synthesis of benzochromene derivatives using nano-KF/clinoptilolite as basic catalyst: study of antioxidant activity. Mol Divers. 2020 24(1):81–91. doi:10.1007/s11030-019-09935-6.

5 Cheaper Transition Metals-Based Nanocatalyzed Organic Transformations and Synthesis of Bioactive Heterocycles
Strategic Approaches and Sustainable Applications

Ravi K. Yadav,[1] Vedant V. Deshmukh,[2] Tushar M. Boralkar,[2] Mukesh Jain,[1] and Sandeep Chaudhary[1,2]

[1] Laboratory of Organic and Medicinal Chemistry, Malaviya National Institute of Technology, Jawaharlal Nehru Marg, Jaipur, India
[2] Department of Medicinal Chemistry, National Institute of Pharmaceutical Education and Research-Raebareli (Transit Campus), Lucknow, India

5.1 INTRODUCTION

Advances in the concept of the term "*catalysis*" have been conferred by the Swedish chemist Jöns Jacob Berzelius in 1836, who defined it as the "catalytic power" of the substance that enhanced the reactivity of the reacting substrate (which were not affected at a particular temperature) simply by its presence and not by its kinships.[1] Catalysis can be subdivided into two classes: (1) homogenous catalysis; and (2) heterogeneous catalysis. Unlike homogeneous catalysts, a heterogeneous catalyst is more important and advantageous because of its easy removal from the reaction mixture and for its recyclable properties. During the last two decades, nanoparticle (NP)-catalyzed synthesis has been recognized as a promising catalyst in organic transformations along with widespread applications in catalysis, sensing, medicine, electronics and photonics. Mainly, all NPs are heterogeneous and can accelerate the synthetic endeavors in co-alignment with the basic fundamentals of green chemistry.[2]

Currently, synthetic organic chemistry is focused on new modern techniques that are focused on environmentally benign features.[3,4] The elements and parameters of the reactions are judged on the basic concept of its being eco-friendly, the use of an inexpensive catalytic system(s), and the involvement of solvent-free synthesis. These are the important sectors in current organic transformations and synthesis, which are required for the synthesis of heterocyclic and aromatic core skeletons and pharmaceutically important bioactive scaffolds, therapeutics, and drugs or molecules.[5–8] Several efficient methodologies, such as conventional ultrasonic (US) and microwave (MW) irradiation have

DOI: 10.1201/9781003141488-5

been reported in the literature for the synthesis of bioactive heterocycles.[9–10] These methodologies have benefits; however, many of them have serious drawbacks, such as inaccessible materials, use of expensive instruments, non-recyclability, and non-selectivity.[11–12] Nanocatalyzed based organic transformations and the synthesis of bioactive heterocycles are novel and advanced methodologies. Nanotechnology driven organic synthesis and research have been based on carbon (C) dot (C_{60}) molecules. Due to their importance in forming complexes in the organic ring core; transition metal-based nanomaterials can enhance reactivity; therefore, playing an important role in nanoscience and nanotechnology. NPs < 0 nm have great importance in nanoscale electronics, catalysis, and optics. However, NPs catalytic activity is altered with the variation in the size of the NPs. Therefore, the ratio of atoms present on the surface changes dramatically with the change in the size of the particle(s).

In green chemistry, NP catalyzed organic transformations are the safest and eco-friendly reactions pathways. Vital applications of NPs and metal oxide NPs have been established for some different reactions such as carbon–hydrogen (C–H) activation,[13–14] C–C bond formation,[15] and various other rare organic transformations.[16] A number of applications for NPs in a large number of organic transformations and functionalization have been mentioned in the literature; however, this chapter will focus on some of the important historical developments and sustainable applications of cheaper transition metal nanoparticles (MNPs), especially iron (Fe), cobalt (Co), nickel (Ni), and copper (Cu), in the synthesis and functionalization of various organic and heterocyclic scaffolds that have reported during the last 7 years (2014–2020). This chapter will cover developments in the most efficient methodologies used for the synthesis of bioactive heterocycles.

5.2 CHEAPER TRANSITION METAL NANOPARTICLE ASSISTED ORGANIC TRANSFORMATIONS

Based on synthetic procedures that have been reported in the literature to date, all the cheaper transition metal (e.g., Fe, Co, Ni, and Cu) NP assisted organic transformations and synthesis of bioactive heterocycles have been divided into four sections as follows.

5.2.1 Cobalt or Cobalt–Ferrite based Nanoparticle Assisted Organic Transformations and Synthesis of Bioactive Heterocycles

Some of the most important organic transformations that are applied in the synthesis of several nitrogen-containing (N) heterocycles of biological interest will be discussed. In addition, the application of Co or Co–ferrite based nanocatalyst (NCs) that have been used in the synthesis of bioactive heterocycles will be discussed. Therefore, some of the promising literature reports are included in this section.

5.2.1.1 N-doped carbon-supported cobalt nanoparticle catalyzed synthesis of N-heterocyclic compounds

Zhang et al. reported the oxidative dehydrogenation (ODH) of various cyclic heterocycles via N-doped C-supported cobalt NPs (Co/MC). This methodology involved the treatment of N-heterocyclic compounds, such as 1,2,3,4-tetrahydroquinoline 1 with Co/MC at 150°C under 2.5 bar oxygen (O_2) using acetonitrile (CH_3CN (ACS)) as a solvent, which was converted into a quinoline 2 skeleton with an 88.4% to 98.8% yield. However, the over-oxidized side-product of quinoline, for instance, quinoline N-oxide 3 was formed with comparable selectivity. The selectivity in the formation of quinoline 2 was based on the solvent system. In different solvents, such as water, methanol (MeOH), acetonitrile (ACN), tetrahydrofuran (THF), toluene, and hexane the selectivity for quinoline N-oxide 3 varied from 39.9% to 77.8 % yield (Scheme 5.1).[17] This methodology provided a green, sustainable, and cost-effective method for the synthesis of heteroarenes via ODH using the high catalytic activity of N-doped Co/MC NPS in excellent yields.[17]

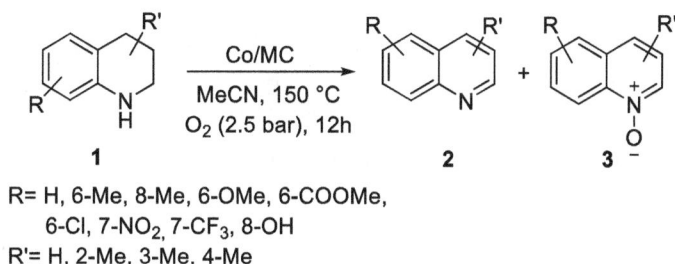

R= H, 6-Me, 8-Me, 6-OMe, 6-COOMe,
6-Cl, 7-NO$_2$, 7-CF$_3$, 8-OH
R'= H, 2-Me, 3-Me, 4-Me

SCHEME 5.1 N-doped C-supported Co/MC-catalyzed synthesis of N-heterocyclic compounds (quinoline **2**)

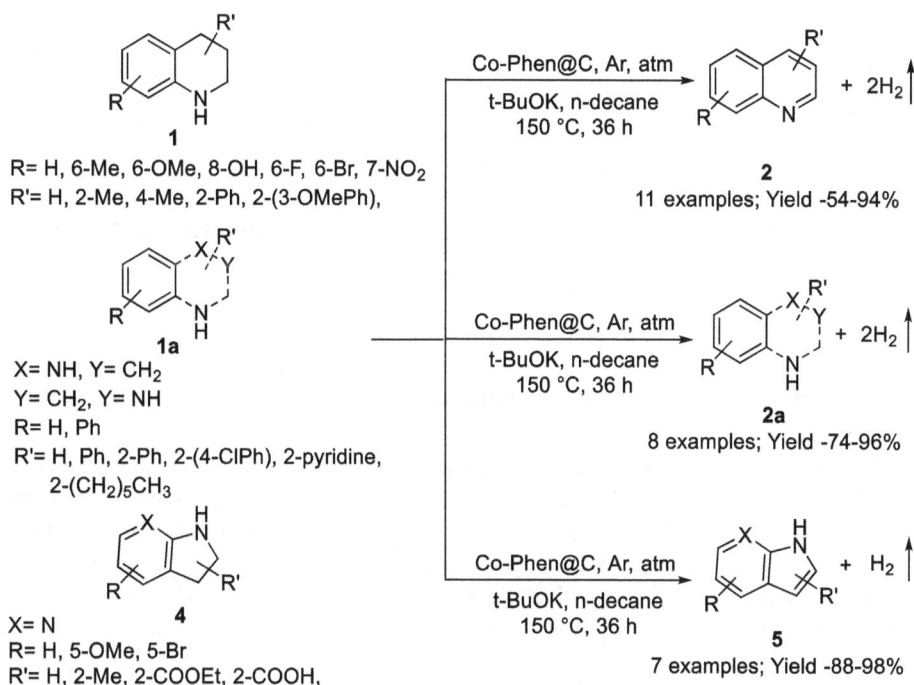

R= H, 6-Me, 6-OMe, 8-OH, 6-F, 6-Br, 7-NO$_2$
R'= H, 2-Me, 4-Me, 2-Ph, 2-(3-OMePh),

2
11 examples; Yield -54–94%

X= NH, Y= CH$_2$
Y= CH$_2$, Y= NH
R= H, Ph
R'= H, Ph, 2-Ph, 2-(4-ClPh), 2-pyridine,
2-(CH$_2$)$_5$CH$_3$

2a
8 examples; Yield -74–96%

X= N
R= H, 5-OMe, 5-Br
R'= H, 2-Me, 2-COOEt, 2-COOH,

5
7 examples; Yield -88–98%

SCHEME 5.2 Co-Phen@C Co NP catalyzed dehydrogenation of various heterocycles

5.2.1.2 Co-Phen@C catalyzed reversible acceptorless dehydrogenation and hydrogenation of various N-heterocycles

Balaraman et al. reported the novel highly competent, vigorous, and recyclable catalytic procedure for the reversible acceptorless dehydrogenation (ADH) and hydrogenation of various N-heterocycles, for example, 1,2,3,4-tetrahydroquinoline **1**, various other substituted heteroaromatics **1a,** and substituted or unsubstituted indolines **4** that used the Co-based NC Co-Phen@C at 150°C in an argon atmosphere for 36 h, which used n-decane as the solvent and produced the corresponding substituted or unsubstituted quinolines **2**, cyclized heteroaromatic **3a,** and substituted or unsubstituted indoles **5**, respectively, with very good to excellent yields. The Co-Phen@C catalyst in the presence of potassium tertiary butoxide (t-BuOK) removed H$_2$ from 1,2,3,4-tetrahydroquinoline **1,** which resulted in the formation of the corresponding dihydroquinoline that on treatment with another molecule of Co-Phen@C and t-BuOK resulted in the formation of the desired product with the simultaneous removal of H$_2$ (Scheme 5.2, Figure 5.1).[18]

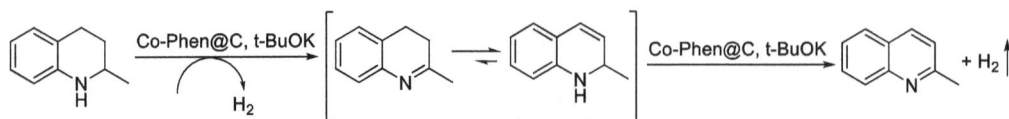

FIGURE 5.1 Mechanistic pathway for the reversible ADH of 2-methyl-1,2,3,4-tetrahydroquinoline

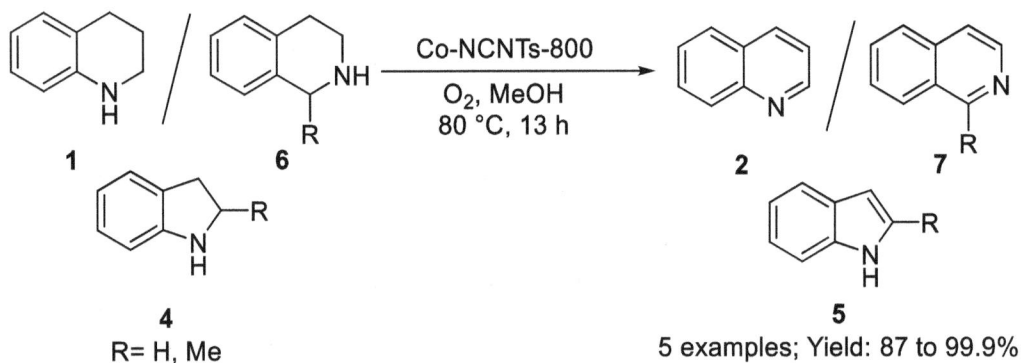

SCHEME 5.3 Co-NCNT-800 Co NP catalyzed ODH of various N-containing heterocyclic systems

5.2.1.3 Co@NCNTs catalyzed oxidative dehydrogenation of various N-containing heterocycles

Xu et al developed another Co NP-based catalyst for the ODH of various N-containing heterocycles, such as 1,2,3,4-tetrahydroquinoline **1**, 1,2,3,4-tetrahydroisoquinoline **6,** and indoline derivatives **4,** which when treated with Co NPs encapsulated by nitrogen-doped carbon nanotubes (Co@NCNTs) in the presence of O_2 at 80°C for 13–25 h produced the corresponding cyclized products quinoline **2**, isoquinoline **7**, and indole **5**, respectively, with ≤99.9% excellent level of selectivity. The Co@ NCNTs were prepared through the pyrolysis of cobalt(II) acetylacetonate ($Co(acac)_2$) and low-cost dicyandiamide (Scheme 5.3).[19]

Xu et al reported high reactivity and reusability of an NC Co-NCNTs-800 for the catalytic transfer hydrogenation (CTH) reactions on various saturated and unsaturated N-containing heterocyclic systems. In this study, 1,2,3,4-tetrahydroquinoline **1**, 1,2,3,4-tetrahydroisoquinoline **6**, phthalazine **8**, indoline **4**, substituted and unsubstituted quinolines **2**, and isoquinolines **7** were reacted with Co NPs encapsulated by NCNTs using formic acid (HCOOH) at 130°C for 0.5–30 h using toluene as the solvent, which produced the corresponding aldehydic products **9, 10, 11, 12, 10a,** and **13**, respectively, in low to excellent selectivity (Scheme 5.4).[19]

5.2.1.4 Co/N–Si–C catalyzed synthesis of (E)-2-alkenyl-azaarenes

Zhang et al reported Co-based NC (Co NCs) supported on N-silica (Si) doped carbon (Co/N–Si–C), which was utilized in the dehydrogenative coupling of aldehydes (**14**) with substituted and unsubstituted (hetero)aryl-fused 2-alkylcyclic amines **15**, which produced the corresponding (E)-2-alkenyl-azaarenes **16** that included substituted quinolines and quinoxalines in good to excellent yields. In this methodology, p-nitro benzoic acid was used as an additive and the reaction was performed in p-xylene at 160°C for 16 h, which produced the corresponding (E)-2-alkenylazaarenes **16** with 25%–95% yield (Scheme 5.5).[20]

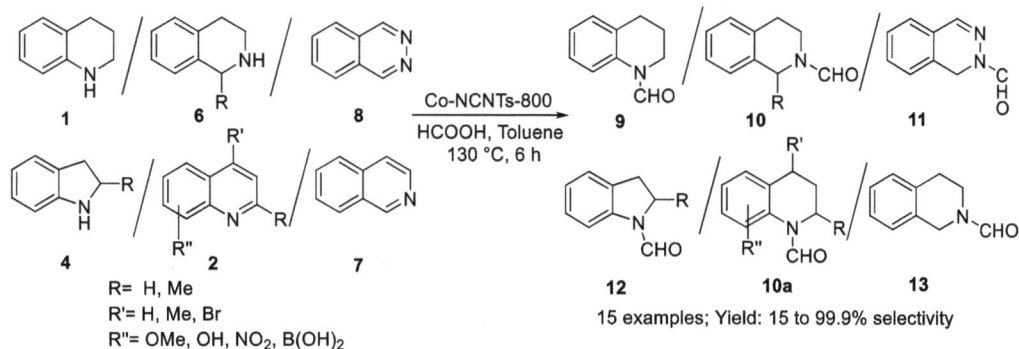

SCHEME 5.4 Co-NCNTs-800 Co NP catalyzed CTH of various heterocycles

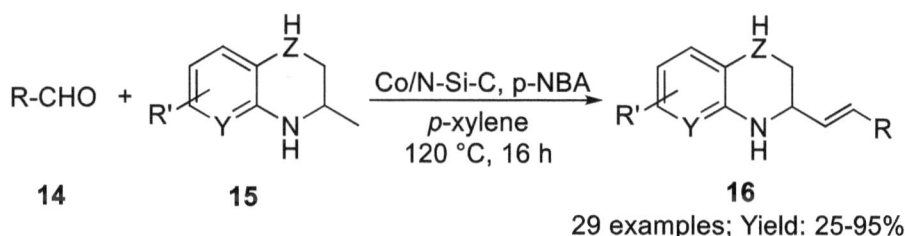

SCHEME 5.5 Co/N–Si–C Co NP catalyzed dehydrogenative coupling for the synthesis of (E)-2-alkenyl-azaarenes

5.2.1.5 Co@NGS-800 catalyzed oxidative dehydrogenation and hydrogenation of quinolones

Li et al discovered a highly efficient bifunctional catalyst with a high degree of stability and reactivity, for instance, Co@N-doped graphene (G) shells (Co@NGS), which were applied for organic conversions with saturated and unsaturated N-containing heterocyclic compounds. This NC was utilized for the ODH and HYD of quinolines. The excellent behavior of NCs is due to the cumulative effect of Co NPs encapsulated with N-doped G shells, which protects them from Co leaching and aggregation from the C shells. In this report, 1,2,3,4-tetrahydroquinoline **1** in the presence of Co@NGS-800 catalyst, potassium carbonate (K_2CO_3) as the base at 80°C for 6 h under aerobic conditions (ODH) using MeOH as solvent was converted into quinoline **2** with 82%–96% yield range. However, quinoline **2** was converted into 1,2,3,4-tetrahydroquinoline **1** in the presence of various Co@NGS (e.g., 700, 800, 800 NL) using H_2 (HYD) and isopropyl alcohol (IPA) at 140°C to achieve a 60%–88% yield range (Scheme 5.6).[21] The catalyst was checked and assessed *via* various chemical and spectroscopic analyses. The poisoning tests with potassium isothiocynate (KSCN) and spectroscopic analysis disclosed that there was a difference between the active sites for ODH and HYD (Scheme 5.6).[21]

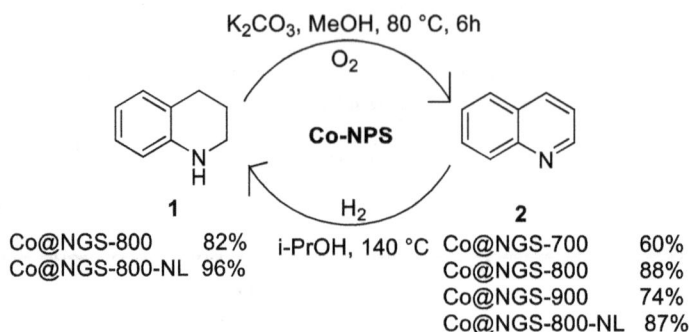

K_2CO_3, MeOH, 80 °C, 6h

O_2

Co-NPS

1

H_2

i-PrOH, 140 °C

2

Co@NGS-800	82%		Co@NGS-700	60%
Co@NGS-800-NL	96%		Co@NGS-800	88%
			Co@NGS-900	74%
			Co@NGS-800-NL	87%

SCHEME 5.6   CoNPS-700/800/900 catalyzed dual functionality

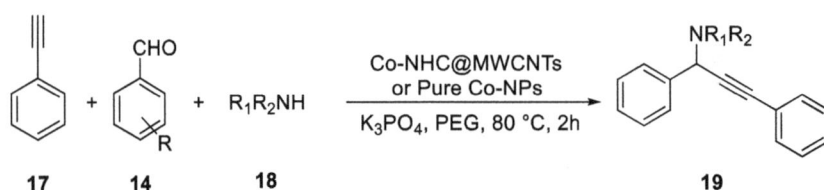

CHO

+   + R_1R_2NH

Co-NHC@MWCNTs
or Pure Co-NPs

K_3PO_4, PEG, 80 °C, 2h

NR_1R_2

17   14   18   19

R = H, 4- NO_2, 4-OH, 2-OH, 4-Cl, 4-NO_2
Amine = 1H-imidazole, N-methylcyclohexanamine,
dicyclohexylamine, pyrrolidine

12 examples; Yield: 85-97% (Co-NHC@MWCNTs)
12 examples; Yield: 68-95% (Pure Co-NP)

SCHEME 5.7   Co–NHC@MWCNTs and pure Co NP catalyzed synthesis of propargylamines **19**

Co@NGS acted as active sites for O_2 activation via electron transfer in ODH, and the underlying Co NPs supported by N dopants favored H_2 activation in HYD. The dual functionality of Co@NGS catalysts has been attributed to the one-pot inclusion of Co sites and N-doped G into 1,2,3,4-tetrahydroquinoline **1** under pyrolyzed conditions (Scheme 5.6).[21]

5.2.1.6   Co–NHC@MWCNTs catalyzed synthesis of various propargylamines and 1,2-diphenylethyne

Mohammadi et al prepared pure Co NPs and a Co N-heterocyclic carbene grafted on CNTs (Co–NHC@MWCNTs) catalyst, which was utilized in the synthesis of various propargylamines **19** via multicomponent reactions and substituted 1,2-diphenylethyne **21** via Sonogashira cross-coupling. In this methodology, phenylacetylene **17**, substituted aromatic aldehydes **14,** and substituted amines **18** were reacted together in the presence of Co–NHC@MWCNTs and in pure Co NPs in the presence of potassium phosphate (K_3PO_4) as the base at 80°C for 2 h in polyethylene glycol (PEG), which produced propargylamines **19** with 85%–97% yield and 68%–95% yield, respectively (Scheme 5.7).[22]

In addition, the catalyst was examined for Sonogashira cross-coupling reaction for the synthesis of substituted 1,2-diphenylethyne **21**. When phenylacetylene **17** reacts with substituted and unsubstituted halobenzene **20** in the presence of Co–NHC@MWCNTs at 80°C for 8–14 h and pure Co NPs at 80°C for 12–24 h, respectively, in ethanol:water (EtOH: H_2O) (1:1) solvent system, it produced substituted 1,2-diphenylethyne **21** at 47%–98% yields using Co–NHC@MWCNTs catalyst and in 66%–91% yields using pure Co NPs (Scheme 5.8).[22]

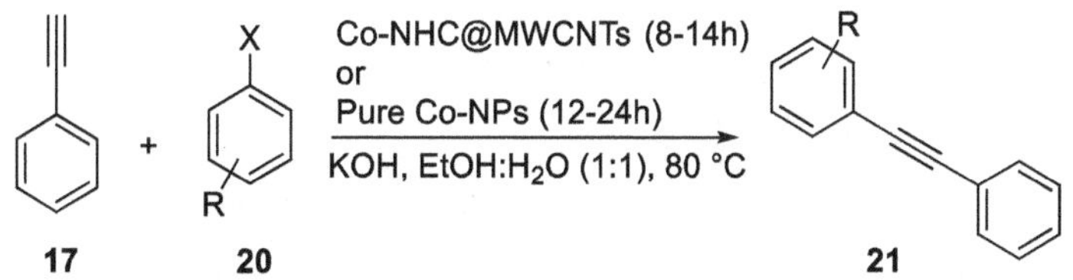

17 **20** **21**

R= H, 4- NO_2, 4-OMe, 4-$COCH_3$, 4-NH_2
X= I, Cl, Br

11 examples; Yield: 47-98% (Co-NHC@MWCNTs)
11 examples; Yield: 66-91% (Pure Co-NP)

SCHEME 5.8 Co–NHC@MWCNTs and pure Co NPs catalyzed synthesis of substituted 1,2-diphenylethynes **21**

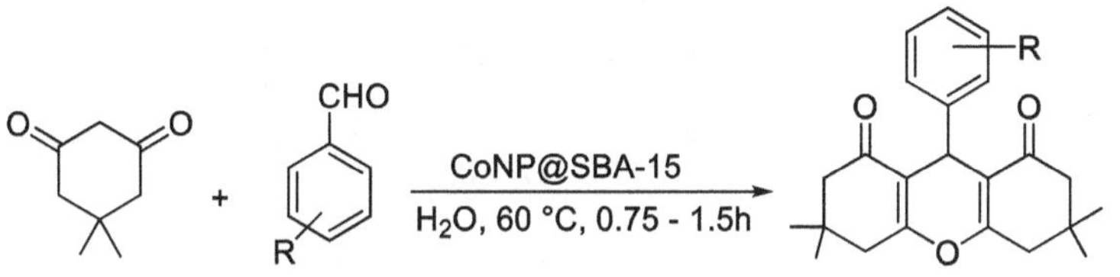

22 **14** **23**

R = H, 4- NO_2, 3-NO_2, 2-NO_2, 4-Cl, 2,4-Cl_2-2- Br, 4-Me, 4-OMe, 2-Cl, 4-OH. 4-F, 3Cl, 4-Br

14 Examples; Yield: 88-99%

SCHEME 5.9 CoNP@SBA-15 and pure Co NP catalyzed synthesis of 1,8-dioxo-octahydroxanthenes **23** in aqueous medium

5.2.1.7 CoNP@SBA-15 catalyzed synthesis of 1,8-dioxo-octahydroxanthenes

Rajabi et al reported a highly efficient aqueous synthetic methodology for the synthesis of 1,8-dioxo-octahydroxanthenes **23** that used a recyclable Co-based catalyst, for instance, Co NPs supported on Si (CoNP@SBA-15). In this methodology, dimedone **22** and substituted and unsubstituted aromatic aldehyde **14** were reacted in presence of CoNP@SBA-15 under aqueous conditions at 60°C for 0.75–1.5 h, which produced 1,8-dioxo-octahydroxanthenes **23** with 88%–99% yields (Scheme 5.9).[23]

5.2.1.8 Cobalt-terephthalic acid metal–organic framework catalyzed hydrogenation of bioactive N-heterocycles

Jagadeesh et al reported the carbon-supported Co-terephthalic acid metal–organic framework (MOF), for instance, Co-terephthalic acid MOF@C-800, which was used in the synthesis and HYD of aliphatic and aromatic nitriles, the chemoselective HYD of nitroarenes, and HYD of nitro heterocycles and nitroalkanes. In this methodology, substituted cyanide molecule **24** was subjected to HYD using a Co-terephthalic acid MOF@C-800 catalyst and H_2 was maintained at 25 bar using toluene as solvent at 120°C for 16 h, which produced the desired primary amine **25** in excellent yields (Scheme 5.10).[24]

In addition, a Co-terephthalic acid MOF@C-800 catalyst was utilized in the reduction of substituted nitroarenes **26** to substituted aniline **27** in the presence of H_2 at 20 bars at 120°C for 20 h in THF: H_2O solvent, which produced substituted anilines **27** with 86%–98% yields (Scheme 5.11).[24]

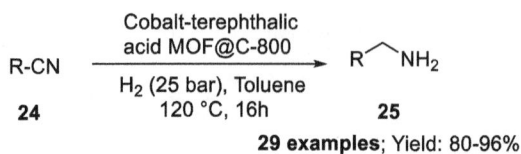

R = napthalene, biphenyl, 4-Me-C_6H_4, 3-Me-C_6H_4, 4-F-C_6H_4, 4-Cl-C_6H_4, 4-Br-C_6H_4,
3-Br-4-Me-C_6H_3, 3-F-4-CH_2OH-C_6H_3, 2-F-3-NH_2-C_6H_3, 3,4,5-F-C_6H_2, 4-CF_3-C_6H_4,
3-,5-CF_3-C_6H_3, 4-OMe-C_6H_4, 3-OMe-C_6H_4, C_6H_4-O-CH_2-Ph, 4-$CONH_2$-C_6H_4,
4-$COOCH_3$-C_6H_4, Pyridine, furan, indole, benzo[d][1,3]dioxole

SCHEME 5.10 Co NP Co-terephthalic acid MOF@C-800 catalyzed reduction of aliphatic and aromatic nitriles **24** to primary amines **25**

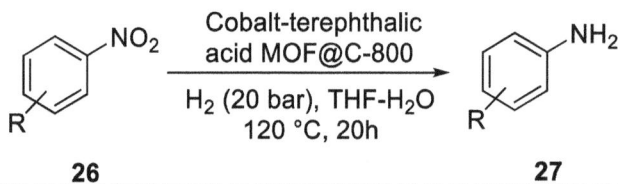

R = H, 4-Me, Ph, 2-Ph, 4-F, 3-Cl, 4-Br, 2,4,6-Cl, 3-Cl-4-F, 4-I, 2,6-Cl-4-NH_2
4-OMe, 4-SMe, 3-N$(CH_3)_2$, 4-Cl-3-NH-Ph, 2-OH, 2-CHO, 4-$COCH_3$,
4-$COOCH_3$, 4-$CONH_2$, 3-O-Ph-4-NH-SO_2Me

SCHEME 5.11 Co NP Co-terephthalic acidMOF@C-800 catalyzed reduction of substituted nitroarenes **26** to substituted aniline **27**.

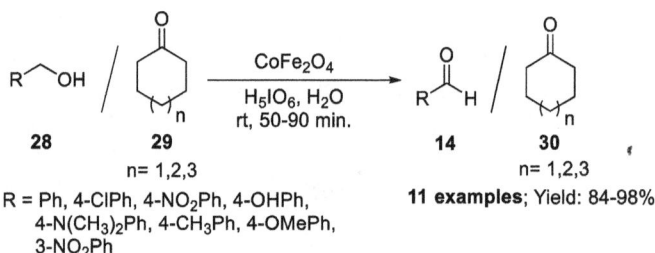

SCHEME 5.12 $CoFe_2O_4$ catalyzed oxidation of alcohols

5.2.1.9 $CoFe_2O_4$-based nanocatalyst for the oxidation of alcohols

Dhar et al prepared magnetically recoverable cobalt–ferrite ($CoFe_2O_4$) based NC, which was used for the oxidation of substituted benzyl and secondary alcohols into their corresponding substituted aldehydes and ketones with excellent yields. In this synthetic strategy, substituted benzyl alcohols **28** and cyclic alcohols **29** were reacted with a $CoFe_2O_4$ catalyst, periodic acid at room temperature for 50–90 min under aqueous condition, which produced substituted aldehydes **14** and cyclic ketones **30** with 84%–98% excellent yields (Scheme 5.12.) [25]

5.2.1.10 CrCoFeO4@G–GO and Zn$_0$.5Co0.5Fe2O4@G–GO as an efficient nanocatalyst for oxidation reactions

In 2016, Shaabani et al reported a new nanocatalyst with high catalytic activity and selectivity, which was composed of chromium (Cr) and zinc (Zn) substituted $CoFe_2O_4$ NPs supported on

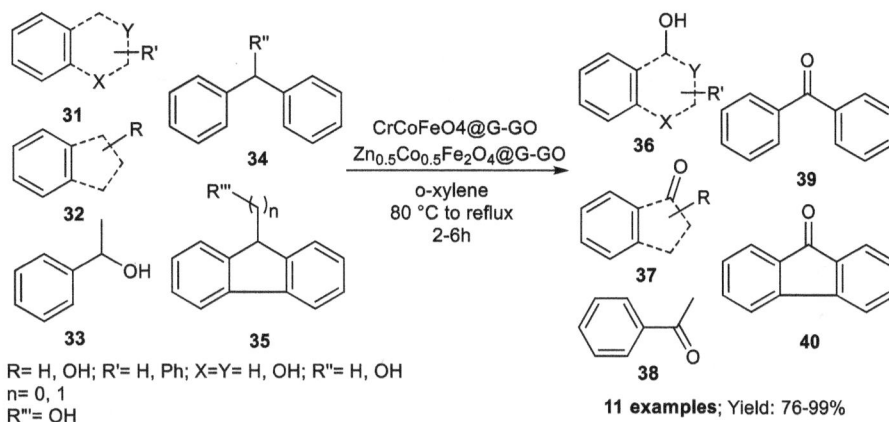

SCHEME 5.13 Cr- and Zn-substituted $CoFe_2O_4$ NPs supported on guanidine-grafted GO nanosheets catalyzed oxidation of arenes

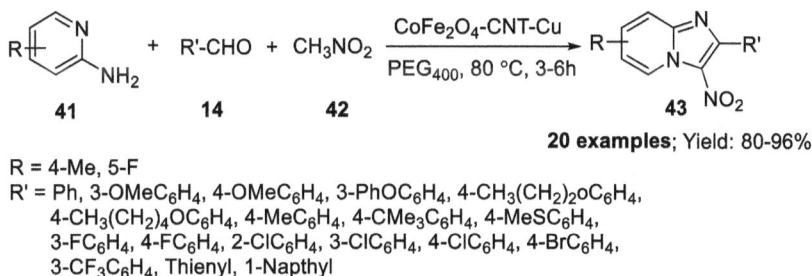

SCHEME 5.14 $CoFe_2O_4$/CNT-Cu catalyzed synthesis of 3-nitro-2-arylimidazo[1,2-a]pyridines via multicomponent reaction

guanidine-grafted graphene oxide (GO) nanosheets, which were used for the oxidation of substituted alkyl arenes and cyclic alcohols into their corresponding ketones efficiently. In this methodology, CrCoFeO4@G–GO and $Zn_{0.}5Co0.5Fe2O4$@G–GO NCs were used in the presence of air as oxidant under reflux conditions that used o-xylene as a solvent and were used for the conversion of various substituted alkyl arenes **31–34** and cyclic alcohols **35** into their analogous ketones **37–40** and alcohols **36** with 76%–99% yields (Scheme 5.13).[25] The catalysts $CrCoFeO_4$@G–GO and $Zn_{0.5}Co_{0.5}Fe_2O_4$@G –GO demonstrated different reactivities, which could directly affect their reaction time, for example, the first catalyst requires 2–4 h reaction time and the second requires 2.5–6 h (Scheme 5.13).[25]

5.2.1.11 CoFe₂O₄/CNT-Cu catalyzed synthesis of 3-nitro-2-arylimidazo [1,2-a]pyridines

Zhang et al reported the synthesis of a fused bioactive heterocyclic imidazo[1, 2-a]pyridine ring via a multicomponent reaction that used magnetically separable, eight-times recyclable $CoFe_2O_4$ NC supported over CNTs Cu (CNT-Cu). Various substituted and unsubstituted 2-aminopyridines **41**, substituted aldehydes **14,** and nitromethane **42** were reacted with $CoFe_2O_4$/CNT-Cu catalyst at 80°C for 3–6 h in PEG_{400} solvent, which produced 3-nitro-2-arylimidazo[1,2-a]pyridines **43** with good to excellent yield (Scheme 5.14).[26]

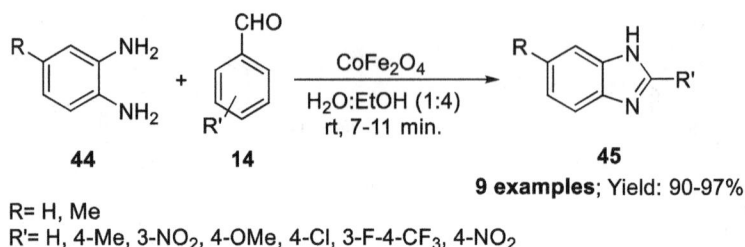

SCHEME 5.15 CoFe$_2$O$_4$ NPs catalyzed multicomponent reaction for the synthesis of substituted benzimidazoles **45**

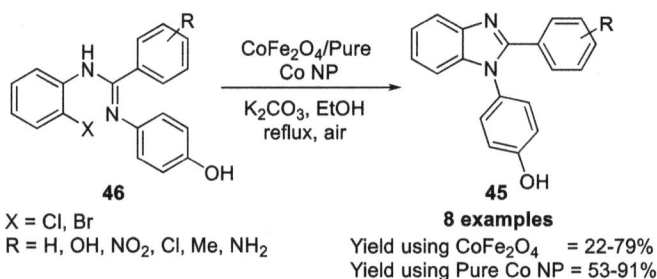

SCHEME 5.16 CoFe$_2$O$_4$ pure Co NPs catalyzed multicomponent synthesis of substituted benzimidazoles **45**

5.2.1.12 Nanoparticle CoFe$_2$O$_4$-catalyzed synthesis of benzimidazoles

In 2018, Borade et al reported the CoFe$_2$O$_4$ catalyzed synthesis of benzimidazoles **45** that used substituted and unsubstituted benzene-1,2-diamines **44** and substituted aldehydes **14** in H$_2$O:EtOH (1:4) for 7–11 min at room temperature, which produced substituted benzimidazoles **45** with 90%–97% excellent yield (Scheme 5.15).[27]

5.2.1.13 CoFe$_2$O$_4$ catalyzed synthesis of benzimidazoles and benzoxazoles

Hajipour et al reported the synthesis of two bioactive heterocycles, for example, substituted benzimidazoles **45** and benzoxazoles **47** from CoFe$_2$O$_4$ catalytic cyclization of o-haloanilides. In this methodology, substituted o-haloanilides **46** was reacted with CoFe$_2$O$_4$ using K$_2$CO$_3$ as a base in EtOH under refluxing conditions for 8–11 h, which produced the substituted benzimidazoles **45** with 22%–75% yield. Furthermore, this transformation was performed with pure Co NPs, which produced substituted benzimidazoles **45** with 53%–91% yield in 6–10 h (Scheme 5.16). [28]

Hajipour et al illustrated the synthesis of substituted benzoxazoles **47** from o-haloanilides **46a** (similar to **46**) that used the same reaction conditions in which substituted benzoxazoles **47** was formed with 23%–79% yield in 10–16 h, which used a CoFe$_2$O$_4$ NC and gave 75%–96% yield under refluxing conditions at 8–16 h, which used pure Co NP (Scheme 5.17).[28]

5.2.1.14 CoFe2O4@SiO2/PrNH2 as an efficient nanocatalytic system for multicomponent reactions

Safaei-Ghomi et al developed an eco-friendly, magnetically separable CoFe$_2$O$_4$@SiO$_2$/PrNH$_2$ nanocatalyst, which efficiently catalyzed the one-pot condensation of aldehydes, aromatic amines, and thioglycolic acids via a multicomponent reaction to produce 1,3-thiazolidin-4-ones **49** in excellent yields. In this methodology, substituted anilines **27**, substituted aldehydes **14,** and 2-mercaptoacetic acid **48** were reacted together in the presence of CoFe$_2$O$_4$@SiO$_2$/PrNH$_2$ in toluene

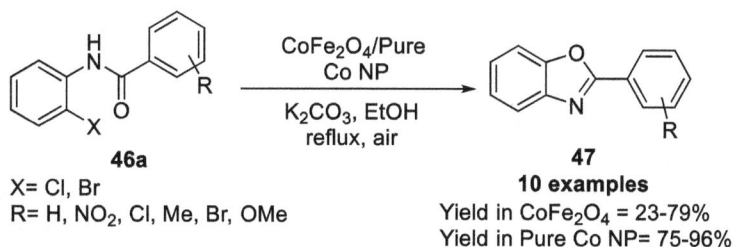

SCHEME 5.17 CoFe$_2$O$_4$ and Co NPs catalyzed multicomponent synthesis of substituted benzoxazoles **47**

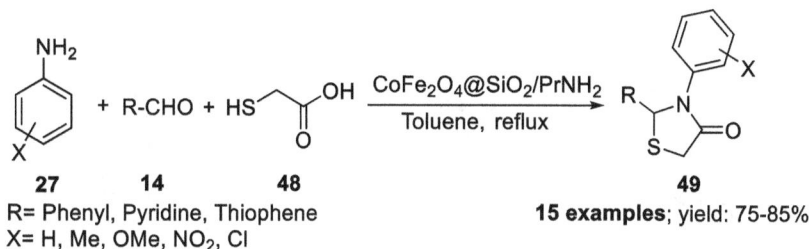

SCHEME 5.18 CoFe2O4@SiO2/PrNH2 NPs catalyzed multicomponent synthesis of 1,3-thiazolidin-4-ones **49**

under refluxing conditions at 120°C–140°C for 120–135 min, which produced substituted 1,3-thiazolidin-4-ones **49** in good to excellent yield (Scheme 5.18).[29]

5.2.1.15 CoFe$_2$O$_4$-GO-SO$_3$H catalyzed synthesis of 3,6-di(pyridin-3-yl)-1*H*-pyrazolo[3,4-b]pyridine-5-carbonitriles

Then, for the synthesis of bioactive N-heterocycles, Zhang et al reported the preparation of a magnetically separable CoFe$_2$O$_4$ and GO anchored sulphonic acid NC (CoFe$_2$O$_4$-GO-SO$_3$H), which was characterized by scanning electron microscopy (SEM), X-ray diffraction (XRD), vibrating sample magnetometry (VSM), and transmission electron microscope (TEM) techniques. This NC was utilized for the synthesis of 3,6-di(pyridin-3-yl)-1H-pyrazolo[3,4-b]pyridine-5-carbonitriles **52** via multicomponent reactions. In this methodology, 1-phenyl-3-(pyridin-3-yl)-1H-pyrazol-5-amine **50**, aldehyde **14** and 3-oxo-3-(pyridin-3-yl)propanenitrile **51** were reacted in the presence of a magnetically separable Fe$_2$O$_4$-GO–SO$_3$H NC under MW irradiation conditions using choline chloride (ChCl)/glycerol (1:3) as a green solvent for 10–15 min, which produced 3,6-di(pyridin-3-yl)-1H-pyrazolo[3,4-b]pyridine-5-carbonitriles **52** in excellent (84%–95%) yield (Scheme 5.19).[30]

5.2.1.16 CoFe$_2$O$_4$ nanoparticles three-component reaction using greener reaction conditions

Sanasi et al reported a novel methodology for the synthesis of 4*H*-pyrano[3,2-h]quinolones through the synthesis of CoFe$_2$O$_4$ NPs that used sol-gel citrate-precursor method that was been characterized by Fourier-transform infrared spectroscopy (FTIR), XRD, TEM, and SEM techniques. The developed NC was utilized in the synthesis of 4-phenyl-4H-pyrano[3,2-h]quinolin-2-amine **55** and 2-amino-4-phenyl-4*H*-pyrano[3,2-h]quinoline-3-carbonitrile **56** derivatives. The three-component reaction involved the treatment of substituted aldehydes **14**, substituted ACS and malononitrile **53,** and 8-hydroxyquinoline **54** dissolved in EtOH (green solvent) with CoFe$_2$O$_4$ NPs under MW irradiations for 2 min, which produced 4-phenyl-4*H*-pyrano[3,2-h]quinolin-2-amines **55** and

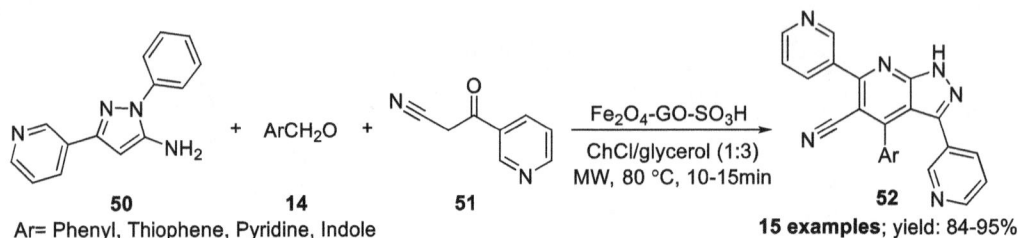

SCHEME 5.19 Fe_2O_4–GO–SO_3H NPs catalyzed multicomponent synthesis of 3,6-di(pyridin-3-yl)-1H-pyrazolo[3,4-b]pyridine-5-carbonitriles **52**

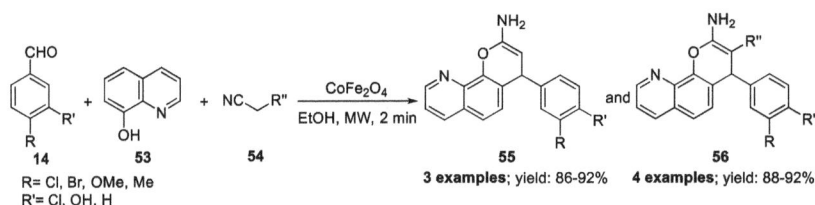

SCHEME 5.20 $CoFe_2O_4$ NPs catalyzed multicomponent synthesis of 4-phenyl-4H-pyrano[3,2-h]quinolin-2-amine **55** and 2-amino-4-phenyl-4H-pyrano[3,2-h]quinoline-3-carbonitriles **56** derivatives

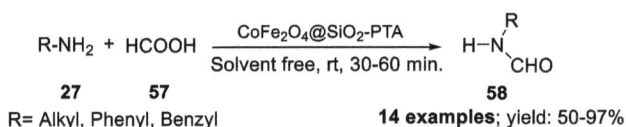

SCHEME 5.21 CoFe2O4@SiO2–PTA NPs catalyzed N-formylation of substituted and unsubstituted anilines **27** with formic acid **57**

2-amino-4-phenyl-4H-pyrano[3,2-h]quinoline-3-carbonitrile **56** derivatives in excellent yields (Scheme 5.20).[31]

5.2.1.17   CoFe$_2$O$_4$@SiO$_2$–PTA catalyzed N-formylation of amines

Kooti and Nasiri established an efficient methodology for the N-formylation of amines via the development of a $CoFe_2O_4$ based NC. In this work, a novel three-component nanocomposite, for instance, $CoFe_2O_4$@SiO$_2$–PTA was prepared by anchoring phosphotungstic acid supported on the surface of Si-coated $CoFe_2O_4$ NPs, which was confirmed by performing characterization by SEM, FTIR, EDX, VSM, inductively coupled plasma mass spectrometry (ICP–AES), and XRD. The reaction involved the treatment of substituted and unsubstituted anilines **27** with formic acid **57** under solvent-free conditions at room temperature for 30–60 min, which produced substituted formylated amines **58** with 50%–97% yield (Scheme 5.21).[32]

5.2.1.18   Co@NGR nanocatalyst hydrogenation of alkynes

Jaiswal et al reported an efficient and nine-run recyclable synthesis of G supported Co NPs NC, which was utilized in the HYD of alkynes. In this report, several internal substituted symmetrical and unsymmetrical alkynes **59** were treated with NH_3-BH_3 using Co@NGR NC at 80°C for 24 h using MeOH as the solvent, which gave 90%–100% yield of substituted Z-alkenes **60** and 0%–10%

R————R' $\xrightarrow[\substack{NH_3-BH_3, MeOH \\ 80\ °C, 24h}]{Co@NGR}$

59

R = Ph, 4-MeC$_6$H$_4$, 4-FC$_6$H$_4$, 4-PhC$_6$H$_4$,
4-OMeC$_6$H$_4$, Thiophene
R' = Ph, 4-MeC$_6$H$_4$, 3-ClC$_6$H$_4$, 3,5-CF$_3$C$_6$H$_3$,
3-F-4-CNC$_6$H$_3$, 4-COOMeC$_6$H$_4$, C4-FC$_6$H$_4$,
3-methylpyridine, -(CH$_2$)$_2$OTBS, -COOMe,
-(CH$_2$)$_3$Me, -CH$_2$OH, -TMS

60

9 examples
Yield: 90-100%

9 examples
Yield: 0-10%   **Symmetrical alkyne**

61

5 examples
Yield: 1-99%

5 examples
Yield: 1-3%   **Unsymmetrical alkyne**

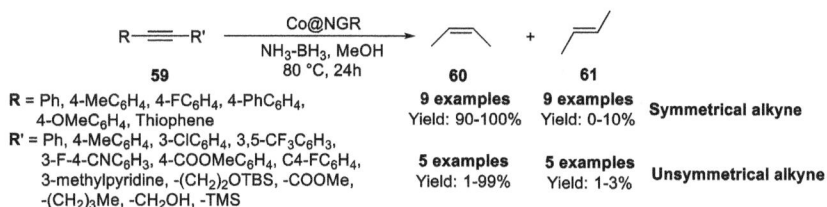

SCHEME 5.22 Co@NGR NPs catalyzed dehydrogenation of internal substituted symmetrical and unsymmetrical alkynes 59

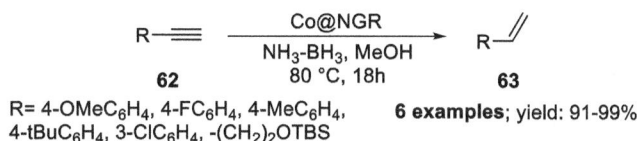

R——— $\xrightarrow[\substack{NH_3-BH_3, MeOH \\ 80\ °C, 18h}]{Co@NGR}$ R

62

R= 4-OMeC$_6$H$_4$, 4-FC$_6$H$_4$, 4-MeC$_6$H$_4$,
4-tBuC$_6$H$_4$, 3-ClC$_6$H$_4$, -(CH$_2$)$_2$OTBS

63

6 examples; yield: 91-99%

SCHEME 5.23 Co@NGR NPs catalyzed dehydrogenation of terminal alkynes

yield of substituted E-alkenes **61** for symmetrical alkynes; and the NC treatment of unsymmetrical alkyne gave 1%–99% yield of substituted Z-alkenes and 1–3% yield of substituted E-alkene (Scheme 5.22).[33]

This methodology was applied on terminal substituted symmetrical and unsymmetrical alkynes **62** under the same reaction conditions for 18–24 h, which gave the corresponding dehydrogenated product, for instance, substituted alkenes **63** with 91%–99% yield (Scheme 5.23).[33]

5.2.1.19 Co Nanoparticles catalyzed hydrogenation of bioactive heterocycles

Jagadeesh et al reported the Co NPs catalyzed HYD of N-heteroarenes, for example, quinoxalines, indole, naphthyridines, phenanthrolines, acridines, and imidazo[1,2-a]pyridines under mild conditions. In this methodology, one or two N-containing heteroarenes and substituted anilines **64** were reported to undergo reduction (HYD) into their corresponding hydrogenated substituted piperidines **65** when subjected to a Co pyromellitic acid@SiO2-800 NC in the presence of H$_2$ at 50 bars at 120°C–135°C, which used i-PrOH: H$_2$O (2:1) as solvent for 24 h with 83%–97% excellent yield range (Scheme 5.24).[34] Then, one N-containing bio heterocycles, such as substituted quinolines **16**, substituted isoquinolines **7**, substituted indoles **5**, and two N-containing heterocycles, such as imidazo[1,2-a]pyridines **43**, quinoxalines **16**, when treated with the same catalyst in the presence of H$_2$ at 10 bar at 70°C that used i-PrOH:H$_2$O (2:1) as the solvent for 24 h gave the corresponding hydrogenated products tetrahydroquinoline **1**, indolines **4**, tetrahydroisoquinoline **6**, 5,6,7,8-tetrahydroimidazo[1,2-a]pyridine **67**, and 1,2,3,4-tetrahydroquinoxaline **68** with good to excellent yield (Scheme 5.24).[34]

5.2.1.20 Co/MA-800 catalyzed hydrogenation of nitroarenes to aminoarenes and some bioactive heterocycles

Natte et al developed a C-supported Co NP catalyst, which was utilized for the HYD of nitroarenes into their corresponding hydrogenated product. In this work, various substituted nitrobenzenes **26** on treatment with a Co-based nanocatalyst (Co/MA-800) in the presence of H$_2$ at 120°C–130°C for 18–24 h that used THF: H$_2$O (10:1) as a solvent gave the corresponding anilines **27** derivatives with good to excellent yield (Scheme 5.25).[35].

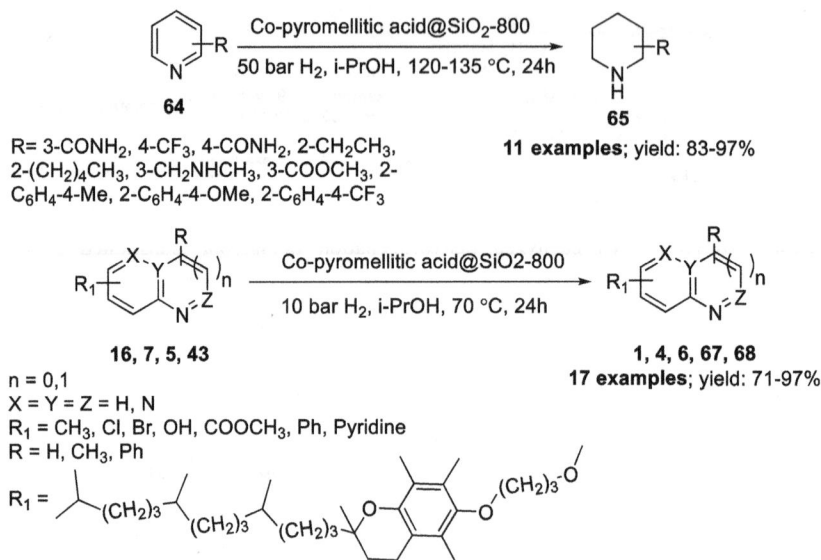

SCHEME 5.24 Co-pyromellitic acid@SiO2-800 nanocatalyzed HYD of N-heteroarenes

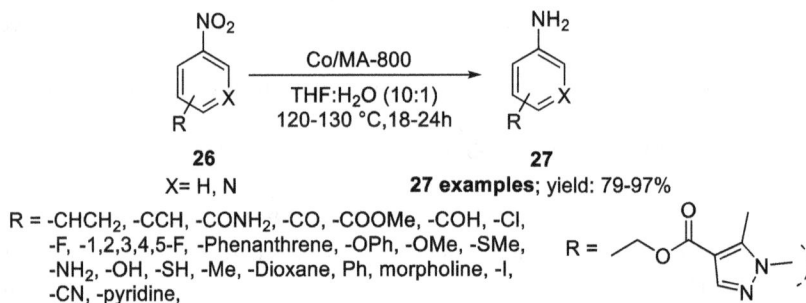

SCHEME 5.25 Co/MA-800 catalyzed HYD of nitroarenes **26**

5.2.2 NICKEL NANOPARTICLE CATALYZED ORGANIC TRANSFORMATIONS AND SYNTHESIS OF BIOACTIVE HETEROCYCLES

In this section, some of the most important organic transformations that are being continuously applied to the synthesis of several N-containing bio heterocycles are discussed. Furthermore, some of the applications for nickel (Ni) NPs, which have been used in the synthesis of bioactive heterocycles are included. Therefore, some of the promising literature reports are considered in this section.

5.2.2.1 Diphenylphosphinated poly(vinyl alcohol-co-ethylene)-nickel nanoparticle catalyzed Mizoroki–Heck reaction

Ebrahimzadeh et al reported the preparation of a Ni-based metallized polymer. The synthesis involved the base-catalyzed reaction of poly(vinyl alcohol-co-ethylene) (PVA-co-PE) with chlorodiphenylphosphine (ClPPh$_2$) followed by treatment with Ni(OAc)$_2$ and NaBH$_4$ reduction gave Ni NPs supported on a diphenylphosphinated poly(vinyl alcohol-co-ethylene) ((DPP-PVA-co-PE)-Ni NP) catalyst. The confirmation of the formation of the catalyst was carried out on TEM, SEM, and XRD. This is one of the best examples of Ni NC that shows the C–C bond forming Mizoroki–Heck reaction. In this methodology, (DPP-PVA-co-PE)-Ni NP catalyzed the reaction of various

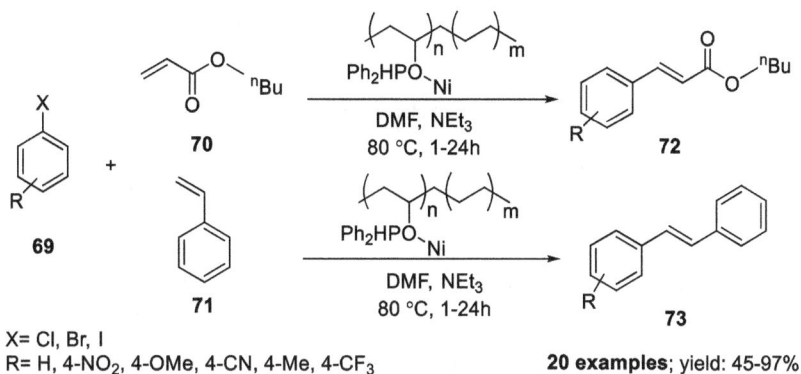

SCHEME 5.26 (DPP-PVA-co-PE)-NiNP catalyzed Mizoroki–Heck reaction of various substituted aromatic haloarenes **69** with various substituted aliphatic **70** and aromatic alkene **71**

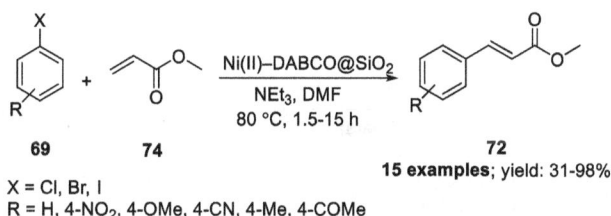

SCHEME 5.27 Ni(II)–DABCO@SiO2 catalyzed Heck reaction

substituted aromatic haloarenes **69** with various substituted aliphatic **70** and aromatic alkene **71** in DMF at 80°C for 1–24 h, which gave the corresponding coupled products, for example, substituted cinnamates **72** and substituted diphenylethene **73** with good to excellent yields (Scheme 5.26).[36]

5.2.2.2 Ni(II)– DABCO@SiO$_2$ as an efficient heterogeneous nanocatalyst for Heck reaction

Hajipour et al prepared a Si-supported Ni(II)– 1,4-Diazabicyclo[2.2.2]octane (DABCO) complex, for example, Ni(II)– DABCO@SiO$_2$ NP, which was utilized in the successful execution of a Heck coupling reaction. In this reaction methodology, substituted haloarenes **69** on treatment with methyl acrylate **74** in the presence of a Ni(II)–DABCO@SiO$_2$ NC in the presence of triethylamine in DMF at 100°C for 1.5–5 h gave the substituted cinnamates **72** with good to excellent yields (Scheme 5.27).[37]

5.2.2.3 Fe$_3$O$_4$@SiO$_2$-EDTA-Ni(0) nanoparticle catalyzed Suzuki-Miyuara and Heck cross-coupling

Inaloo et al reported an Fe$_3$O$_4$@SiO$_2$-EDTA-Ni(0) NP catalyzed Suzuki and Heck reaction. In this reaction, various haloarenes **69**, substituted aryl carbamates **75**, and substituted aryl sulfamates **76** were reacted with coupling partners, for example, substituted boronic acid **77** dissolved in ethylene glycol solvent in the presence of Fe$_3$O$_4$@SiO$_2$-EDTA-Ni(0) NC that used using potassium hydroxide (KOH) as the base at 120°C for 6 h, which produced the furnished corresponding biaryls coupled product **78** in low to excellent yields (Scheme 5.28).[38]

Similarly, substituted aryl carbamates **75** and substituted aryl sulfamates **76** when reacted with activated substituted aromatic and aliphatic alkenes **79** dissolved in ethylene glycol solvent in the presence of Fe$_3$O$_4$@SiO$_2$-EDTA-Ni(0) NC that used KOH as the base at 120°C for 6 h produced

R   + R_1-B$\begin{smallmatrix}OH\\OH\end{smallmatrix}$ $\xrightarrow[\substack{KOH,\ Ethylene\ glycol\\120\ ^\circ C,\ 6h}]{Fe_3O_4@SiO_2\text{-}EDTA\text{-}Ni(0)}$ R-R_1

69/75/76   **77**   **78**

R = Phenyl carbamate, aryl R_1 = C_6H_5, 4-MeC_6H_4, 4-OHC_6H_4,   **47 examples**; yield: 0-94%
sulfamates, I-C_6H_5, (Br, Cl, OMe,   4-FC_6H_4, 4-C$F_3C_6H_4$,
OPiv, OCO$_2^t$Bu, OMs, OTs, OTf,   thiophene
Me, CHO, COCH$_3$, NO$_2$, NC, CF$_3$)
C_6H_5, pyridine, pyrimidine,
naphthalene, quinoline,

R-X   + $=\!\!\!-R_2$ $\xrightarrow[\substack{KOH,\ Ethylene\ glycol\\120\ ^\circ C,\ 6h}]{Fe_3O_4@SiO_2\text{-}EDTA\text{-}Ni(0)}$ R$\diagdown\!\!=\!\!\diagup^{R_2}$

75/76   **79**   **78**

X = carbamate, Sulfamates R_2 = C_6H_5,4 -MeC_6H_4, 4-OMeC_6H_4,   **20 examples**; yield: 0-92%
R = C_6H_4, 4 -MeC_6H_4,   4-CNC_6H_4, 4-NO$_2C_6H_4$,
4-OMeC_6H_4, 4-CNC_6H_4,   4-COCH$_3C_6H_4$, -COO^{n}Bu,
4-NO$_2C_6H_4$, pyridine,
primidine, thiophene

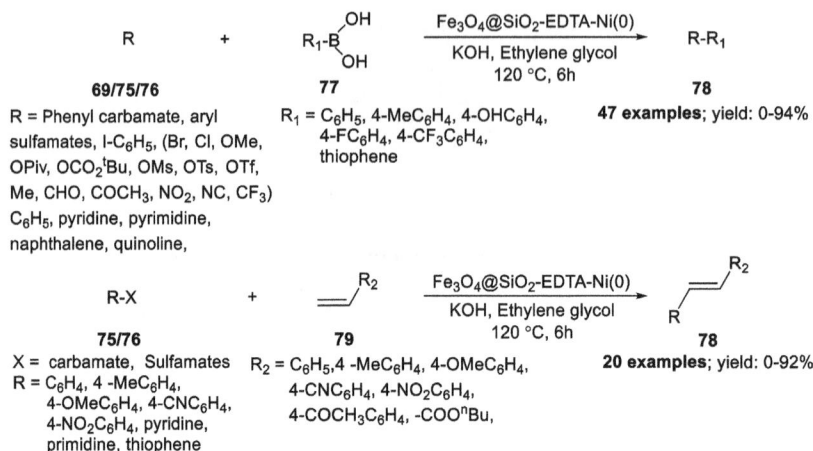

SCHEME 5.28   Fe3O4@SiO2-EDTA-Ni(0) NP catalyzed Suzuki-Miyuara and Heck reaction

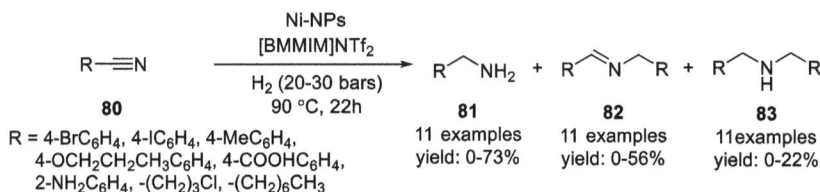

R—≡N $\xrightarrow[\substack{[BMMIM]NTf_2\\H_2\ (20\text{-}30\ bars)\\90\ ^\circ C,\ 22h}]{Ni\text{-}NPs}$ R$\diagup$NH$_2$ + R$\diagup$N$\diagdown$R + R$\diagup$N(H)$\diagdown$R

80   **81**   **82**   **83**

R = 4-BrC_6H_4, 4-IC_6H_4, 4-MeC_6H_4,   11 examples   11 examples   11examples
4-OCH$_2$CH$_2$CH$_3C_6H_4$, 4-COOHC_6H_4,   yield: 0-73%   yield: 0-56%   yield: 0-22%
2-NH$_2C_6H_4$, -(CH$_2$)$_3$Cl, -(CH$_2$)$_6$CH$_3$

SCHEME 5.29   Ni NPs in (BMMIM)NTf$_2$ catalyzed nitrile HYD

the corresponding biaryls or substituted aralkyls of prototype **78** in low to excellent yields (Scheme 5.28).[38]

5.2.2.4 Nickel nanoparticles in [BMMIM]NTf$_2$ catalyzed nitrile hydrogenation

In 2017, Konnerth et al reported nitrile HYD that used Ni NPs implanted in imidazolium based ionic liquids (ILs). The Ni NPs in 1-butyl-2,3-dimethylimidazolium bis((trifluoromethyl)sulfonyl)imide ([BMMIM]NTf$_2$) NC was the universal catalyst for nitrile HYD and showed good selectivity. In this work, substituted aliphatic and aromatic nitriles **80** were treated with Ni NPs in IL [BMMIM]NTf$_2$ at 90°C for 22 h in the presence of H$_2$ at 20–30 bar, which gave the corresponding hydrogenated product substituted primary amines **81**, substituted imines **82**, and substituted secondary amines **83** in low to moderate yields (Scheme 5.29).[39]

5.2.2.5 Nano-NiFe$_2$O$_4$ catalyzed synthesis of alkoxyimidazo[1,2-a]pyridines

Payra et al described the efficient synthesis of alkoxyimidazo[1,2-*a*]pyridines in the presence of nickel ferrite (NiFe$_2$O$_4$)-based NPs under a MW-assisted condensation reaction.

In this methodology, various substituted and unsubstituted 2-aminopyridine **41**, β-nitrostyrene **84** and substituted aliphatic alcohol **85** were treated with a nano NiFe$_2$O$_4$ catalyst at 80°C for 4 h or in MW condition for 5 min, which gave the cyclized product alkoxyimidazo[1,2-*a*]pyridines **43** in good to excellent yields (Scheme 5.30).[40]

5.2.2.6 Nickel nanoparticle catalyzed multicomponent reaction for the synthesis of pyrrole

Moghaddam et al reported Ni NP catalyzed pyrrole synthesis via a multicomponent pathway. In this strategy, substituted cyclic and acyclic amines **27**, 1,3-diketone **86**, aromatic aldehydes **14,** and

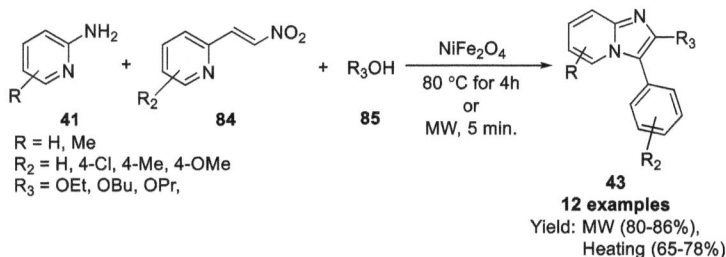

SCHEME 5.30   Synthesis of alkoxyimidazo[1,2-a]pyridines using $NiFe_2O_4$ NC

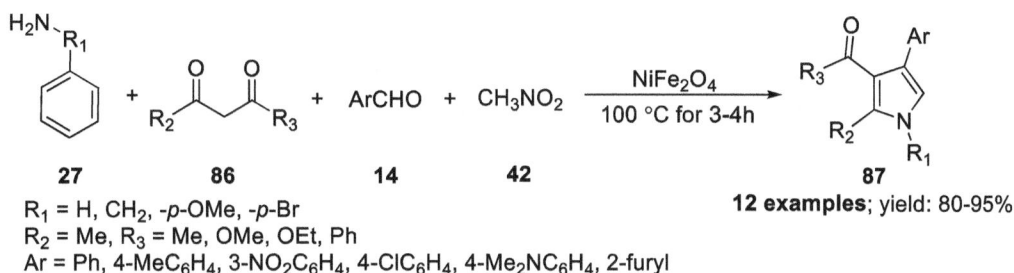

SCHEME 5.31   Ni NP catalyzed multicomponent reaction for pyrrole synthesis

nitromethane **42** were reacted in a one-pot method in the presence of $NiFe_2O_4$ NPs at 100°C for 3–4 h under neat conditions, which produced substituted pyrrole **87** derivatives in good to excellent yields (Scheme 5.31).[41]

5.2.2.7   Nickel nanoparticle catalyzed stereo- and chemo-selective semihydrogenation of functionalized alkynes of structurally diverse

Jagadeesh et al. prepared a highly stable, selective, and recyclable monodisperse Ni NP captured in G shells as sustainable HYD catalysts, which utilized immobilization and pyrolysis of fructose as low-cost monosaccharides and nickel(II) acetate ($Ni(OAc)_2$) on Si for its controlled preparation. These NPs were applied in the HYD of several structurally diverse substituted aromatic, heterocyclic, and aliphatic alkynes to the corresponding substituted alkenes with a high order of stereoselectivity and chemoselectivity. In this methodology, substituted internal alkynes **59** in the presence of Ni-fructose@SiO_2-800 NPs under 10 bars H_2 at 110°C for 15 h in the presence of ACN gave the corresponding hydrogenated substituted alkene product **60** (Z-alkene) as a major product (i.e., 98%–100% Z-alkene formation) along with the formation of the minor product **61** (E-alkene). Similarly, substituted terminal alkyne **62** in the presence of the previously mentioned reaction conditions gave the corresponding substituted alkenes as hydrogenated product **63** (Scheme 5.32).[42]

5.2.2.8   Resin-encapsulated Nickel nanocatalyst for the reduction of nitroarenes

Rani et al reported the utilization of an impregnation method for the synthesis of resin-encapsulated Ni NC by the treatment of Ni(II) acetate tetrahydrate ($Ni(OAc)_2.4H_2O$) in the presence of sodium borohydride ($NaBH_4$). The synthesized NC was confirmed by various spectroscopic techniques, such as field emission scanning electron microscope (FESEM), transmission electron microscope (TEM), and inductively coupled plasma mass spectroscopy (ICP–MS). The resin-encapsulated Ni NC was applied in the synthesis of aniline via the reduction of nitrobenzene that used Ni NPs. In this methodology, substituted nitroarenes **26** in the presence of the NC underwent reduction, which produced the corresponding substituted amines **27** with excellent yield in the presence of $NaBH_4$ as co-catalyst at 50°C for 0.5–2 h under MeOH: H_2O (3:7) solvent conditions (Scheme 5.33).[43]

$$R_1 \!\!=\!\!\! R_2 \quad \xrightarrow[\substack{\text{10 bar } H_2,\ \text{ACN} \\ 110\ ^\circ\text{C, 15h}}]{\text{Ni-fructose@SiO}_2\text{-800}} \quad \overset{R_1}{\diagup}\!\!\diagdown_{R_2} \quad + \quad R_1\!\!\diagdown\!\!\diagup^{R_2}$$

59   **60**   **61**

24 examples; yield: 82-95%

R₁ = Ph, 4-MePh, 4-NH₂Ph, 4-FPh, 4-ClPh, 4-BrPh, 4-OMePh,
    4-COHPh, 4-COMePh, 4-CH₂CH₃Ph, benzo[*b*]thiophene,
    -(CH₂)₈OH, -(CH₂)₈OMe
R₂ = Ph, 4-CH₂CH₃Ph, 4-NH₂Ph, 3-CNpyridine, 4-BoranePh,
    pyridine, 4-Si(CH₃)₃Ph, dihydrofuran-2,5-dione, isobenzofuran-1,3-dione,
    4-MePh, -CH₂OH, -C(CH₂)₂OH, -CH₂NHCH₂CH₂CH₃, 4-C₉H₁₇Ph, -CH₂CH₃

$$R_1\!\!=\!\!\! \quad \xrightarrow[\substack{\text{10 bar } H_2,\ \text{ACN} \\ 110\ ^\circ\text{C, 15h}}]{\text{Ni-fructose@SiO}_2\text{-800}} \quad R_1\!\!\diagdown\!\!\diagup\!\!\parallel$$

62   **63**

12 examples; yield: 83-94%

R₁ = Ph, 2-MePh, 2-FPh, 4-CH₂OHPh, 4-(CH₃)₃Ph, 4-CF₃Ph,
    2-OMeNaphthalene, 4-CNPh, pyridine, -4-(CH₂)₄CH₃Ph, Cyclohexyl

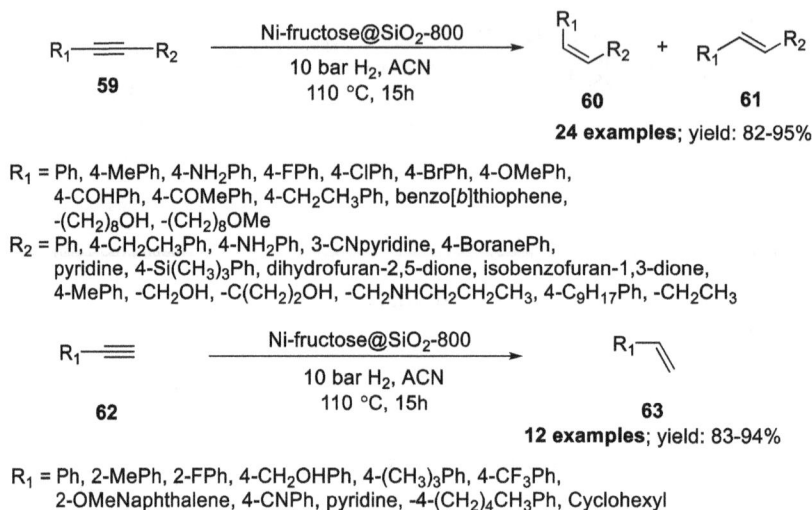

SCHEME 5.32 Ni-fructose@SiO2-800 stereo and chemoselective semi-HYD of functionalized alkynes

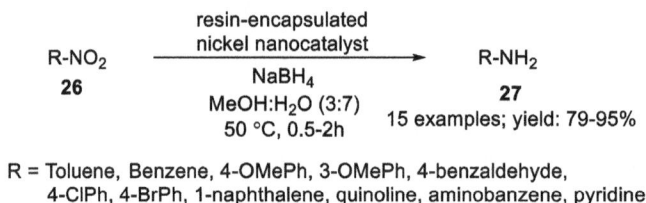

$$\text{R-NO}_2 \quad \xrightarrow[\substack{\text{NaBH}_4 \\ \text{MeOH:H}_2\text{O (3:7)} \\ 50\ ^\circ\text{C, 0.5-2h}}]{\substack{\text{resin-encapsulated} \\ \text{nickel nanocatalyst}}} \quad \text{R-NH}_2$$

26   **27**

15 examples; yield: 79-95%

R = Toluene, Benzene, 4-OMePh, 3-OMePh, 4-benzaldehyde,
    4-ClPh, 4-BrPh, 1-naphthalene, quinoline, aminobanzene, pyridine

SCHEME 5.33 Resin-encapsulated Ni NC for the reduction of nitroarenes

5.2.2.9 NiFe2O4@SiO2–H₃PW₁₂O₄₀ catalyzed synthesis of tetrahydrobenzo[b]pyran and pyrano[2,3-c]pyrazoles

In 2015, Maleki et al reported a highly efficient and magnetically separable, Keggin (H₃PW₁₂O₄₀) heteropoly acid (HPA) supported on Si-coated NiFe₂O₄ NPs, for instance, NiFe₂O₄@SiO₂–H₃PW₁₂O₄₀ NC that was confirmed by various spectroscopic techniques, such as XRD, TEM, SEM, VSM, and FT-IR. The NC was efficiently recycled up to six times without any substantial loss of catalytic activity. The catalyst was utilized in the synthesis of tetrahydrobenzo[*b*]pyrans **91** and pyrano[2,3-*c*] pyrazoles **92** derivatives. In this methodology, substituted aldehydes **14**, substituted acetate **88,** and cyclic 1, 3-dicarbonyl **89** or 3-methyl-1-phenyl-1*H*-pyrazol-5(4*H*)-one **90** were reacted together in a one-pot multicomponent reaction that used NiFe₂O₄@SiO₂–H₃PW₁₂O₄₀ NC under reflux conditions for 5–60 min, which produced substituted tetrahydrobenzo[b]pyrans **91** and pyrano[2,3-*c*]pyrazoles **92** with 76%–95% yield (Scheme 5.34).[44]

5.2.2.10 PdRuNi@GO NPs assisted synthesis of Hantzsch 1, 4-dihydropyridines

Demirci et al reported the synthesis of 1, 4-dihydropyridines that used Ni NPs of PdRuNi furnished on GO (PdRuNi@GO NPs). In this methodology, cyclic 1,2-diketones that included dimedone **89**, substituted cyclic aldehydes **14,** and substituted β-keto acetate **88** were used in a one-pot in the presence of PdRuNi@GO NPs and ammonium acetate (NH₄OAc) at 70°C for 45 min using DMF as a solvent and produced Hantzsch dihydropyridines **93** with good to excellent yield (Scheme 5.35).[45]

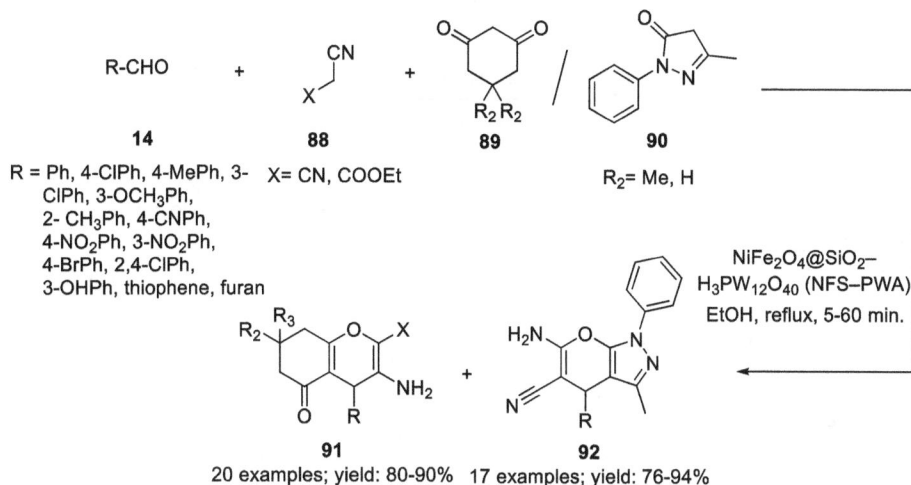

SCHEME 5.34 NiFe2O4@SiO2–H$_3$PW$_{12}$O$_{40}$ catalyzed synthesis of tetrahydrobenzo[b]pyrans **91** and pyrano[2,3-c]pyrazoles **92**

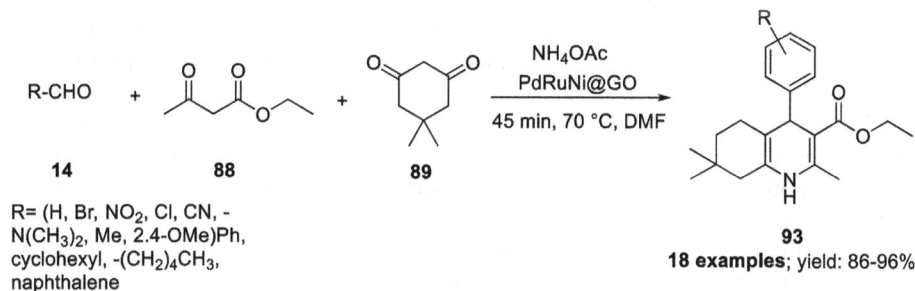

SCHEME 5.35 PdRuNi@GO NPs assisted synthesis of Hantzsch 1, 4-dihydropyridines

5.2.3 COPPER NANOPARTICLE CATALYZED ORGANIC TRANSFORMATIONS AND SYNTHESIS OF BIOACTIVE HETEROCYCLES

In this section, some of the most important organic transformations that are being continuously applied in the synthesis of several N-containing bioheterocycles using that used Cu NPs are incorporated. Furthermore, the application of Cu NPs, which have been used in the synthesis of bioactive heterocycles will be discussed. Therefore, literature on structurally diverse examples were considered for discussion in this section.

5.2.3.1 Heterogenous recyclable Copper(0) nanoparticle deposited on nanoporous polymer catalytic system for Ullman reaction in water

Mondal et al reported the development of a highly efficient Cu^{0}NP catalytic system that carried out Ullman cross-coupling of various substituted aryl halides and with substituted amines under aqueous conditions. The synthesis of Cu NPs involved the reaction of divinylbenzene with acrylic acid under a hydrothermal environment, which underwent polymerization in an organic environment. The resultant adduct was subjected to Cu^0 NP deposition that led to the formation of a Cu–Boron NC. Similarly, another Cu–A NC (i.e., Cu^0 NP loaded with porous C) was prepared to compare the reactivity of the NC toward Ullman cross-coupling reactions under aqueous conditions. Several

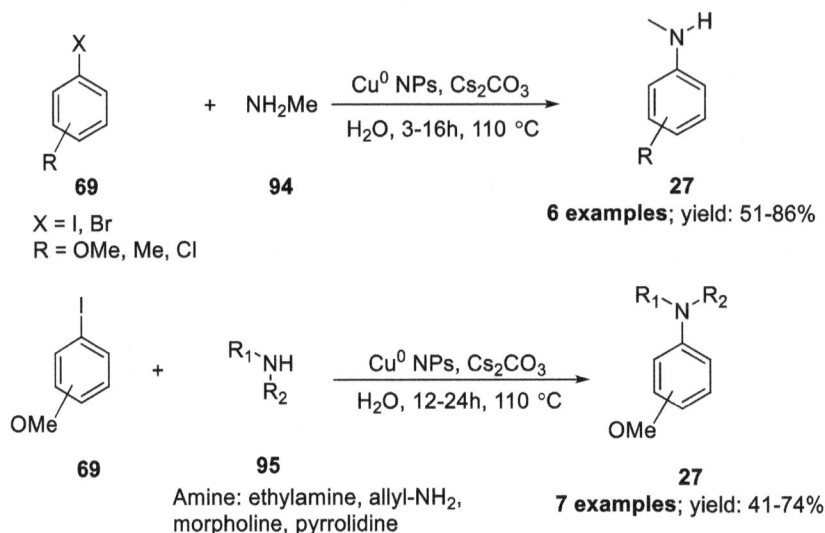

SCHEME 5.36 Cu⁰ NP deposited on nanoporous polymer catalyzed Ullman reaction in H₂O

characterization techniques, such as TEM, SEM, XRD, and XPS were utilized for the synthesized NCs. Furthermore, this Ullman coupling methodology used a Cu-B nanocatalyst involved the reaction of substituted aryl halide **69** with substituted methyl amine **94** in the presence of Cu–B NC and cesium (Ce) carbonates as the base in H₂O under continuous heating at 110°C for 3–16 h produced the corresponding substituted methyl anilines **27** with excellent yields (Scheme 5.36). In addition, the Ullman reaction performed with other NCs, such as Cu–A, Cu⁰NPs, Cu⁰-Carbon black, and nanoporous polymer DVAC-1 (i.e., developed by the nonaqueous polymerization of acrylic acid) either gave the Ullman product at a lower yield or the reaction did not occur. The high catalytic efficiency of the Cu–B NC was shown due to its high Brunauer–Emmett–Teller (BET) surface area and unique sea-urchin-like nanostructure.[46]

Similarly, substituted aryl iodide **69** reacted with various secondary amines, such as ethylamine, allyl-NH₂, morpholines, and pyrrolidines **95** in the presence of Cu–B NC and Ce carbonates as the base in H₂O under continuous heating at 110°C for 3–16 h, which produced the corresponding substituted arylated anilines **27** with a good yield (Scheme 5.36).[46]

5.2.3.2   Solvent-Dependent CuNPs/C catalyzed multicomponent synthesis of indolizines and Chalcones

Alonso et al reported the multicomponent synthesis of indolizines that used a Cu NC. In this methodology, Cu-based NPs supported on activated charcoal (i.e., CuNPs/C, 0.5 mol% catalyst loading) was utilized as an efficient NC in a multicomponent reaction in which various substituted heteroaromatic aldehydes i.e., (nicotinimide) **97**, substituted secondary amine **95,** and substituted terminal alkynes **62** were subjected to a one-pot multicomponent reaction at 70°C for 3–20 h in DCM, which produced substituted cyclized indolizines **98** with good to high yields (Scheme 5.37A). In addition, the reaction worked well with Cu NPs compared with commercial copper catalyst, such as copper(I) chloride (CuCl), copper(II) chloride (CuCl₂), copper(I) bromide (CuBr), copper(I) iodide (CuI), copper(II) oxide CuO, cuprous oxide (Cu₂O), copper(II) acetate (Cu(OAc)₂), copper(I) acetate (CuOAc), copper(I) bromide dimethyl sulfide complex (CuBr.SMe₂), and copper(II) triflate (CuOTf).[47]

Similarly, various substituted hetero and aromatic aldehydes **14** and substituted terminal alkynes **62** were reacted together in the presence of Cu NPs/C (0.5 mol% catalyst loading) using piperidine

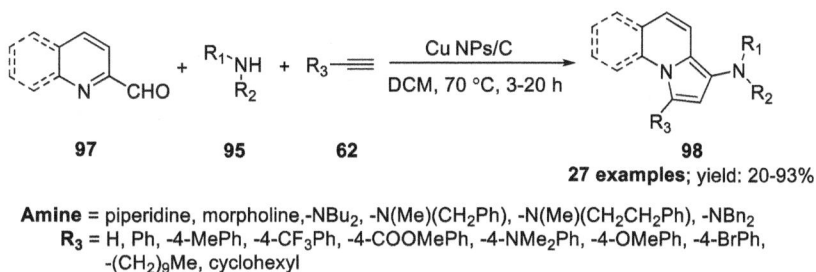

Amine = piperidine, morpholine,-NBu$_2$, -N(Me)(CH$_2$Ph), -N(Me)(CH$_2$CH$_2$Ph), -NBn$_2$
R$_3$ = H, Ph, -4-MePh, -4-CF$_3$Ph, -4-COOMePh, -4-NMe$_2$Ph, -4-OMePh, -4-BrPh,
      -(CH$_2$)$_9$Me, cyclohexyl

SCHEME 5.37A   CuNPs/C catalyzed multicomponent synthesis of indolizines in DCM

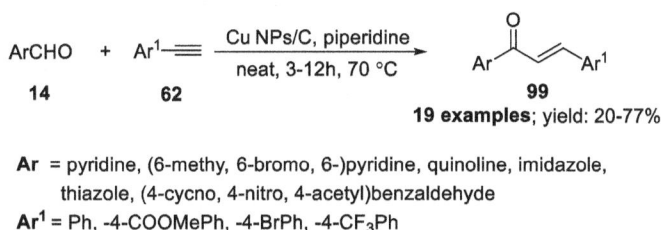

Ar = pyridine, (6-methy, 6-bromo, 6-)pyridine, quinoline, imidazole,
      thiazole, (4-cycno, 4-nitro, 4-acetyl)benzaldehyde
Ar^1 = Ph, -4-COOMePh, -4-BrPh, -4-CF$_3$Ph

SCHEME 5.37B   CuNPs/C catalyzed synthesis of Chalcones under neat conditions

(1 equiv.) as a base in the absence of any solvents, for instance, neat conditions at 70°C for 3–12 h produced substituted chalcones with good to excellent yields (Scheme 5.37B).[47]

5.2.3.3   Cu$_3$(BTC)$_2$ derived CuNPs immobilized on activated charcoal as an efficient nanocatalyst for the synthesis of unsymmetrical chalcogenides under ligand-, base-, and additive-free conditions via Se(Te)-Se(Te) bond activation

Mohan et al reported the synthesis of highly porous [Cu$_3$(BTC)$_2$] (BTC=benzene-1,3,5-tricarboxylate) MOF-based Cu NPs. The structure of the NP was confirmed by various XRD, EDX, TEM, SEM, and BET techniques. Without further treatment, under US conditions, the synthesized Cu NPs were immobilized onto activated charcoal (AC). The prepared heterogeneous Cu NPs/AC NC was utilized for the cross-coupling of substituted diphenyl diselenide/ditelluride **100** with several substituted boronic acids **77** in dimethyl sulfoxide (DMSO) at 100°C for 3–6 h and produced diphenyl selenides and tellurides **101** in good to very high yields via selenium (tellurium)–selenium (tellurium) bond activation under ligand-, base-, and additive-free conditions. This methodology referred to Se–C bond formation in which Cu NPs formed a bis(phenylselenyl)Cu intermediate **102,** which could be converted into the final product. The copper NPs/AC that had high catalytic activity and low catalyst loading were well-suited with a diverse substituent on diphenyl selenides in DMSO under atmospheric air as oxidant through selenium–carbon (sp^3-, sp^2-, and spcarbon) bond formation (Scheme 5.38).[48]

5.2.3.4   Cu/CuNPs catalyzed synthesis of aryl nitrile and 1,2,3-triazoles

Nasrollahzadeh et al reported a novel Cu immobilized on Cu NPs methodologies for the preparation of aryl nitrile and 1,2,3-triazoles. This methodology was composed of the reaction of substituted aryl iodide **69** with potassium ferrocyanide (K$_4$Fe(CN)$_6$) **103** as the source of nitrile groups in the presence of C-supported Cu NPs catalyst, which produced aryl nitrile **104**. The Cu NPs catalyzed methodology occurred in DMF in the presence of K$_2$CO$_3$ as the base at 120°C for 12 h. Similarly, substituted benzyl halides **105**, substituted benzoyl halides **106** and/or substituted alkyl halides **107** on treatment with substituted terminal alkynes **62** in the presence of sodium azide **108** and C/Cu

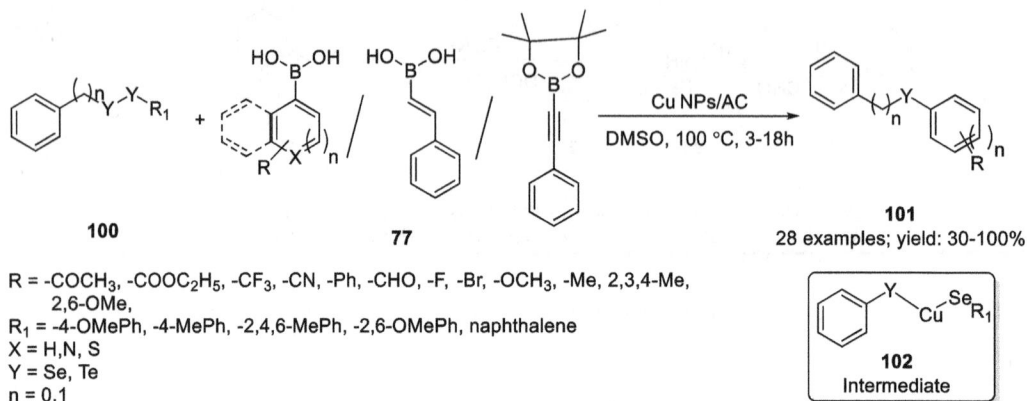

SCHEME 5.38 $Cu_3(BTC)_2$ derived Cu NPs immobilized on AC catalyzed synthesis of unsymmetrical chalcogenides via Se(Te)-Se(Te) bond activation

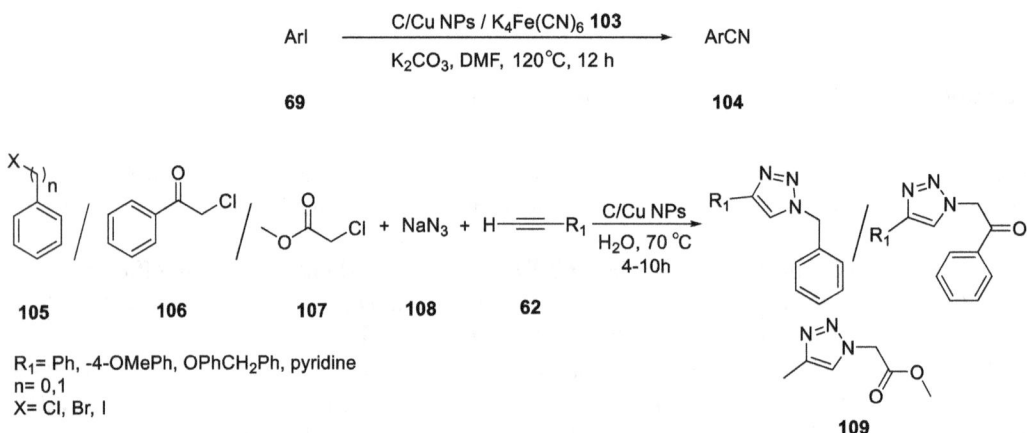

SCHEME 5.39 Cu/CuNPs catalyzed synthesis of aryl nitrile **104** and 1,2,3-triazoles **109**

NPs in water at 70°C for 4–10 h gave the corresponding substituted 1,2,4-triazoles **109** as the major product. In this reaction, the sodium azide **108** acted as a source of azole (Scheme 5.39).[49] Compared with the reported synthesis of alkyl nitriles; the salient features of this methodology includes the exclusion of metal (e.g., Pd and Cu) homogeneous catalysts, toxic reagents, ligand-free approach, high yielding reaction, operationally simple and cost-effective process, reusable and recyclable catalyst, use of $K_4Fe(CN)_6$ as a nonexplosive, non-flammable, cheap and less toxic cyanide source, and its application to large-scale synthesis, etc. (Scheme 5.39).[49]

5.2.3.5   Cu–Ferrite NPs catalyzed direct, one-pot redox synthesis of 2-substituted benzoxazoles

Sarode et al reported a practical, green, and sustainable protocol for the synthesis of 2-substituted benzoxazoles that used Cu–ferrite $CuFe_2O_4$ NPs. This reaction methodology incorporated the reaction of substituted and unsubstituted benzyl amine **110** with substituted and unsubstituted 2-nitrophenol **111** in the presence of Cu Fe_2O_4 NPs at 130°C for 16 h in N-methyl-2-pyrrolidone (NMP) and produced 2-substituted benzoxazole **47** in good to excellent yield (Scheme 5.40).[50]

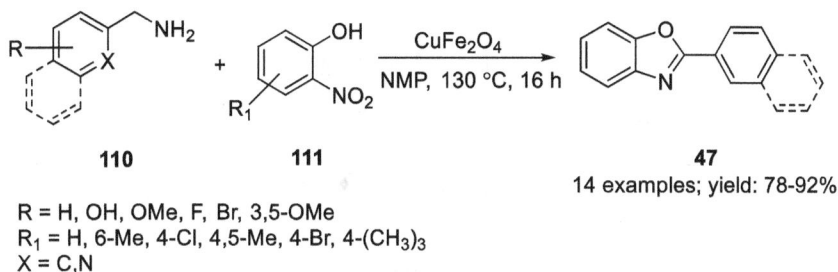

SCHEME 5.40 $CuFe_2O_4$ NPs catalyzed direct, one-pot redox synthesis of 2-substituted benzoxazoles

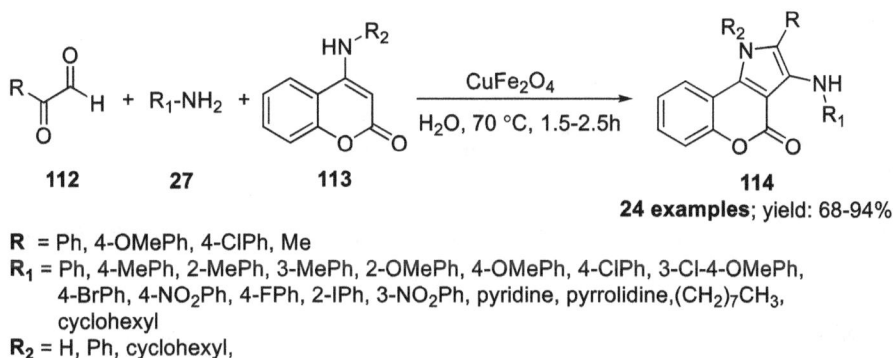

SCHEME 5.41 $CuFe_2O_4$ catalyzed multicomponent synthesis of chromeno[4,3-b]pyrrol-4(1H)-one in aqueous media

5.2.3.6 $CuFe_2O_4$ catalyzed multicomponent synthesis of chromeno[4,3-b]pyrrol-4(1H)-one in aqueous media

Saha et al reported an efficient green protocol that involved Cu NPs in multicomponent reactions toward the synthesis of chromeno[4,3-b]pyrrol-4(1*H*)-one **114**. The methodology was composed of a one-pot reaction of substituted glyoxals **112**, substituted primary amines **27**, and various substituted 4-aminocoumarins **113** in H_2O at 70°C for 1.5–2.5 h, which produced the corresponding chromeno[4,3-b]pyrrol-4(1*H*)-one **114** with good to excellent yield (Scheme 5.41).[51] The magnetically separable NPs of $CuFe_2O_4$ ferrite were prepared by the citric acid complex method and were characterized by several spectroscopic techniques, such as FTIR, TEM, XRD, and high-resolution transmission electron microscopy (HRTEM). Mechanistically, it involved the reaction of primary amine **27** with phenyl glyoxals monohydrate **112** that were activated by Fe^{3+} ions of $CuFe_2O_4$ NPs to form intermediate imine. The imine intermediate, activated and held by the Cu^{2+} ion of $CuFe_2O_4$ NPs, was then attacked by the Michael reaction donor C–3 center of 4-aminocoumarin **113** to form the imino–amine unstable intermediate, which after intramolecular cyclization and dehydration produced the chromeno[4,3-b]pyrrol-4(1*H*)-one **114** core (Scheme 5.41).[51]

5.2.3.7 $CuFe_2O_4$ nanoparticle catalyzed synthesis of Naphthoxazinones

Ghaani et al demonstrated the novel MW-assisted coprecipitation protocol for the synthesis of $CuFe_2O_4$ NPs. The NPs were characterized by various spectroscopic techniques, such as FTIR, XRD, and SEM. The ferromagnetic property of the synthesized $CuFe_2O_4$ NPs were confirmed by VSM. The synthesized NPs showed excellent properties in the one-pot three-component synthesis of naphthoxazinones, where 2-naphthols **115**, substituted aromatic aldehydes **14**, and urea **116** were

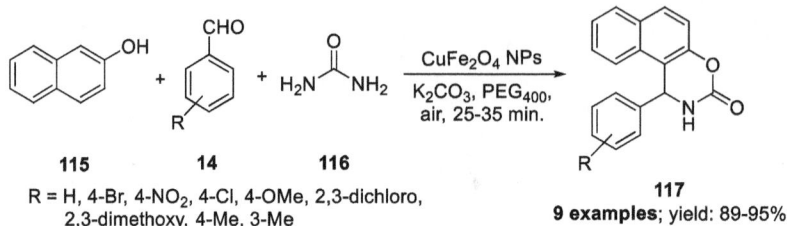

SCHEME 5.42 CuFe$_2$O$_4$ NP catalyzed synthesis of naphthoxazinones

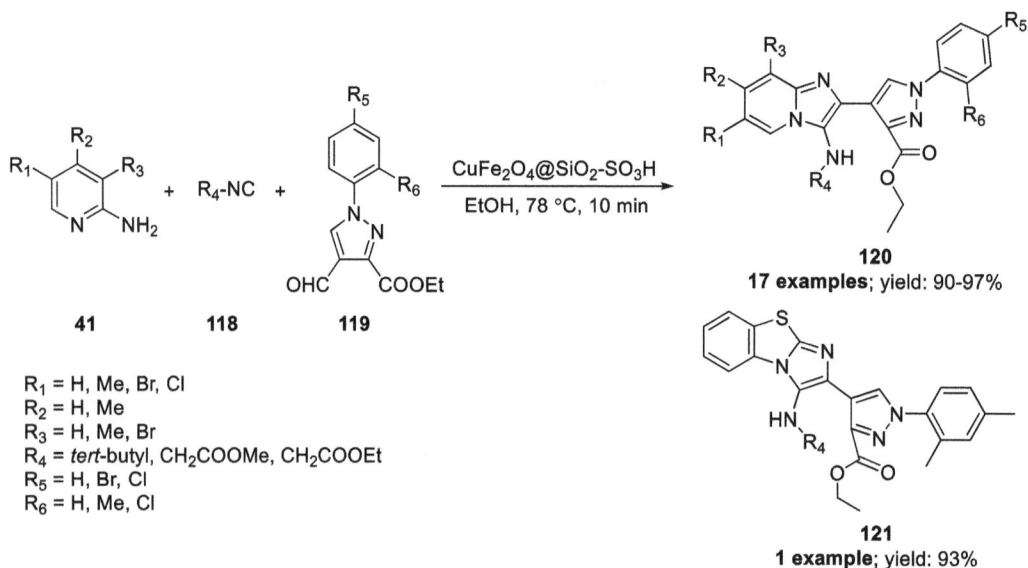

SCHEME 5.43 CuFe$_2$O$_4$@SiO2-SO3H NPs catalyzed synthesis of substituted 2-pyrazole-3-amino-imidazo[1,2-a]pyridines **120** and pyrazole-benzo[d]imidazo[2,1-b]thiazole **121**

reacted together along with CuFe$_2$O$_4$ NPs in the presence of K$_2$CO$_3$ in PEG$_{400}$ in air for 25–35 min, which gave substituted naphthoxazinones **117** with 89%–95% yields (Scheme 5.42).[52]

5.2.3.8 CuFe2O4@SiO2-SO3H nanoparticles catalyzed synthesis of 2-pyrazole-3-amino-imidazo[1,2-a]pyridines-based heterocycles

Swami et al reported the synthesis of Si-coated CuFe$_2$O$_4$ NPs functionalized with sulphonic acid, which was utilized in the synthesis of 2-pyrazole-3-amino-imidazo[1,2-a]pyridines and their congeners. The synthesized NPs were characterized by various spectroscopic techniques, such as FTIR, TEM, XRD, SEM, VSM, and EDX. In this protocol, various substituted and unsubstituted 2-aminopyridines **41**, substituted isocyanides **118**, and ethyl 4-formyl-1-phenyl-1H-pyrazole-3-carboxylate **119** were subjected to a one-pot reaction in the presence of CuFe$_2$O$_4$@SiO$_2$-SO$_3$H NPs under reflux conditions at 7 °C for 10 min, which gave substituted 2-pyrazole-3-amino-imidazo[1,2-a]pyridines **120** with 90%–97% yields and pyrazole-benzo[d]imidazo[2,1-b]thiazole **121** with a 93% yield (Scheme 5.43).[53]

5.2.3.9 Cu-ACP-Am-Fe3O4@SiO2 catalyzed Huisgen 1,3-dipolar cycloaddition reaction

Vibhute et al demonstrated the use of a novel Cu-based heterogeneous nanocatalyst, for instance, Cu-ACP-Am-Fe$_3$O$_4$@SiO$_2$ (i.e., acetylpyridine immobilized on amine-functionalized Si-coated

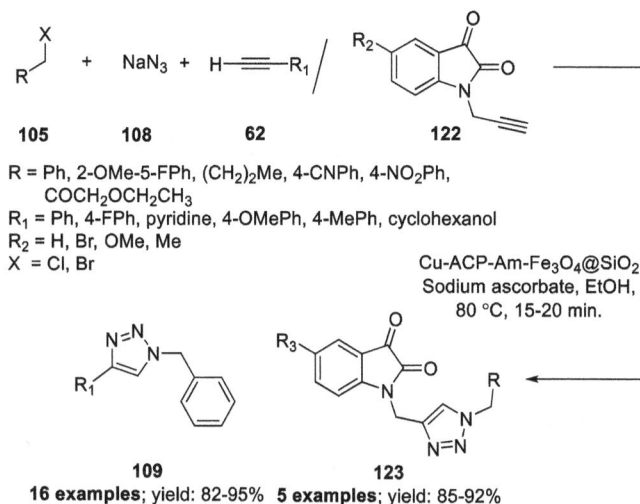

SCHEME 5.44   Cu-ACP-Am-Fe3O4@SiO2 catalyzed Huisgen 1,3-dipolar cycloaddition reaction

magnetite NPs) in a Huisgen 1,3-dipolar cycloaddition reaction for the preparation of triazoles. The characterization of the NC was carried out by various physicochemical methods, such as FTIR, thermal gravimetric analysis–differential scanning calorimetry (TGA–DSC), XPS, SEM, EDS, VSM, XRD, and TEM. The recyclable NP driven Huisgen 1,3-dipolar cycloaddition reaction involved the multicomponent reaction of substituted aromatic and aliphatic halide **105**, terminal alkyne **62**, and sodium azide **108** in EtOH that used Cu-ACP-Am-Fe$_3$O$_4$@SiO$_2$ catalyst, sodium ascorbate at 80°C for 15–20 min, which gave 1,4-disubstituted-1,2,3-triazoles **109** with 82%–95% yields (Scheme 5.44).

Indoline-2,3-dione **122** had been used as a starting precursor to perform an NP catalyzed Huisgen 1,3-dipolar cycloaddition reaction that used the Cu-ACP-Am-Fe$_3$O$_4$@SiO$_2$ catalyst, sodium ascorbate at 80°C for 20–24 min, which produced indoline-2,3-dione linked substituted 1,2,3-triazoles **123** with 85%–92% yields (Scheme 5.44).[54] Considering the environmental aspects, this protocol was proved to be an environmentally benign and efficient protocol that had milder reaction conditions, was less hazardous, and proceeded with a high turnover frequency and turnover number (TON), which made this protocol a competent strategy (Scheme 5.44).

5.2.3.10   Cu@TiO2 nanocatalyzed C-2 amination of benzothiazoles, benzoxazoles, and thiazoles

Dutta et al prepared a titanium oxide (TiO$_2$) encapsulated Cu NC (Cu@TiO$_2$) that demonstrated C-2 amination of benzothiazoles, benzoxazoles, and thiazoles **126** with ≤95% yield. In this report, the C-2 amination reaction of benzothiazoles **124** or benzoxazoles **47** occurred either with substituted secondary amine **95** or with formamides **125** in the presence of Cu@TiO$_2$ NC that used silver acetate (AgOAc) as an oxidant and sodium tert-butoxide (NaO^{t}Bu) as a base at 120°C for 5 h, which gave the desired C$_2$ aminated benzothiazoles and benzoxazoles **126** with 54%–95% yields (Scheme 5.45).[55]

The recyclable multipurpose robust protocol was feasible under solvent- and ligand-free conditions with moderate to excellent yields of various secondary amines and their corresponding formamides. The control and kinetic experiments supported the putative mechanism of the reaction. The synthetic utility of the NC had was exemplified by large-scale synthesis of the bioactive benzoxazoles **127** (Scheme 5.45).[55]

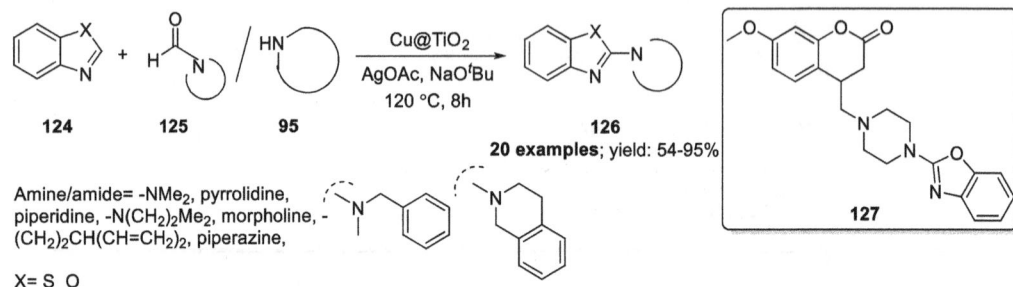

SCHEME 5.45 Cu@TiO2 nanocatalyzed C-2 amination of benzothiazoles, benzoxazoles, and thiazoles

5.3 DISCUSSION AND SUMMARY

NC-driven organic transformations and synthesis of bioactive heterocycles is an advanced novel strategy in medicinal and pharmaceutical chemistry. Transition metal-based nanomaterials are reported in the literature to augment reactivity and selectivity in nanoscience and nanotechnology. However, the variation in the size of the NPs affects the catalytic activity of the NPs. Therefore, the ratio of atoms present on the surface changes dramatically with the change in the size of the particle(s). NP catalyzed organic transformations were identified as the safest, most eco-friendly reaction pathway. In addition, NPs/metal oxide-based NPs play an important role in C–C bond formation via C–H activation and other organic transformations. Many reports had been published in the literature on the preparation of NP catalyzed organic transformations and bioactive heterocycles. However, in the last two to three decades, environmentally benign, fast and efficient green synthesis has been a focus and nanoparticle assisted organic synthesis has been an integral part of the green and sustainable developments in chemical synthesis. In particular, this chapter included some of the important recent developments and sustainable applications of NP driven organic synthesis, especially with the cheaper transition metal(s)-NPs, such as Fe, Co, Ni, and Cu over the last 7 years (2014–2020). This chapter included the developments of the most efficient methodologies that are practiced in the synthesis of bioactive heterocycles.

Therefore, Co or Co-Fe NPs, such as N-doped Co/MC (Scheme 5.1); Co-Phen@C (Scheme 5.2); Co@NCNTs and Co-NCNTs-800 (Scheme 5.3); N-Si doped carbon (Co/N–Si–C) (Scheme 5.4); Co@N-doped G shells (Co@NGS) (Scheme 5.5); Co N-heterocyclic carbene grafted on CNTs (Co–NHC@MWCNTs) (Scheme 5.6); Co NPs supported on Si (CoNP@SBA-15) (Scheme 5.7); Co-terephthalic acid MOF@C-800 (Scheme 5.8); $CoFe_2O_4$ (Scheme 5.9); CrCoFeO4@G–GO and $Zn_0.5Co0.5Fe2O4@G$–GO (Scheme 5.10); $CoFe_2O_4$/CNT-Cu (Scheme 5.11); $CoFe_2O_4$ (Scheme 5.11) and CoFe2O4@SiO2/PrNH2 (Scheme 5.13 and 5.14); GO anchored sulphonic acid nanocatalyst ($CoFe_2O_4$-GO-SO_3H) (Scheme 5.15); CoFe2O4@SiO2–PTA (Scheme 5.17); and Co@ NGR (Scheme 5.18) have been utilized extensively for various types of organic transformations in an highly efficient manner.

Similarly, several Ni-based NPs, such as Ni NPs supported on diphenylphosphinated poly(vinyl alcohol-co-ethylene), for instance, (DPP-PVA-co-PE)-NiNP catalyst (Scheme 5.26); Si-supported Ni(II)–DABCO complex, for instance, Ni(II)–DABCO@SiO2 NP (Scheme 5.27); Fe3O4@ SiO2-EDTA-Ni(0) NP (Scheme 5.28); Ni NPs in [BMMIM]NTf$_2$ NC (Scheme 5.29); $NiFe_2O_4$ NC (Scheme 5.30 and 5.31); Ni-fructose@SiO2-800 (Scheme 5.32); resin-encapsulated Ni NC (Scheme 5.33); NiFe2O4@SiO2–$H_3PW_{12}O_{40}$ (Scheme 5.34); PdRuNi@GO NPs (Scheme 5.35) were utilized for Mizoroki–Heck reactions; Suzuki-Miyuara cross-coupling, nitrile HYD, synthesis of alkoxyimidazo[1,2-*a*]pyridines, pyrrole synthesis, stereo and chemoselective semihydrogenation of functionalized alkynes, reduction of nitroarenes, synthesis of tetrahydrobenzo[*b*]pyran and pyrano[2,3-*c*]pyrazoles, and synthesis of Hantzsch 1, 4-dihydropyridines.

In addition, Cu NPs have been utilized extensively for various organic transformations and synthesis of bio heterocycles. For example, Cu⁰NP (Scheme 5.36); CuNPs/C (Scheme 5.37); Cu$_3$(BTC)$_2$ derived CuNPs immobilized on AC (Scheme 5.38); Cu/Cu NPs (Scheme 5.39); Cu-Fe$_3$O$_4$ NPs (Schemes 5.40 and 42); CuFe2O4@SiO2-SO3H NPs (Scheme 5.43); Cu-ACP-Am-Fe$_2$O$_4$@SiO$_2$ (Scheme 5.44); Cu@TiO2 (Scheme 5.45) was applied in Ullman reactions; synthesis of indolizines, chalcones, unsymmetrical chalcogenides, aryl nitrile, 1,2,3-triazoles, 2-substituted benzoxazoles, chromeno[4,3-b]pyrrol-4(1*H*)-one, naphthoxazinones, 2-pyrazole-3-amino-imidazo[1,2-*a*] pyridines, pyrazole-benzo[*d*]imidazo[2,1-*b*]thiazole, Huisgen 1,3-dipolar cycloaddition reaction, C-2 amination of benzothiazoles, benzoxazoles, and thiazoles with good to excellent yields.

5.4 CONCLUSION

This chapter demonstrated the latest developments in cheaper transition metal-nanocatalyzed synthetic organic reactions and transformation to develop new bioactive scaffolds, heterocycles, drugs, therapeutics, and increased the reactivity of synthesized ones. Transition metal-catalyzed organic reactions, in particular, C–C bond forming reactions via C–H bond activations were the first choice of organic chemist. However, the use of excess metal in stochiometric amounts is not considered an environmentally friendly procedure; therefore, the scope to develop various reactions in the presence of NCs, especially with cheaper transition metals (e.g., Fe, Co, Ni, Cu based nanocatalyst) reached the position to develop C–H activation and C–C bond formation reactions during the last two decades. Therefore, this chapter illustrated the importance of cheaper transition metal NCs in organic synthesis. Several specific reactions, such as the Mizoroki–Heck reaction, Suzuki-Miyuara cross-coupling, Ullman coupling, Hantzsch 1, 4-dihydropyridines synthesis, Huisgen 1,3-dipolar cycloaddition reaction, ADH and HYD of various N-heterocycles, ODH and HYD, N-formylation of amines, multicomponent reaction, HYD of alkynes, and HYD of nitroarenes to aminoarenes are some of the best examples of NP catalyzed synthesis illustrated in this chapter. These NP assisted methodologies could offer medicinally important cores very efficiently and could be utilized to generate more bioactive heterocycles for faster medicinal chemistry and drug discovery.

5.5 DECLARATIONS

AUTHORS' CONTRIBUTIONS

SC conceived and designed the concept. RKY, VVD, TMB, and MJ carried out all the literature searches. SC and RKY wrote the chapter manuscript. All the authors have read and approved the final version of the chapter.

ACKNOWLEDGMENTS

RKY acknowledges UGC, Delhi for the financial assistance in terms of Senior Research Fellowship. VVD and TMB acknowledges the Department of Pharmaceuticals, Ministry of Chemicals and Fertilizers for the financial assistance for M.S. Pharm fellowships. The NIPER-Raebareli manuscript communication number is NIPER-R/Communication/263.

LIST OF ABBREVIATIONS

NPs   Nanoparticles
US   Ultrasonic
MW   Microwave
nm   Nanometer
MNPs   Transition metal nanoparticles

ACN	Acetonitrile
THF	Tetrahydrofuran
ADH	Acceptorless hydrogenation
t-BuOK	Potassium tertiary butoxide
ODH	Oxidative dehydrogenation
CTH	Catalytic transfer hydrogenation
Co NCs	Cobalt based nanocatalyst
HYD	Hydrogenation
IPA	Isopropyl alcohol
KSCN	Potassium Isothiocynate
MOF	Metal–organic Framework
PEG_{400}	Polyethylene glycol
CNT	Carbon nanotubes
SEM	Scanning electron microscopy
XRD	X-ray diffraction
VSM	Vibrating sample magnetometry
TEM	Transmission electron microscope
EDX	Energy dispersive X-ray analysis
ICP–AES	Inductively coupled plasma atomic emission
Ni NPs	Nickel nanoparticles
DPP-PVA-co-PE	Diphenylphosphinated poly(vinyl alcohol-co-ethylene) =
DABCO	1,4-Diazabicyclo[2.2.2]octane
[BMMIM]NTf$_2$]	1-butyl-2,3-dimethylimidazolium bis((trifluoromethyl)sulfonyl)imide =
DMSO	Dimethyl sulfoxide
XPS	X-ray photoelectron spectroscopy
DCM	Dichloromethane
AC	Activated charcoal
$K_4Fe(CN)_6$	Potassium ferrocyanide
NMP	N-methyl-2-pyrrolidone
VSM	Value stream mapping
TGA–DSC	Thermal gravimetric analysis–differential scanning calorimetry
AgOAc	Silver acetate
NaO^{t}Bu	Sodium tert-butoxide
TON	Turnover number
FTIR	Fourier-transform infrared spectroscopy
HRTEM	High-resolution transmission electron microscopy
BTC	benzene-1,3,5-tricarboxylate
DVAC	developed by nonaqueous polymerization of acrylic acid
ICP–MS	Inductively coupled plasma mass spectrometry

REFERENCES

1. Roberts MW. Preface. Catal Lett. (2000) 67: 0. doi.10.1023/A:1016600921086.
2. Duan H, Wang D, Li Y. Green chemistry for nanoparticle synthesis. Chem Soc Rev. 2015. 44:5778–52. doi.10.1039/c4cs00363b.
3. Roopan SM, Khan FRN. ZnO nanoparticles in the synthesis of AB ring core of camptothecin. Chemical Papers. 2010. 64:812–17. doi.10.2478/s11696-010-0058-y.
4. Madhumitha G, Roopan SM. Devastated crops: multifunctional efficacy for the production of nanoparticles. J Nanomater. 2013. 2013: 1–12. doi.10.1155/2013/951858.
5. Lee S-B, Park YI, Dong M-S, Gong Y-D. Identification of 2,3,6-trisubstituted quinoxaline derivatives as a Wnt2/β-catenin pathway inhibitor in non-small-cell lung cancer cell lines. Bioorg Med Chem Lett. 2010. 20: 5900–4. doi.10.1016/j.bmcl.2010.07.088.

6. Sabry NM, Mohamed HM, Khattab ESAEH, Motlaq SS, El-Agrody AM. Synthesis of 4*H*-chromene, coumarin, 12*H*-chromeno[2,3-*d*]pyrimidine derivatives and some of their antimicrobial and cytotoxicity activities. Eur J Med Chem. 2011. 46: 765–72. doi.10.1016/j.ejmech.2010.12.015.

7. Raj R, Singh P, Singh P, Gut J, Rosenthal PJ, Kumar V. Azide-alkyne cycloaddition en route to 1*H*-1,2,3-triazole-tethered 7-chloroquinoline-isatin chimeras: synthesis and antimalarial evaluation. Eur J Med Chem. 2013. 62: 590–6. doi.10.1016/j.ejmech.2013.01.032.

8. Sitonio MM, De Carvalho Jr. CHR, Campos IDA, Silva JBNF, De Lima MDCA, Goes AJS et al. Antiinflammatory and anti-arthritic activities of 3, 4-dihydro-2, 2- dimethyl-2*H*-naphthol[1,2-*b*]pyran-5, 6-dione (*β*-lapachone). Inflamm Res. 2013. 62: 107–13. doi:10.1007/s00011-012-0557-0.

9. Lak A, Mazloumi M, Mohajerani MS, Zanganeh S, Shayegh MR, Kajbafvala A. et al. Rapid formation of mono-dispersed hydroxyapatite nanorods with narrow-size distribution via Microwave Irradiation. J Am Ceram Soc. 2008. 91:3580–4. doi.10.1111/j.1551-2916.2008.02690.x.

10. Mohajerani MS, Mazloumi M, Lak A, Kajbafvala A, Zanganeh S, Sadrnezhaad SK. Self-assembled zinc oxide nanostructures via a rapid microwave-assisted route. J Cryst Growth. 2008. 310:3621–5. doi.10.1016/j.jcrysgro.2008.04.045.

11. Narayanan R. Synthesis of green nanocatalysts and industrially important green reactions. Green Chem Lett Rev. 2012. 5:707–25. doi.10.1080/17518253.2012.700955.

12. Mohamed RM, McKinney DL, Sigmund WM. Enhanced nanocatalysts. Mater Sci Eng R. 2012. 73:1–13. doi.10.1016/j.mser.2011.09.001.

13. Pla D, Gomez M. Metal and metal oxide nanoparticles, a lever for C–H functionalization. ACS Catal. 2016. 6:3537–52. doi.10.1021/acscatal.6b00684.

14. Saha D, Mukhopadhyay C. Metal Nanoparticles: An Efficient Tool for Heterocycles Synthesis and Their Functionalization via C-H Activation. *Curr Organocatal*. 2019. 6:79–91. doi.10.2174/2213337206666181226152743.

15. Yasukawa T, Miyamura H, Kobayashi S. Chiral Ligand-Modified Metal Nanoparticles as Unique Catalysts for Asymmetric C–C Bond-Forming Reactions: How Are Active Species Generated? ACS Catal. 2016 6:7979–88. doi.10.1021/acscatal.6b02446.

16. Wang Q, Astruc D. State of the Art and Prospects in Metal–Organic Framework (MOF) Based and MOF-Derived Nanocatalysis. Chem Rev. 2020. 120:1438–511. doi.10.1021/acs.chemrev.9b00223.

17. Liao C, Li X, Yao K, Yuan Z, Chi Q, Zhang Z. Efficient Oxidative Dehydrogenation of N-Heterocycles over Nitrogen-Doped Carbon-Supported Cobalt Nanoparticles. ACS Sustain Chem Eng. 2019. 7:13646–54. doi.10.1021/acssuschemeng.8b05563.

18. Jaiswal G, Subaramanian M, Sahoo MK, Balaraman E. A Reusable Cobalt Catalyst for Reversible Acceptorless Dehydrogenation and Hydrogenation of N-Heterocycles. ChemCatChem. 2019. 11:2449–57. doi.10.1002/cctc.201900367.

19. Xu D, Zhao H, Dong Z, Ma J.Cobalt Nanoparticles Apically Encapsulated by Nitrogen-doped Carbon Nanotubes for Oxidative Dehydrogenation and Transfer Hydrogenation of N-heterocycles. ChemCatChem. 2019. 11: 5475–86. doi.10.1002/cctc.201901304.

20. Zhou C, Tan Z, Jiang H, Zhang M. Synthesis of (*E*)-2-Alkenylazaarenes via Dehydrogenative Coupling of (Hetero) aryl-fused 2-Alkylcyclic Amines and Aldehydes with a Cobalt Nanocatalyst. ChemCatChem. 2018. 10:2887–92. doi.10.1002/cctc.201800202.

21. Li J, Liu G, Long X, Gao G, Wu J, Li F. Different active sites in a bifunctional Co@N-doped graphene shells based catalyst for the oxidative dehydrogenation and hydrogenation reactions. J Catal. 2017. 355:53–62. doi:10.1016/j.jcat.2017.09.007.

22. Hajipour AR, Khorsandi Z, Mohammadi B. Cobalt-Catalyzed Three-Component Synthesis of Propargylamine Derivatives and Sonogashira Reaction: A Comparative Study between Co-NPs and Co-NHC@MWCNTs. ChemistrySelect. 2019. 4: 4598 –603. doi.10.1002/slct.201803586.

23. Rajabi F, Dios M P, Abdollahi M, Luque R. Aqueous synthesis of 1,8-dioxo-octahydroxanthenes using supported cobalt nanoparticles as a highly efficient and recyclable nanocatalyst. Catal Comm. 2018. 120:95–100. doi.10.1016/j.catcom.2018.10.004.

24. Murugesan K, Senthamarai T, Sohail M, Alshammari AS, Pohl M-M. et al. Cobalt-based nanoparticles prepared from MOF–carbon templates as efficient hydrogenation catalysts Chem Sci. 2018. 9:8553–60. doi.10.1039/C8SC02807A.

25. Paul B, Purkayastha DD, Dhar SS. One-pot hydrothermal synthesis and characterization of $CoFe_2O_4$ nanoparticles and its application as magnetically recoverable catalyst in oxidation of alcohols by periodic acid. Mater Chem Phys. 2016. 181:99–105. doi.10.1016/j.matchemphys.2016.06.039.

26. Zhang M, Lu J, Zhang JN, Zhan ZH. Magnetic carbon nanotube supported Cu (CoFe$_2$O$_4$/CNT-Cu) catalyst: A sustainable catalyst for the synthesis of 3-nitro-2-arylimidazo[1,2-*a*]pyridines. Catal Comm. 2016. 78:26–32. doi.10.1016/j.catcom.2016.02.004.

27. Borade RM, Shinde PR, Kale SB, Pawar RP. Preparation, characterization and catalytic application of CoFe$_2$O$_4$ nanoparticles in the synthesis of benzimidazoles. *2nd International Conference on Condensed Matter and Applied Physics*. AIP Conference Proceedings **1953**, 030194 (2018). 10.1063/1.5032529.

28. Hajipour AR, Khorsandi Z. A comparative study of the catalytic activity of Co- and CoFe$_2$O$_4$-NPs in C–N and C–O bond formation: Synthesis of benzimidazoles and benzoxazoles from o-haloanilides. New J Chem. 2016. 40:10474–481. doi.10.1039/C6NJ02293F.

29. Ghomi JS, Navvab M, Alavi HS. CoFe$_2$O$_4$@SiO$_2$/PrNH$_2$ nanoparticles as highly efficient and magnetically recoverable catalyst for the synthesis of 1,3-thiazolidin-4-ones. J Sulfur Chem. 2016. 37:601–12. doi.10.1080/17415993.2016.1169533.

30. Zhang M, Liu P, Liu YH, Shang Z-R, Hu H-C, Zhang Z-H. Magnetically separable graphene oxide anchored sulfonic acid: a novel, high efficient and recyclable catalyst for one-pot synthesis of 3,6-di(pyridin-3-yl)-1*H*-pyrazolo[3,4-*b*]pyridine-5-carbonitriles in deep eutectic solvent under microwave irradiation. RSC Adv. 2016. 6:106160–70. doi.10.1039/C6RA19579B.

31. Bandaru S, Majji RK, Bassa S, Chilla PN, Yellapragada R, Vasamsetty S. et al. Magnetic Nano Cobalt Ferrite Catalyzed Synthesis of 4*H*-Pyrano[3,2-*h*]quinolone Derivatives under Microwave Irradiation. Green Sustain Chem. 2016. 6, 101–. doi.10.4236/gsc.2016.62009

32. Kooti M, Nasiri E.Phosphotungstic acid supported on silica-coated CoFe$_2$O$_4$ nanoparticles: An efficient and magnetically-recoverable catalyst for *N*-formylation of amines under solvent-free conditions. J Molec Catal A: Chem. 2015. 406:168–77. doi.10.1016/j.molcata.2015.05.009.

33. Jaiswal G, Landge VG, Subaramanian M, Kadam RG, Zboril R, Gawande MB. et al. N-Graphitic Modified Cobalt Nanoparticles Supported on Graphene for Tandem Dehydrogenation of Ammonia-Borane and Semihydrogenation of Alkynes. ACS Sustain Chem Eng. 2020. 8:11058–68. doi.10.1021/acssuschemeng.9b07211.

34. Murugesan K, Chandrashekhar VG, Kreyenschulte C, Beller M, Jagadeesh RV.A General Catalyst based on Cobalt Core-shell Nanoparticles for Hydrogenation of *N*-Heteroarenes including Pyridines. Angew Chem Int Ed. 2020. 59:17408–12. doi.10.1002/anie.202004674.

35. Goyal V, Sarki N, Singh B, Ray A, Poddar M, Bordoloi Aet al. Carbon-Supported Cobalt Nanoparticles as Catalysts for the Selective Hydrogenation of Nitroarenes to Arylamines and Pharmaceuticals. ACS Appl Nano Mater. 2020. 3:11070–9. doi.10.1021/acsanm.0c02254.

36. Ebrahimzadeh F. Nickel nanoparticles supported on diphenylphosphinated poly(vinyl alcoholcoethylene) as a new heterogeneous and recyclable catalyst for Mizoroki-Heck reactions. J Chem Res. 2017. 41:541–6. doi.10.3184/174751917X15040898434417.

37. Hajipour AR, Abolfathi P.Silica-Supported Ni(II)–DABCO Complex: An efficient and Reusable Catalyst for the Heck Reaction. Catal Lett. 2017. 147:188–95. doi.10.1007/s10562-016-1880-9.

38. Inaloo ID, Majnooni S, Eslahi H, Esmaeilpour M. Air-Stable Fe$_3$O$_4$@SiO$_2$-EDTA-Ni(0) as an Efficient Recyclable Magnetic Nanocatalyst for Effective Suzuki-Miyaura and Heck Cross-Coupling via Aryl Sulfamates and Carbamates. Appl Organometal Chem. 2020. 34:e5662. doi.org/10.1002/aoc.5662.

39. Konnerth H, Prechtl MHG.Nitrile hydrogenation using nickel nanocatalysts in ionic liquids. New J Chem. 2017. 41:9594–7. doi.10.1039/C7NJ02210G.

40. Payra S, Saha A, Banerjee S. Nano-NiFe$_2$O$_4$ catalyzed microwave assisted one pot regioselective synthesis of novel 2-alkoxyimidazo[1,2-a]pyridines under aerobic conditions. RSC Adv. 2016. 6:12402–7. doi.10.1039/C5RA25540F.

41. Moghaddam FM, Foroushani BK, Rezvani HR. Nickel Ferrite Nanoparticles: An Efficient and Reusable Nanocatalyst for a Neat, One-Pot and Four-component Synthesis of Pyrroles. RSC Adv. 2015. 5:18092–6. doi.10.1039/C4RA09348H.

42. Murugesan K, Alshammari AS, Sohail M, Beller M, Jagadeesh RV.Monodisperse nickel-nanoparticles for stereo- and chemoselective hydrogenation of alkynes to alkenes. J Catal. 2019. 370:372–7. doi.10.1016/j.jcat.2018.12.018.

43. Rani P, Singh KN, Kaur A. Synthesis, characterization, and application of easily accessible resin-encapsulated nickel nanocatalyst for efficient reduction of functionalized nitroarenes under mild conditions. J Chem Sci. 2018. 130:160. doi.10.1007/s12039-018-1548-7.

44. Maleki B, Eshghi H, Barghamadi M, Nasiri N, Khojastehnezhad A, Ashrafi SS. et al. Silica-coated magnetic NiFe$_2$O$_4$ nanoparticles supported H$_3$PW$_{12}$O$_{40}$: Synthesis, preparation, and application as an efficient, magnetic, green catalyst for one-pot synthesis of tetrahydrobenzo[*b*]pyran and pyrano[2,3-*c*] pyrazole derivatives. Res Chem Intermed. 2016. 42:3071–93. doi.10.1007/s11164-015-2198-8.

45. Demirci T, Celik B, Yildiz Y, Eris S, Arslan M, Sen F. et al. One-Pot Synthesis of Hantzsch Dihydropyridines Using Highly Efficient and Stable PdRuNi@GO Catalyst. RSC Adv. 2016. 6:76948–56. doi.10.1039/C6RA13142E.

46. Mondal J, Biswas A, Chiba S, Zhao Y.Cu^0 Nanoparticles Deposited on Nanoporous Polymers: A Recyclable Heterogeneous Nanocatalyst for Ullmann Coupling of Aryl Halides with Amines in Water. Sci Rep. 2015. 5:8294. doi.10.1038/srep08294.

47. Albaladejo MJ, Alonso F, Gonzalez-Soria MJ.Synthetic and Mechanistic Studies on the Solvent-Dependent Copper-Catalyzed Formation of Indolizines and Chalcones ACS Catal. 2015. 5:3446–56. doi.10.1021/acscatal.5b00417.

48. Mohan B, Yoon C, Jang S, Park KH. Copper Nanoparticles Catalyzed Se(Te)–Se(Te) Bond Activation: A Straightforward Route Towards Unsymmetrical Organochalcogenides from Boronic Acids. ChemCatChem. 2015. 7:405–12. doi.10.1002/cctc.201402867.

49. Nasrollahzadeh M, Jaleh B, Fakhri P, Zahraei A, Ghadery E.Synthesis and catalytic activity of carbon supported copper nanoparticles for the synthesis of aryl nitriles and 1,2,3-triazoles. RSC Adv. 2015. 5:2785–2793. doi.10.1039/C4RA09935D

50. Sarode S A, Bhojane JM, Nagarkar JM. An efficient magnetic copper ferrite nanoparticle: For one pot synthesis of 2-substituted benzoxazole via redox reactions. Tetrahedron Lett. 2015. 56:206–10. doi.10.1016/j.tetlet.2014.11.065.

51. Saha M, Pradhan K, Das AR. Facile and eco-friendly synthesis of chromeno[4,3- b]pyrrol-4(1*H*)-one derivatives applying magnetically recoverable nano crystalline CuFe$_2$O$_4$ involving a domino three-component reaction in aqueous media. RSC Adv. 2016 6:55033–8. doi.10.1039/C6RA06979G.

52. Ghaani M, Saffari J. Synthesis of CuFe$_2$O$_4$ Nanoparticles by a new co-precipitation method and, using them as Efficient Catalyst for the one pot synthesis of Napthoxazinones. J Nanostruct. 2016. 6:172–8. doi.10.7508/jns.2016.02.010.

53. Swami S, Agarwala A, Shrivastava R. Sulfonic acid functionalized silica-coated CuFe$_2$O$_4$ core-shell nanoparticles: An efficient and magnetically separable heterogeneous catalyst for syntheses of 2-pyrazole-3-aminoimidazo-fused polyheterocycles. New J Chem. 2016. 40:9788–94. doi.10.1039/C6NJ02264B.

54. Vibhute SP, Mhaldar PM, Korade SN, Gaikwad DS, Shejawal RV, Pore DM.Synthesis of magnetically separable catalyst Cu-ACP-Am-Fe$_3$O$_4$@SiO$_2$ for Huisgen 1,3-dipolar cycloaddition. Tetrahedron Lett. 2018. 59:3643–52. doi.10.1016/j.tetlet.2018.08.045

55. Dutta PK, Sen S, Saha D, Dhar B.Solid Supported Nano Structured Cu-Catalyst for Solvent/Ligand Free C2 Amination of Azoles. Eur J Org Chem. 2018. 2018:657–65. doi.10.1002/ejoc.201701669.

6 Nanocatalysis
An Efficient Tool for the Synthesis of Triazines and Tetrazines

A. B. Kanagare,[1] D. N. Pansare,[1] Ajit K. Dhas,[1] Rajita D. Ingle,[1] R. N. Shelke,[2] Keshav Lalit Ameta,[3] and R. P. Pawar[4]

[1] Department of Chemistry, Deogiri College, Aurangabad, Maharashtra, India
[2] Department of Chemistry, Sadguru Gadage Maharaj College Karad, Maharashtra, India
[3] Department of Chemistry, School of Liberal Arts and Sciences, Mody University of Science and Technology, Lakshmangarh, Rajasthan, India
[4] Department of Chemistry, Shiv Chattrapati College, Aurangabad, Maharashtra, India

6.1 TRIAZINES

Polyazines, similar to tetrazine and triazines, are derivatives of nitrogen (N) containing heterocyclic compounds that are extremely electron-deficient aromatic systems because of the availability of electronegative N atoms. Therefore, they are highly reactive toward a variety of electron-rich dienophiles and nucleophiles in the Diels–Alder cycloaddition reaction and nucleophilic addition or substitution reactions. Because of the scope of these reactions, which permit the synthesis of a broad range of heterocyclic systems and functionalized polyazines and others that produce new materials. These compounds show diverse properties and applications that take advantage of nanoparticle (NP) synthesis. In addition, bioactive compounds, such as polyazines, which are aza-analogs of natural metabolites, might demonstrate several kinds of biological activity. Similarly, their high reactivity means that they are suitable for use in bioorthogonal chemistry. Apart from their electrophilic behavior, the presence of N atoms means that they can be exploited as donor aza ligands for the complexation of transition metals in coordination chemistry. Similar azine-based organometallic derivatives have many applications in design, synthesis, sensing, catalytic, luminescent, and other kinds of materials. All of these could be applied as a template for the synthesis of nanosize frameworks.

The chemical compound 1,3,5-triazine here is known as s-triazine. It is an organic compound that has a chemical structure containing a six-membered aromatic heterocyclic ring, which has three N atoms and three carbon (C) atoms.

1,3,5-triazine

DOI: 10.1201/9781003141488-6

6.1.2 Synthesis

The symmetrical 1,3,5-triazines are produced by the trimerization of certain nitrile compounds, such as cyanimide or cyanogen chloride. The benzoguanamine (with two amino and one phenyl substituent) was synthesized from dicyandiamide and benzonitrile.[1] In the Pinner triazine synthesis,[2] the reactants were an aryl or alkyl phosgene and amidine.[3,4] The introduction of an N–hydrogen (N–H) group inside the hydrazide using a copper (Cu) carbenoid, followed by treatment with ammonium chloride could give the triazine core.[5] The amino-substituted triazines are called guanamines, which can be synthesized by the condensation of a cyanoguanidine with the respective nitrile.[6]

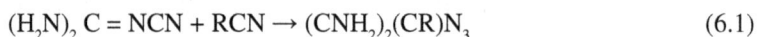

$$(H_2N)_2 C = NCN + RCN \rightarrow (CNH_2)_2(CR)N_3 \qquad (6.1)$$

The reaction of benzohydrazide, 4,4′-dimethoxybenzyl, ammonium acetate, and GO@N-Ligand-Cu nanocomposites catalyst under solvent-free conditions at specific temperature resulted in the product. This work explored the performance of graphene oxide (GO) catalysts for the synthesis of triazines from benzhydrazides, benzyl derivatives, and ammonium acetate (Scheme 6.1).

Comparison with other catalysts, the GO@N-Ligand-Cu required a shorter reaction time by offering thermal stability and being environmentally friendly. Various methods and different catalysts have been used for the synthesis of the triazine compounds; however, this method has received interest for synthesis.[7]

Based on the versatility and increased efficiency of solid-supported iron (III) chloride (FeCl$_3$), and the importance of the derivatives of the 1,2,4-triazines, Emami-Noril et al reported a one-pot synthesis for a series of 1,2,4-triazines that treated thiosemicarbazide with different α,β-dicarbonyl compounds under reflux conditions in presence of the FeCl$_3$@silicon dioxide (FeCl$_3$@SiO$_2$) catalyst (Scheme 6.2).

The reaction rate and the yield were improved if the reaction was carried out in the presence of the catalyst. In addition, supplying support of FeCl$_3$ on SiO$_2$ and reducing the particle size of SiO$_2$, the reaction time decreased. Therefore FeCl$_3$@SiO$_2$ is the best solid catalyst for the synthesis of 1,2,4-triazine derivatives. These nanocatalysts (NCs) produce quantitative yields with shorter reaction times to obtain the products compared with other reported methods.[8]

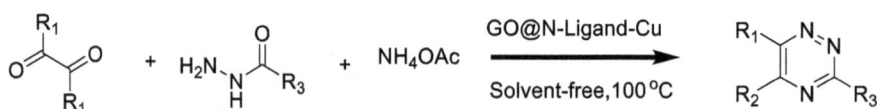

SCHEME 6.1 Synthesis of triazine derivative with multiple substitutions.

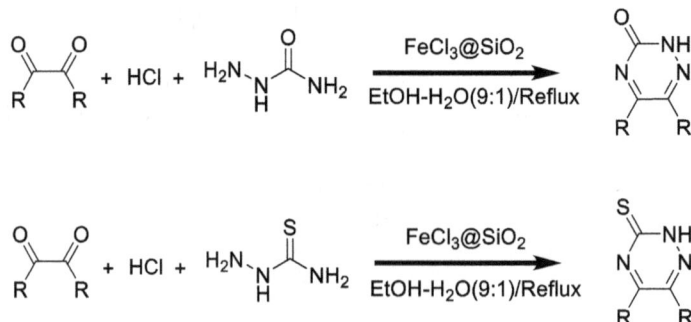

SCHEME 6.2 Production of the 1,2,4-triazine derivatives.

Saad et al. synthesized palladium (Pd) NPs supported on 1,2,3-triazoles from alkyne derivatives of 1,3,5-triazine complexes, designed using click chemistry. The foundation for the use of the maximum support of the surface area was to achieve excellent scattering of the NC and to increase its catalytic activity. The reduction of 4-nitrophenol into aminophenol using sodium borohydride (NaBH$_4$) as the reducing agent and Pd as a catalyst was carried out to measure the catalytic performance of a hybridized silica-immobilized (Si) novel metal NC.

This work represents the dual-functional click-generated triazole-triazine/SBA-15 mesoporous silica sieve system, which acted as a unique hybrid platform designed for the immobilization of Pd NCs and for in situ synthesis. High surface area and strong attachment of Pd NPs are due to the role of the dendron-like structure that is offered by triazole and triazine heterocycles. This SBA-15/nitrogen heterocycle/Pd NP catalytic system was used for the reduction of p-nitrophenol and could be used in the catalysis of other reactions.[9]

In the construction of a high surface area polymer material, Modak et al used 4,4',4''-(1,3,5-triazine-2,4,6-triyl) tris(oxy) tribenzaldehyde as the cross-linker pattern for the extensive aromatic substitution under acidic hydrothermal conditions on pyrrole (Scheme 6.3). This synthesis was carried out in a high pressure Teflon lined autoclave under experimental conditions. Because the highly acidic reaction medium favored initial protonation of the aromatic aldehyde followed by the electrophilic aromatic substitution at the pyrrole, it produced free aldehyde (–CHO) that contained the three porphyrin centers for each triazine unit, which was further condensed with pyrrole and formed a complete porous polymeric network of novel triazine-functionalized porphyrin-based porous organic polymer, TPOP-1 as shown in (Scheme 6.4).

Triazine functionalized porous organic polymer material can act as a good carbon dioxide (CO$_2$) storage material and support Pd NC for C–C cross-coupling reactions. The material act as a very efficient catalyst in the Sonogashira cross-coupling reaction.[10]

In this work, Hasanpour et al showed the catalytic efficiency of a new triazine (TA)-based vitamin B5 Cu(II) complex [Cu(II)-TA/B5] in the aerobic oxidation of benzyl alcohols. This complex acted as an eco-friendly and efficient catalyst for the selective aerobic oxidation of benzylic alcohols to aldehydes followed by coupling with the indole molecules through C–C bonds to give the bis(indolyl)methane with no side reactions (Scheme 6.5).

The reaction of cyanuric chloride (CC) with pantothenic acid (vitamin B5) was carried out in tetra hydro furan (THF) under ultrasonic agitation to replace the chlorine atoms of CC to give TA/B5 as a star-shaped ligand that was used for complex formation with Cu(II) to form Cu(II)-TA/B5 as shown in (Scheme 6.6).

A new star-shaped Cu(II)-TA/B5 NC was synthesized by the incorporation of copper(II) acetate (Cu(OAc)$_2$) in 2,4,6-tripantothenate-1,3,5-triazine in ultrasonic agitation. This catalytic oxidation system produced excellent selectivity, along with easy isolation of organic products.[11]

Shafiee et al developed a resourceful, sustainable, and greener method for organic transformation reactions, and reported an easy way for the synthesis of a new dicationic ionic liquid (IL) with 1,3,5-triazine core anchor for nano-super ferromagnetic particles, which were used in the Betti reaction to synthesize b-amido alkyl naphthols using a one-pot multicomponent reaction. For the catalyst, the synthetic pathway is shown in Scheme 6.7. The free-dicationic IL (Cl-ACl$_2$) was initially synthesized using the reaction of 1,3,5-trichlorotriazine (TCT) with two equimolar N-methyl imidazole in the presence of dry dioxane. The important factor in the synthesis was a nucleophilic substitution reaction between the TCT and N-methyl imidazole to generate the required bis-imidazolium salt. Finally, the IL was anchored for the superparamagnetic iron oxide nanoparticles using (SPIONs) using an ipso-substitution reaction by the hydroxyl (OH) group of Si-encapsulated iron (III) oxide (Fe$_3$O$_4$) NPs.[12]

Sadeghzadeh et al reported the reaction between the primary amines (1) and alkyl methyl pyruvates (arylmethylidene) (2) with dialkyl acetylene dicarboxylates (3) for the synthesis of 1,4-dihydropyridines (4) (Scheme 6.8). To develop sustainable and greener methods for the organic

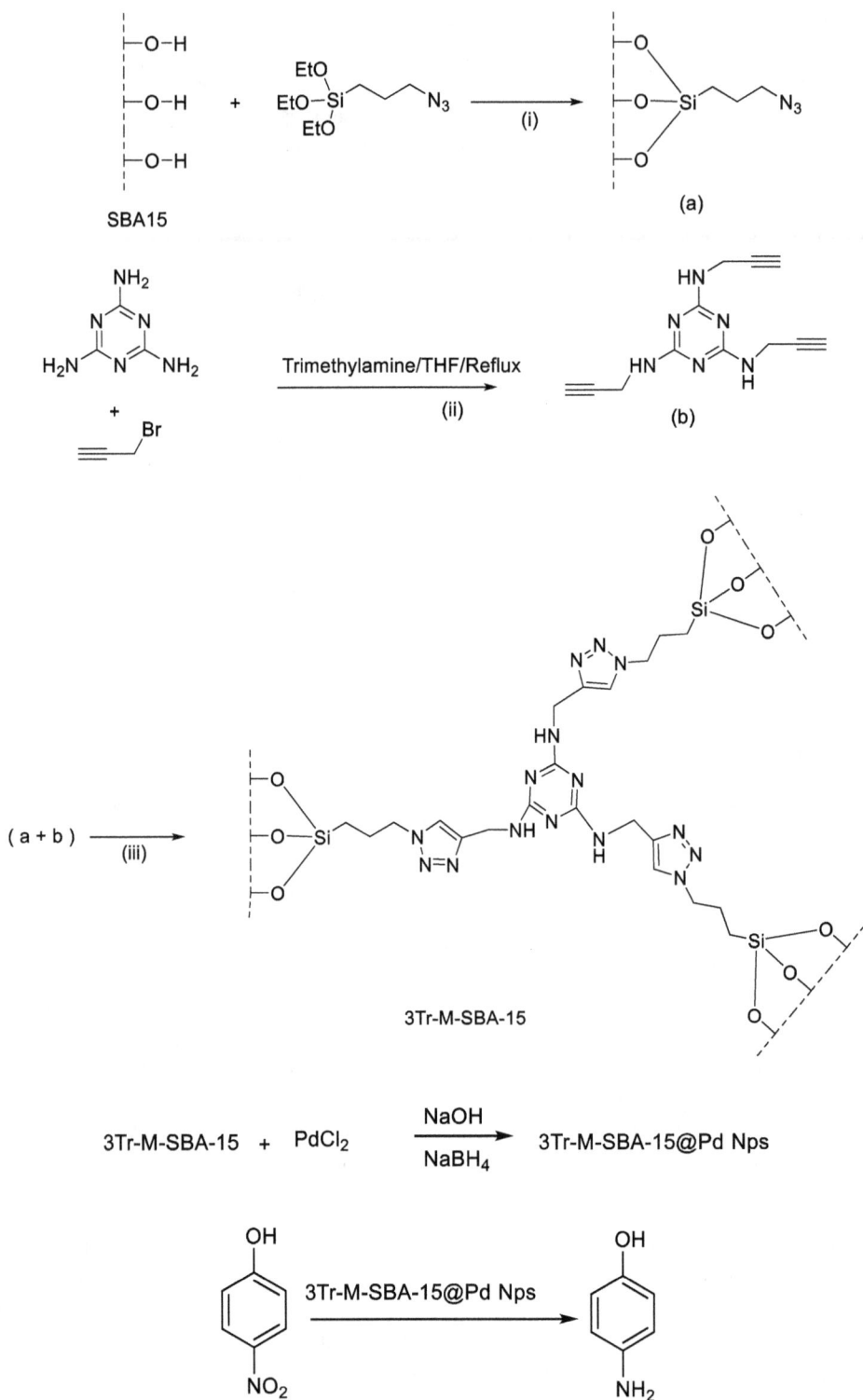

SCHEME 6.3 Synthesis of 1,2,3-triazoles using alkyne derivatives of the 1,3,5-triazines supported on mesoporous Si-Pd complex.

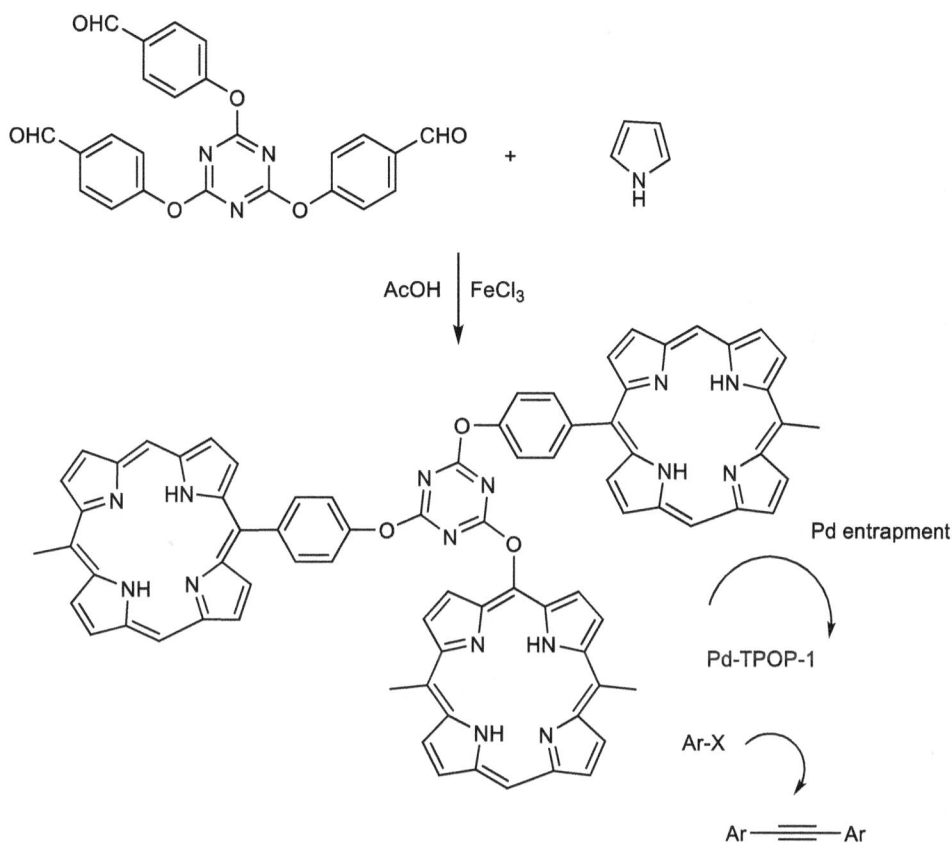

SCHEME 6.4 Synthesis of Pd-TPOP-1.

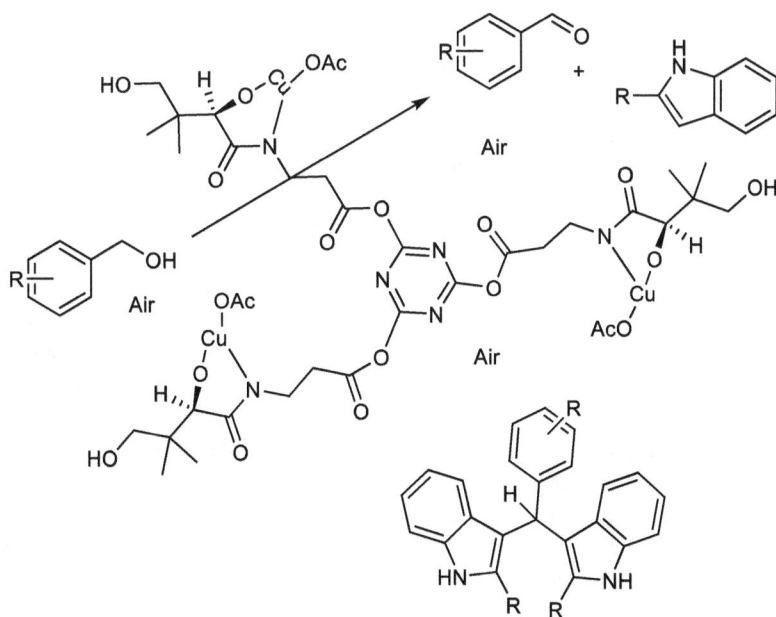

SCHEME 6.5 One-pot synthesis of bis(indolyl)methanes using an aerobic oxidation of benzylic alcohols catalyzed by Cu(II)-TA/B5.

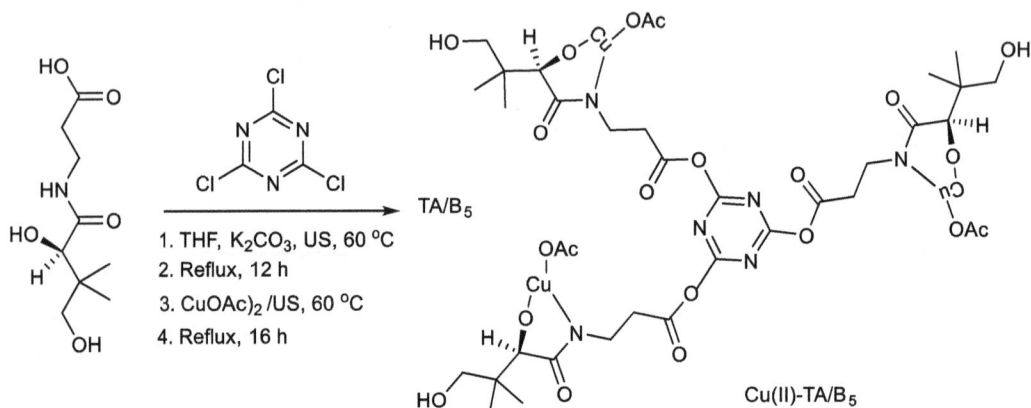

SCHEME 6.6 Synthetic route for Cu(II)-TA/B5.

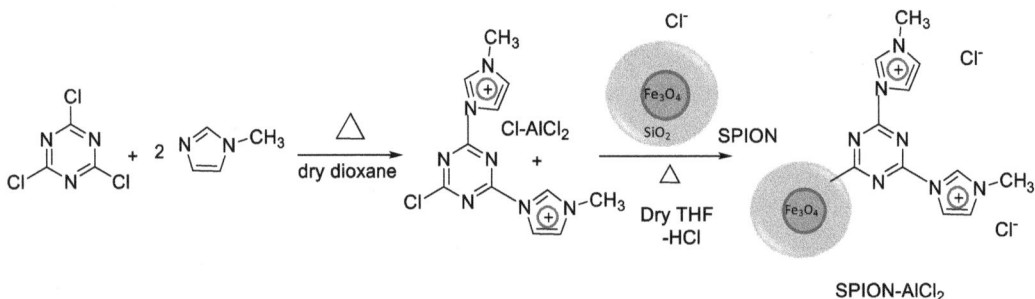

SCHEME 6.7 Synthesis of 1,3,5-triazine functionalized bisimidazolium dichloride tethered to SPIONs.

transformation reactions, nanocatalysis, and nanomaterials, an easy and efficient production method for a magnetically recyclable, nano- Fe_3O_4 supported and low cost pyridine catalyst and study of the performance of fibrous nano-silica (KCC-1) efficiency for a novel magnetic catalyst was reported. The excellent performance of the Fe_3O_4/KCC-1/ bis(4-pyridylamino) triazine(BPAT) catalyst was due to the triazine (BPAT) units, which can catalyze the 1,4-dihydropyridines (4) in aqueous media.[13]

The development of non-noble metal catalysts that have analogous stability and activity toward noble metals is of major importance in renovation and the consumption of clean energy. A transition metal with the most favorable electronic composition that bonds H_2O and –OH in intermediate strengths would support the hydrolysis of ammonia borane (AB). Using a covalent triazine framework (CTF), a newly synthesized porous material that could donate electrons from the lone pairs on N. The density of the electron on nanosized Ni and Co that hold the CTF have increased their catalytic activities.

The kinetic isotope effects (KIE) measurements illustrate that the rate determining step (RDS) for AB hydrolysis is the cleavage of the O–H bond in H_2O. The d-block metals with the most favorable electron structure that bonds to H_2O and –OH with transitional strengths might assist the hydrolysis of AB. The newly developed CTF-1, which was rich in N content, had an electron-donating effect that significantly increased the electron density of the nickel (Ni) or cobalt (Co) support on it. Because of this, the catalytic activity was significantly enhanced in AB hydrolysis. Therefore, the homolytic activation of H_2O might occur and then react with activated AB to form H_2 and B–OH. The catalytic hydrolysis of AB on Co/CTF-1 is shown in Scheme 6.9.[14]

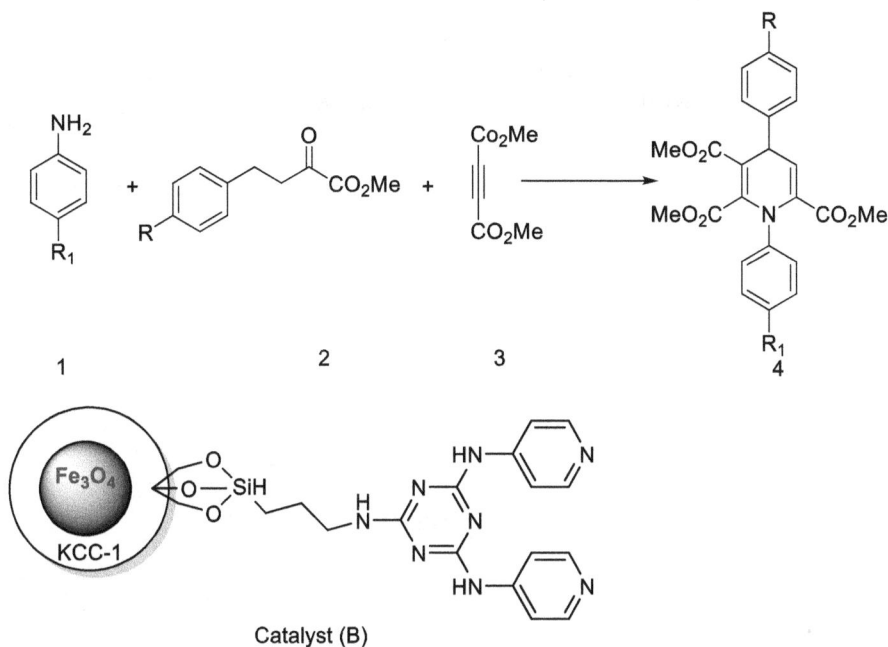

SCHEME 6.8 Production of N-substituted 1,4-dihydropyridines using Fe$_3$O$_4$/KCC-1/BPAT.

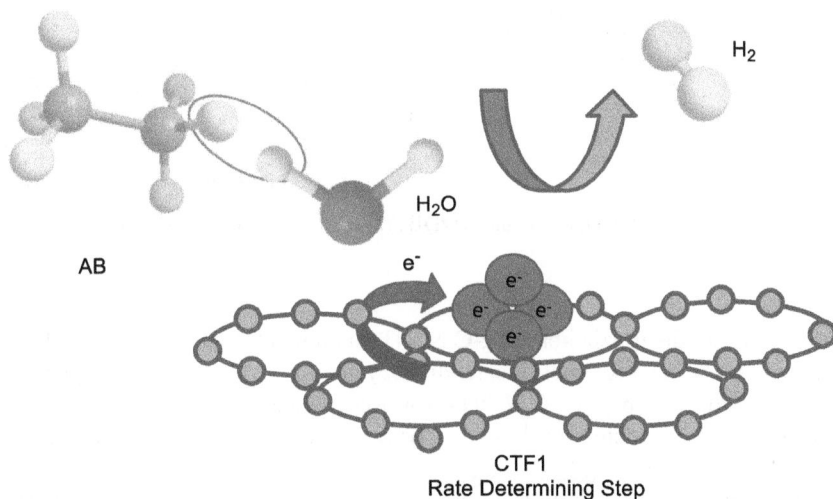

SCHEME 6.9 Proposed mechanism for catalytic hydrolysis of AB using Co/CTF-1.

Wang et al prepared Pd/triazine-based graphitic carbon nitride (g-C$_3$N$_4$) NTs by the immobilization of Pd NPs within the triazine-based g-C$_3$N$_4$ NTs through the metal–support interaction, which acted as a heterogeneous catalyst in the Knoevenagel condensation–reduction tandem reaction (Scheme 6.10). The huge catalytic activity of the Pd/triazine-based g-C$_3$N$_4$ NTs was due to the confinement effect of the nanotube structure. Therefore, the structure of these nanotubes adjusted the size of the Pd particle catalysts and offered spatial control the on metal catalyst encapsulated on their channels, which could load the particles aggregations throughout the reaction; therefore, retaining the good catalytic activity and stability. Furthermore, the stabilization and anchor effects of

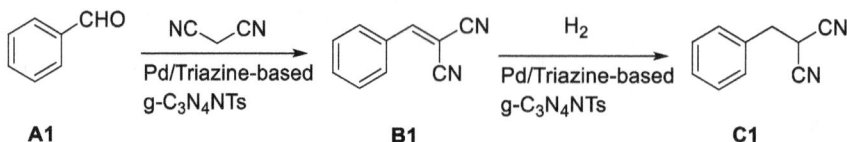

SCHEME 6.10 One-pot novel condensation–reduction reaction using the Pd/triazine-based g-C$_3$N$_4$ NTs.

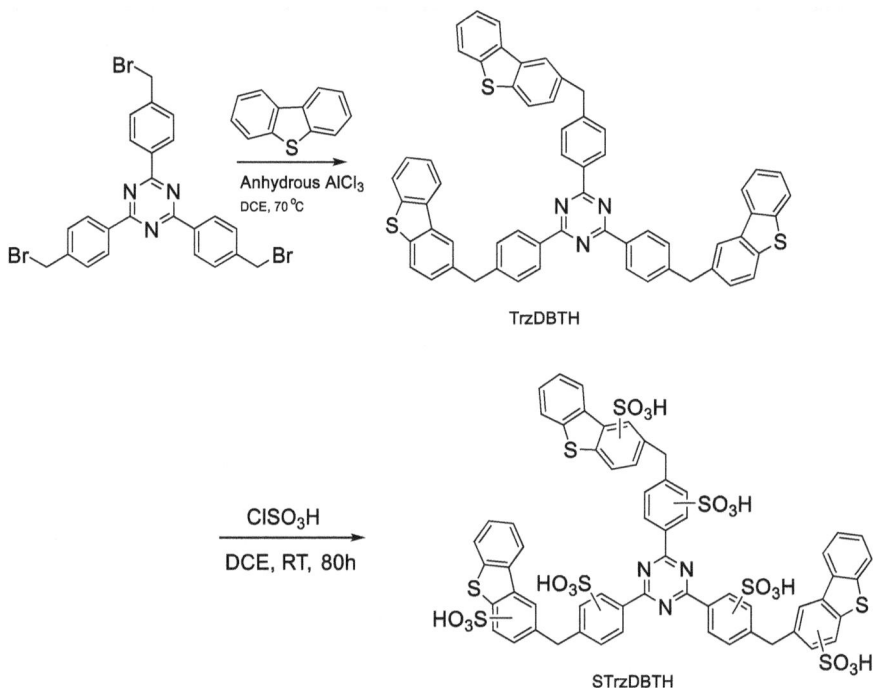

SCHEME 6.11 Synthesis of STrzDBTH and TrzDBTH using the Friedel-Craft alkylation followed by sulfonation.

the pyridine N atoms of the triazine-based g-C$_3$N$_4$ NTs inhibited the aggregation and leaking of the active sites; therefore, achieving superior catalytic recyclability in the tandem reaction.

Therefore, the Pd/triazine-based g-C$_3$N$_4$ NTs was used as an efficient catalyst in the Knoevenagel condensation–reduction tandem reaction of benzaldehyde and its substituted derivatives benzylmalononitrile.[15]

Functionalized organic porous polymers are extremely promising materials for heterogeneous catalysis because of their easy synthesis and flexible framework composition. In addition, they have reasonable porosity, a more specific surface area, simplicity in functionalization, and chemical stability. This class of porous polymers have massive potential to be employed in catalysis. Das et al reported a novel triazinethiophene supported porous organic polymers N-rich triazinethiophene-based microporous polymer (Scheme 6.11), which could be used as a base catalyst for the one-pot synthesis of multicomponent reactions (MCR) of 2-amino-4H chromene derivatives under microwave heating conditions (Scheme 6.12).

Das et al reported an N-rich triazinethiophene base microporous polymer TrzDBTH using the Friedel-Craft alkylation reaction of the dibenzothiophene (DBTH) with a tripodal building block 2,4,6-tris[4-(bromomethyl)phenyl]-1,3,5-triazine. They were used as the heterogeneous base catalyst for the one-pot synthesis of biologically significant chromene derivatives. In addition, the

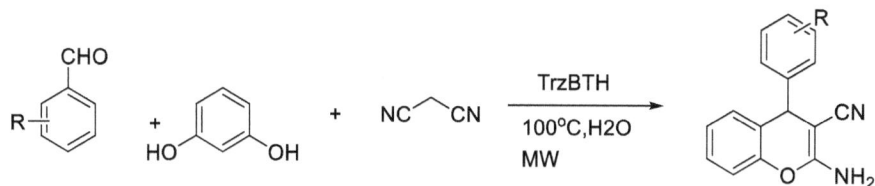

SCHEME 6.12 Synthesis of chromene derivatives.

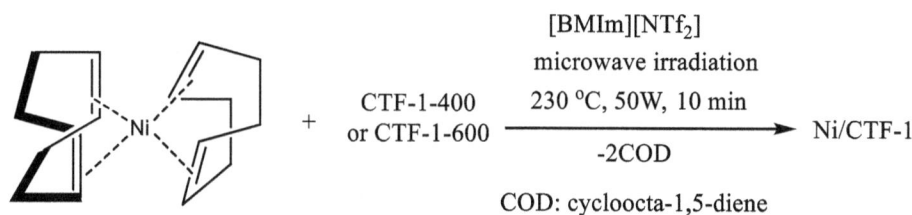

SCHEME 6.13 Ni/CTF-1 composite synthesis using microwave-assisted thermal disintegration of Ni(COD)$_2$ in the presence of IL [BMIm][NTf$_2$] and CTF-1.

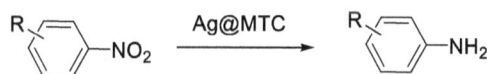

SCHEME 6.14 Catalytic reduction of nitroaromatic compounds via Ag@MTC.

sulfonation of TrzDBTH gave the sulfonated hyper-crosslinked porous polymer STrzDBTH, which could be used as a solid acid catalyst for the synthesis of a precious chemical intermediate, for instance, 5-hydroxymethylfurfural (HMF) from different biomass-derived carbohydrates. Therefore, the setriazine–thiophene supported porous organic polymers provided an extremely cost-effective, scalable, and green route for the synthesis of HMF, and chromene derivatives.[16]

Limited research has been carried out on CTFs; however, they could be used in electrocatalysis, particularly for the oxygen evolution reaction (OER). Therefore, for the synthesis of Ni NPs onto CTFs, the precursor bis(cycloocta-1,5-diene)nickel(0) (Ni(COD)$_2$) and the CTF were spread in 1-butyl-3-methylimidazolium bis(trifluoromethylsulfonyl)imide by shaking under inert conditions for 12 h. A homogenized suspension was irradiated with microwaves and produced Ni NPs immobilized on the CTFs using the disintegration of the metal precursor present in the IL (Scheme 6.13). Therefore, the CTFs are potential candidates for electrochemical OER and could be improved[17]

Vahedi-Notash et al. reported an effective technique for the synthesis of a novel mesoporous triazine-based carbon (MTC) substrate and its application as a recoverable and green catalyst for the synthesis of organic compounds. The porous C provides a substrate for silver (Ag) active species by modifying its surface using chloroacetonitrile (Ag@MTC). This Ag@MTC catalyst was useful in the reduction of nitroaromatic compounds within aqueous media with the help of NaBH$_4$ (a reducing agent) at room temperature. This NC can be readily recovered and regenerated for at least nine runs without a notable decrease in its effectiveness. The catalytic efficiency study showed that Ag@MTC NC had excellent activity in reduction reactions.

Vahedi-Notash et al reported a facile and efficient process for the synthesis of Ag@MTC NC. The synthesized Ag@MTC has good catalytic performance in the reduction of nitroaromatic compounds and has attractive reusability (Scheme 6.14). The major advantages of this catalyst include short reaction time, low cost, low reaction temperature, and recyclability without decreasing the catalytic activity, and is not toxic.[18]

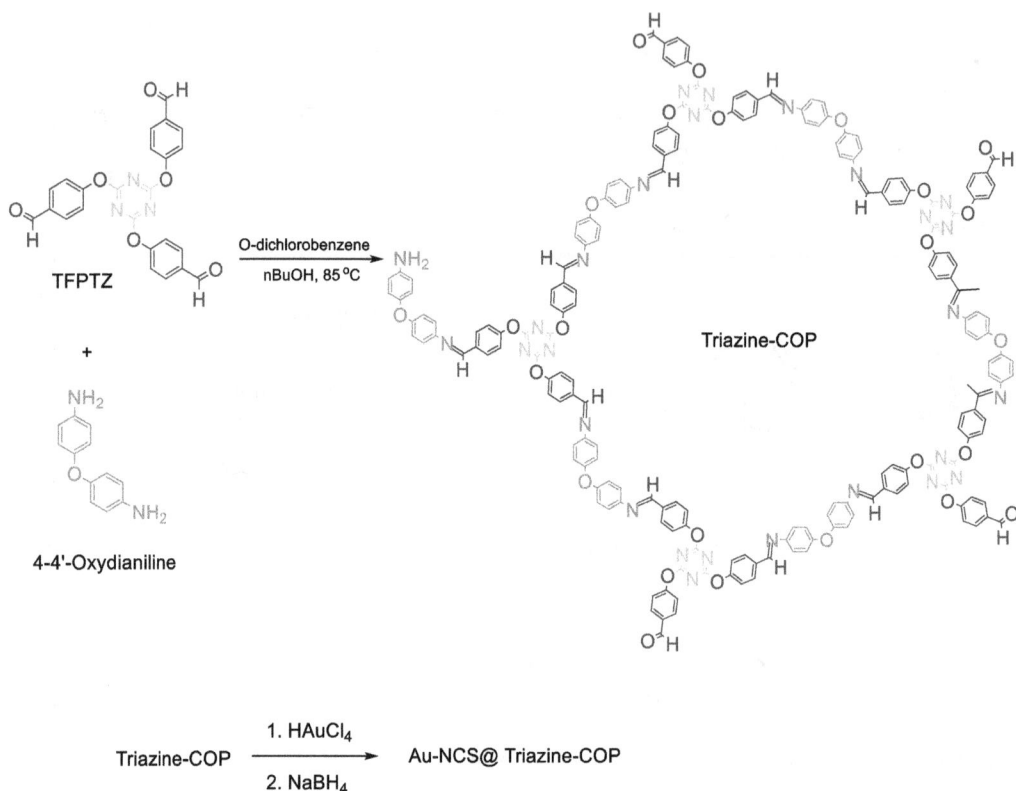

SCHEME 6.15 Au-nano-clusters intercalated triazine-COP.

A novel porous triazine-based covalent organic polymer (triazine-COP) was synthesized using the Schiff base condensation of 4,4-oxydianiline and 2,4,6-tris(4-formyl phenoxy)- 1,3,5-triazine under sonication. The prepared triazine-COP had a high surface area and was stable in organic solvents and H$_2$O. Then, Au (III) ions were immobilized on the N-rich triazine-COP, which on reduction with NaBH$_4$ generated the heterogeneous catalyst of nanosize gold (Au) clusters (Au-NCs@Triazine-COPs), which is shown in Scheme 6.15.

This system can be used as an efficient catalyst for the A3 coupling reaction of aldehydes and alkynes with amines. The electron-releasing and withdrawing groups generate the subsequent propargylamines with maximum yields. In this reaction, the NCs@Triazine-COPs produced high activity of the Au, because the nanoporous structure gave support that permitted an unhindered open environment and high dispersion for the NCs. The catalyst was recycled up to seven times with no significant loss in activity from the three-component reaction of piperidine, 4-methylbenzaldehyde, and phenylacetylene under reflux conditions using the Au-NCs@Triazine-COP catalyst selected as the model reaction (Scheme 6.16).

A novel triazine-based COP was synthesized through Schiff base condensation under sonication. Furthermore, a facile in situ approach was developed to synthesize the Au NCs encapsulated inside the triazine-COP via metal ion doped COPs as the precursors during the in situ reductions. The Au-NCs@Triazine-COP generated nanocomposites showed high catalytic performances in the A3 coupling reaction of amines, aldehydes, and a terminal alkyne. The high catalytic activity was observed because of the synergism of the porous spherical structure and homogeneously distributed Au NCs.[19]

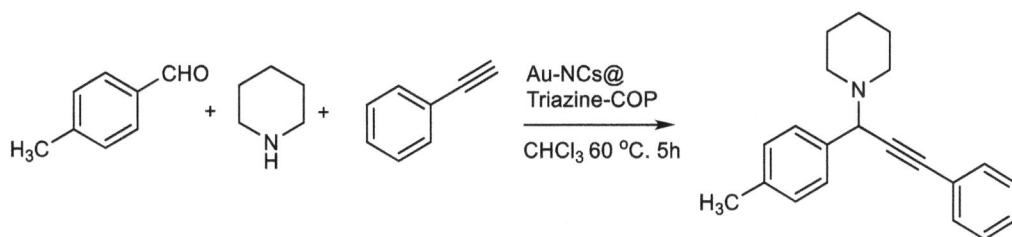

SCHEME 6.16   A3-coupling reaction via Au-NCs@Triazine-COP.

6.2   TETRAZINE

Tetrazine is a compound that consists of a six-membered aromatic ring with four N atoms with the molecular formula $C_2H_2N_4$. The name tetrazine is used in the nomenclature of derivatives of this compound. Three core-ring isomers exist: 1,2,3,4-tetrazines, 1,2,3,5-tetrazines, and 1,2,4,5-tetrazines, respectively which are known as v-tetrazines, as-tetrazines and s-tetrazines.[20]

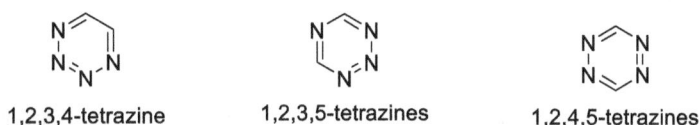

6.2.1   SYNTHESIS

Jain et al synthesized a novel and extremely capable platform for the modification of polymers, based on the inverse electron demand Diels–Alder reaction (iEDDA).[21] In addition, this was useful for the functionalization of materials, such as Au nanoparticles (AuNPs).[22] Miomandre used this reaction for the functionalization of dispersed functional graphene sheet nanocomposite (FGSx). Then, the nanocomposite was coated on the electrode surface and the polypyrrole was deposited using electropolymerization. The material produced had small resistance and large capacitance. The reaction with tetrazine allowed the modification of graphene's surface without disturbing its electrical properties.[23] This study expanded the application of β-lactam carbenes in the synthesis of complex heterocycles (Scheme 6.17).

Jain et al examined the nucleophilic addition of 2-azetidinon-4-ylidenes (ambiphilic β-lactam carbenes) with 3,6-di(2-thienyl) tetrazines. Triazaspiro [3,4 octa-5,7-dien-2-ones **5** and pyrrol-2(1H)-ones **9** were obtained. This study expanded the application of β-lactam carbenes in organic synthesis by providing a synthetic approach for heterocyclic compounds.[24]

Testa et al proposed an exciting method for the ortho-functionalization of 3,6-diphenyl-s-tetrazine. A Pd-catalyzed ortho-CdH activation reaction provided by the N present in tetrazine. The halogens or the acetyl substituents could be introduced using reactants, such as N-chloro-, N-bromo-, N-iodosuccinimide (NCS, NBS, NIS), N-fluorobenzenesulfonimide, or phenyliodine(III) diacetate (PhI(OAc)$_2$). The degree of substitution was controlled by the number of halogen sources introduced (Scheme 6.18).

The Pd-catalyzed cross-coupling reaction for aromatic C–C bond formation (Scheme 6.19) was recently adapted for the tetrazine series but had very limited scope. Testa et al reported the ortho – C–H activation of s-tetrazines, a reaction that permits the introduction of a variety of functional groups in the tetrazine core. A novel and powerful methodology was developed for the electrophilic ortho fluorination of tetrazines via microwave irradiation and N-fluorobenzenesulfonimide (NFSI), within 10 min by keeping it open to the air. Therefore, this work gave a resourceful and practical entrance to access more substituted derivatives of tetrazine. This method assisted the expansion of

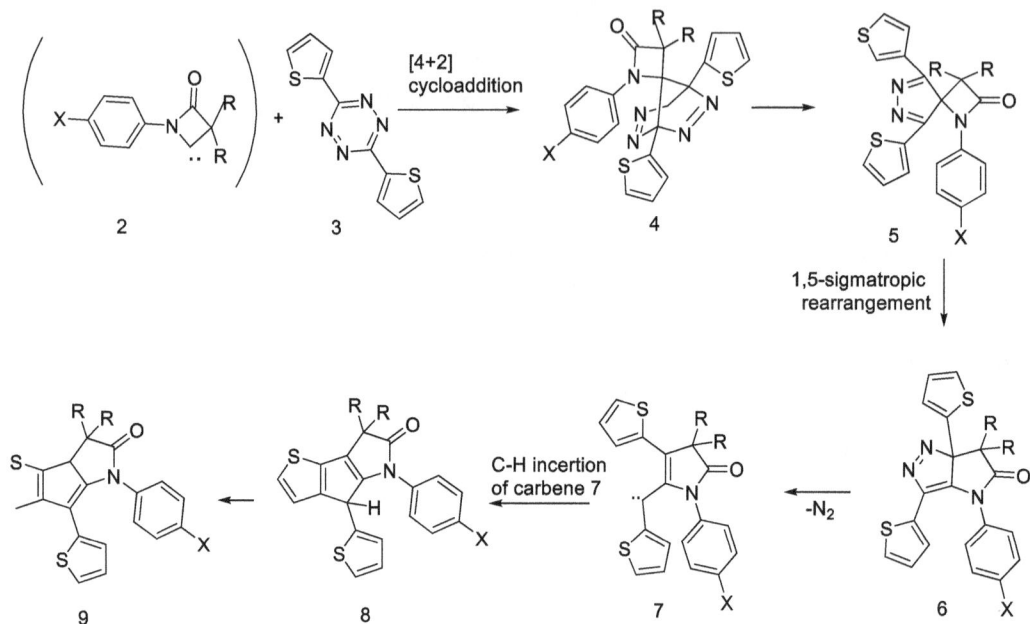

SCHEME 6.17 Predicted mechanisms for 3,6-di-(2-thienyl)-tetrazine with β-lactam carbene reactions.

ortho-functionalized aryl tetrazines as a useful precursor for the synthesis of bioactive compounds and materials that are not easy to obtain using the usual Pinner-like synthesis.[25]

The 1,2,4,5-tetrazine derivatives can be used in a variety of supramolecular approaches. Audebert and Cosnier synthesized NPs through a β-cyclodextrin(CD)–polystyrene diblock copolymer in the presence of a naphthalimide–tetrazine that formed an addition complex with cyclic polycarbohydrate on the shell of the nanoobject in H2O (Scheme 6.20A). The NPs formed in the presence of the tetrazine derivative were smaller and extra stable over time compared with those prepared without the NPs. The tetrazine holds its electroactivity, and tetrazine and naphthalimide produced fluorescence.[26]

Similarly, the same group prepared by modifying an electrode with a polypyrrole functionalized with the β-CD. The surface immobilized the similar tetrazine derivative by the construction of an enclosure complex (Scheme 6.20B). The 1,8-naphthalimide could form an enclosure complex with β-CD. A glucose base oxidase modified using β-could therefore be immobilized on the film for the preparation of a model biosensor during supramolecular interactions.

The derivatives of tetrazine were immobilized onto an electrogenerated polypyrrole-β-CD film that had advantages of the host–guest connections between tetrazine derivatives and β-CD as mentioned previously. Once immobilization occurred, the tetrazine derivatives were very stable and maintained their electrochemical and emission properties. These new unique molecular architectures allowed the competent immobilization of proteins modified by β-CD, such as glucose oxidizes. It could be a novel approach for the construction of biosensors. This novel design that was obtained by supramolecular interactions on the electrode surface illustrated the potential for improvements in biomolecular architectures with fluorescence and electrochemical properties.[27]

The ability to quickly diagnose Gram-positive pathogenic bacteria could have a lot of technological and biomedical applications. Fritea et al illustrated the bioorthogonal modification of small molecule antibiotics (e.g., daptomycin and vancomycin), which could bind with the cell wall of Gram-positive bacteria. The antibiotics conjugates that were bound could react orthogonally with modified tetrazine NPs, using an almost instant cycloaddition, which could detect the bacteria by

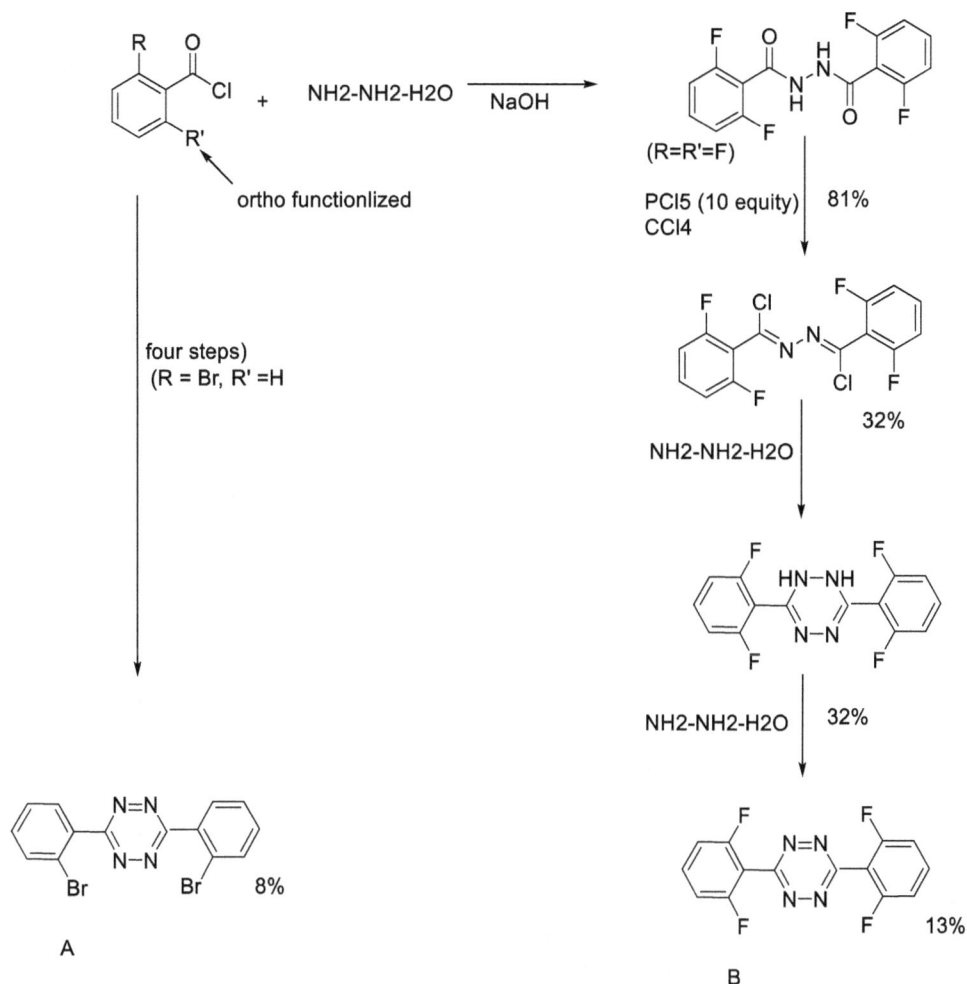

SCHEME 6.18 Multistep synthesis of ortho-functionalized aryl tetrazines: useful for haloaryl tetrazines using palladation.

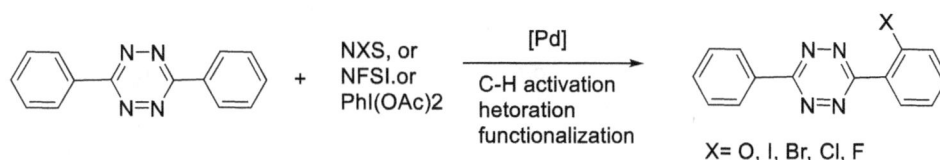

SCHEME 6.19 Pd-catalyzed tetrazine functionalizations.

magnetic or optical sensing. This approach is selective, specific, biocompatible, and fast. In addition to this, it could be adapted for the detection of intracellular pathogens.

The labeling mechanism with vancomycin trans-cyclooctene (vanc-TCO) as a targeting ligand is shown in Scheme 6.21. The binding of the vanc-TCO to Gram-positive bacteria was achieved using an H bond interaction between the drug and the D-Ala-D-Ala units of the N-acetylmuramic acid (NAM) and N-acetylglucosamine (NAG) peptides. The tetrazine-modified magneto-fluorescent nanoparticles (MFNP-Tz) were applied, which resulted in the magnetic and fluorescent labeling of

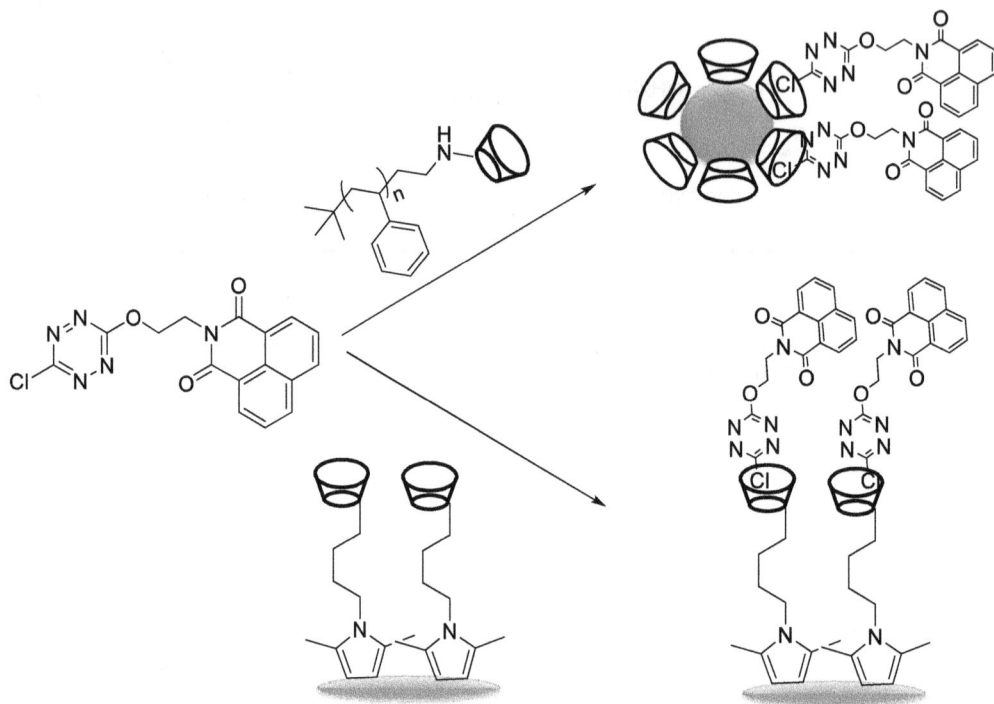

SCHEME 6.20   3-chloro-1,2,4,5-tetrazin-6-oxy-unit can produced using β-cyclodextrin units.

the microbes through a bioorthogonal cycloaddition reaction. By applying the proper Tz-modified nanoprobe, detection could be carried out using magnetic, optical, or any other sensing modality.[28]

The NPs were focused on as key materials for biomedical sensing applications because of their tunable and unique multivalent targeting capability, physical properties, and elevated cargo capacity. Haun et al proposed a new NP objective platform that could be used as a fast, no catalyst, cycloaddition reaction using a coupling mechanism. Haun et al proved that this technique was chemoselective, fast, scalable for biomedical use, and adaptable for metal nanomaterials. This method supported biomarker signals, which make it superior to substitute techniques that contain avidin or biotin. Scheme 6.22 shows the chemistry, relative molecular species dimensions, and experimental approaches for the different bioorthogonal nanoparticle detection (BOND) techniques. They used MFNPs to measure the performance of BOND using well-known fluorescence techniques and a new miniaturized diagnostic magnetic resonance detector system that was designed for clinical point-of-care use.[29]

Since the first report by Hilderbrand and Fox separately in 2008, the utilization of 1,2,4,5-tetrazine in bioorthogonal reactions has undergone remarkable development, due mainly to its high selectivity in reactions and most significantly, the very high reaction rate in an aqueous medium. This tetrazine is utilized in the bioorthogonal reactions from a well-defined iIEDDA reaction. This reaction included in vivo and in vitro fluorescent imaging, nuclear imaging, prodrug releasing system, and MFNP labeling for clinical diagnostics. Lai et al studied a proline-mediated iEDDA of aldehyde and tetrazine as a potential bioorthogonal reaction (Scheme 6.23). This biocompatible reaction was extremely fast and has been used in an aqueous medium for labeling bovine serum albumin.[30]

The production of 3,6-di(pyridin-2-yl)-1,2,4,5-s-tetrazine (pytz) capped AgNPs was accomplished by reacting 3,6-di(pyridin-2-yl)-1,4-dihydro-1,2,4,5-tetrazine with an aqueous silver nitrate (AgNO_3) solution in ethanol (EtOH)without a reducing agent. The pytz capped Ag NPs could be used for the selective and sensitive detection of Cu^{2+}, Ag^+ and Ni^{2+} in an aqueous medium. The

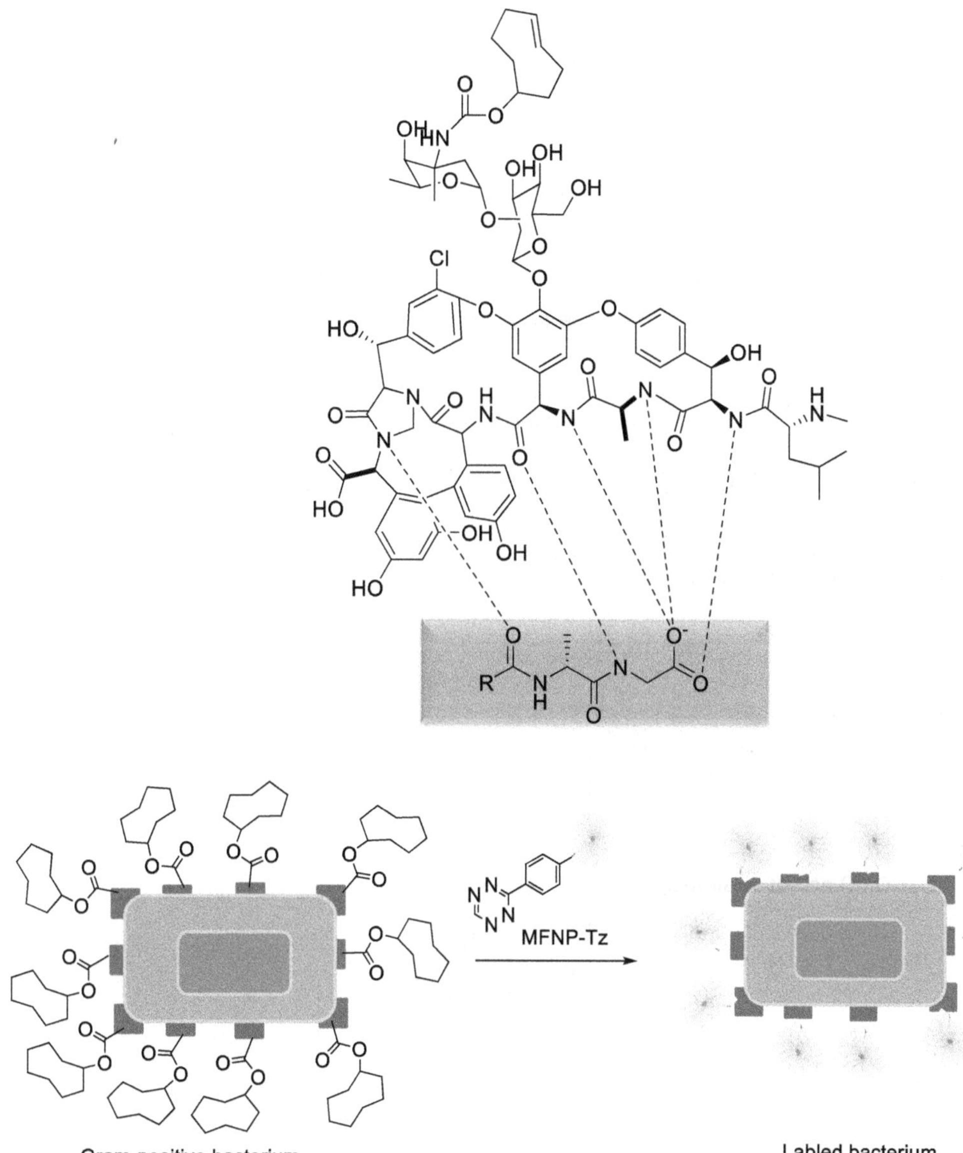

SCHEME 6.21 Vancomycin-transcyclooctene(vanc-TCO) targeted Gram-positive bacteria by binding with their membrane subunits.

sensor was fast and the measurements could occur within 3 min of additional time for the test solution using an AgNPs–pytz hybrid (TzAgNPs). Furthermore, this AgNPs–pytz hybrid sensor could be used for the detection of Cu^{2+}, Ag^+ and Ni^{2+} with the naked eye.

The synthesis of 3,6-di(pyridin-2-yl)-1,4-dihydro-1,2,4,5-tetrazine (H2pytz) was carried out using Pinner synthesis. This synthesis occurred by reacting 2-cyano pyridine with hydrazine (Scheme 6.24). The dihydro tetrazine was produced, which further oxidized using hydrochloric acid and sodium nitrite mixture inside the aromatic pytz. Audebert et al proposed a potential mechanism for the improvement in the synthesis that contained sulfur addition along with hydrazine (Scheme 6.25).[31]

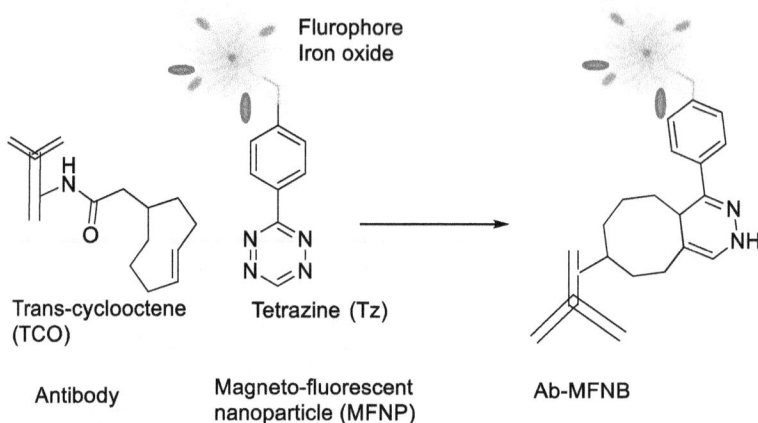

SCHEME 6.22 Conjugation chemistry between NP and antibody.

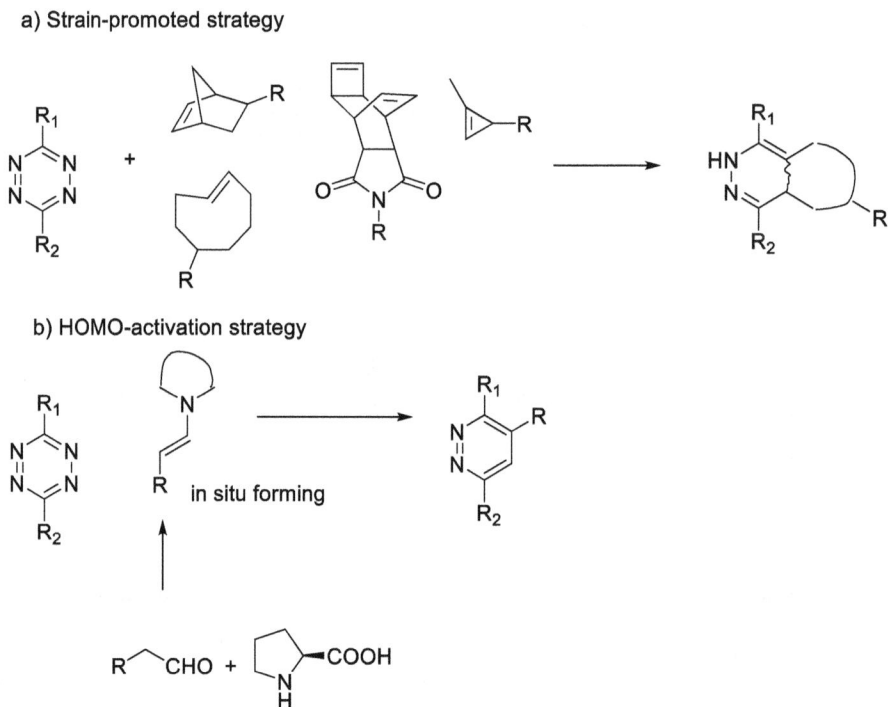

SCHEME 6.23 Showing: (a) strain-promoted iEDDA reaction; and (b) highest occupied molecular orbital (HOMO)-activated iEDDA.

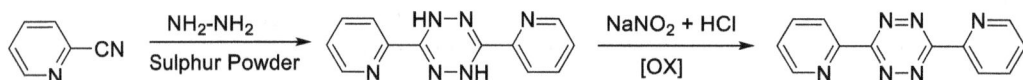

SCHEME 6.24 Synthesis of pytz and H₂pytz.

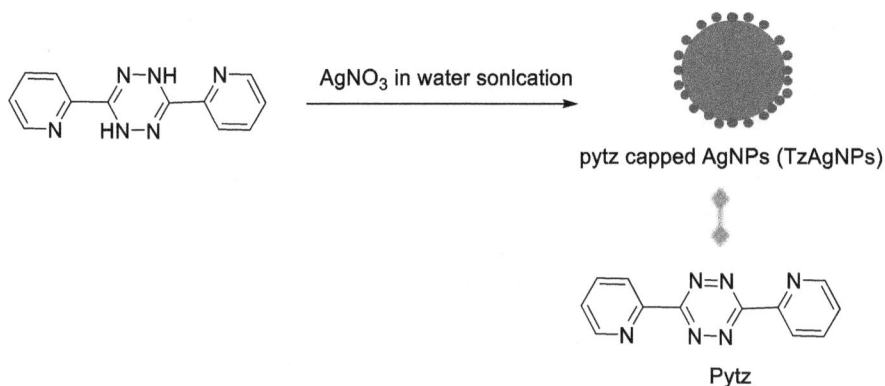

SCHEME 6.25 Synthesis of pytz capped TzAgNPs.

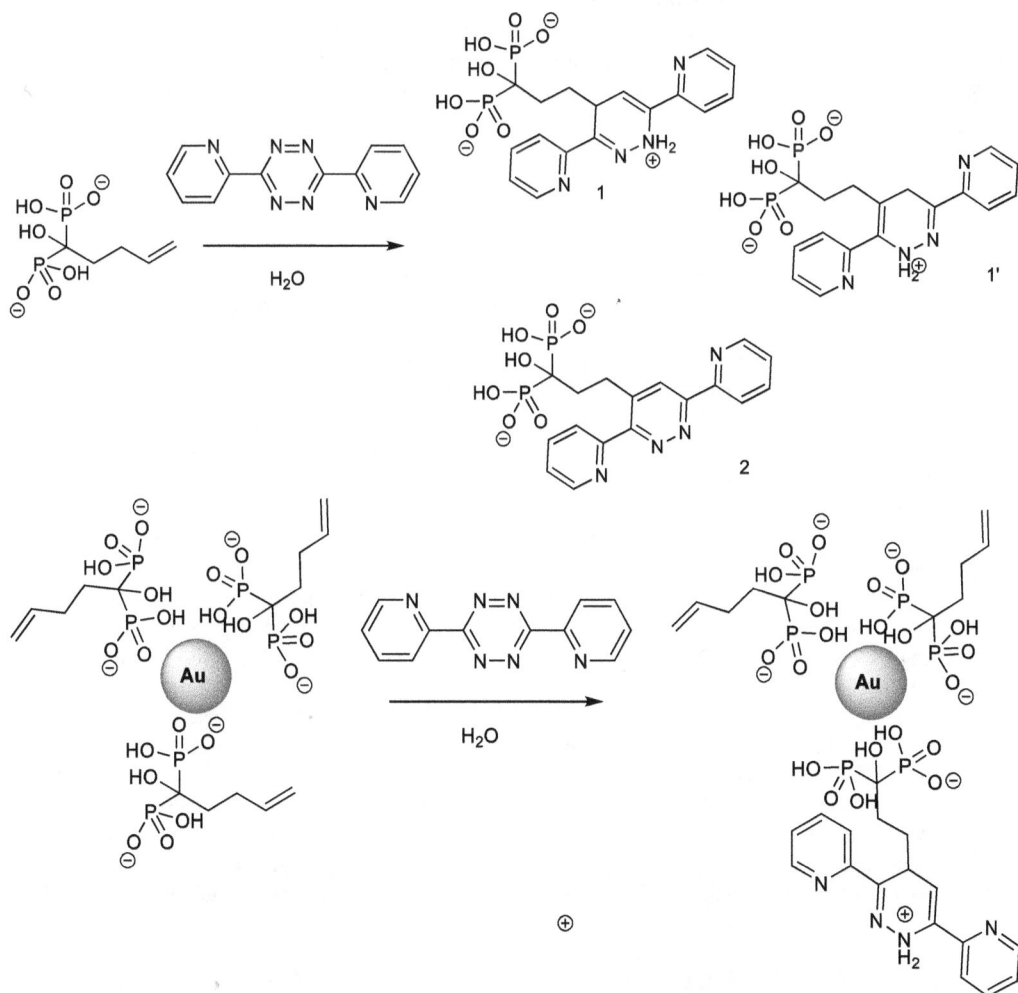

SCHEME 6.26 HMPBene reaction with tetrazine and surface modification of HMBPene functionalized Au NPs.

The iEDDA reaction was evaluated for the functionalization of Au NPs. This reaction was first modeled with molecules with free coating, for instance, 1- hydroxy-1,1-methylene bisphosphonate with an alkene functionality (HMBPene). The reaction was then transposed at the NP surface. Au NPs bearing the alkene functionality was obtained using a one-pot synthesis method with tetrazine and HMBPene click chemistry, which was evaluated at their surface using pytz. Noril et al estimated the effectiveness of the iEDDA reaction for the conversion of an alkene functionalized HMBP and its application at the surface of Au NPs (Scheme 6.26). This click methodology was extended for the conjugation of a near-infrared (NIR) probe at the surface of the NP. This type of bioorthogonal reaction and click chemistry could be used to determine an innovative path for fast and easily affordable surface-modified nanosystems.[32]

6.3   CONCLUSION

The versatility and increased efficiency of solid supported $FeCl_3$, and the importance of the derivatives of 1,2,4-triazines were reported using a one-pot synthesis of a series of the 1,2,4-triazines from the reactions between thiosemicarbazide with different α,β-dicarbonyl compounds under reflux conditions, in presence with the $FeCl_3 \cdot SiO_2$ catalyst. This triazine functionalized porous organic polymer material could act as an outstanding CO_2 storage material and support to design Pd NCs for C–C cross-coupling reactions. The material showed very efficient catalysis in the Sonogashira cross-coupling reaction.

REFERENCES

1. Simons JK, Saxton MR. Benzoguanamine. Or`g Synth. 1953. 33:13. doi.10.15227/orgsyn.033.0013.
2. Schroeder H, Grundmann C. The Extension of the Pinner Synthesis of Monohydroxy-s-triazines to the Aliphatic Series. 2,4-Dimethyl-s-triazine1-3 Hansjuergen. J Am Chem Soc. 1956. 78:2447–2451. doi.10.1021/ja01592a028.
3. Mundy BP, Ellerd M, Favaloro FG. Name reactions and reagents in organic synthesis, J Chem Educ. 2005. 82(12):1780. doi.10.1021/ed082p1780.2.
4. Schroeder H, Grundmann C. The Extension of the Pinner Synthesis of Monohydroxy-s-triazines to the Aliphatic Series. 2,4-Dimethyl-s-triazine1-3 Hansjuergen. J Am Chem Soc. 1956. 78:2447. doi.10.1021/ja01592a028.
5. Shi B, Lewis W, Campbell IB, Moody CJ. A Concise Route to Pyridines from Hydrazides by Metal Carbene N–H Insertion, 1,2,4-Triazine Formation, and Diels–Alder Reaction. Org Lett. 2009.11(16):3686–8. doi.10.1021/ol901502u.
6. Simons JK, Saxton MR. Benzoguanamine. Org Synth. 1953. 33(13).doi.10.15227/orgsyn.033.0013.
7. Emami-Nori A, Karamshahi Z, Ghorbani-Vaghei R. Efficient Synthesis of Multiply Substituted Triazines Using GO@N-Ligand-Cu Nano-Composite as a Novel Catalyst, J Inorg Organomet PolymMat. 2021. 31. 1801–10. doi./10.1007/s10904-020-01830-0.
8. Habibi D, Vakili S. Nano-sized silica supported $FeCl_3$ as an efficient heterogeneous catalyst for the synthesis of 1,2,4-triazine derivatives. Chinese J Catal. 2015. 36: 620–5. doi.10.1016/S1872-2067(15)60829-4.
9. Saad A, Vard C, Abderrabba M, Chehimi MM. Triazole/triazine-functionalized mesoporous silica as a hybrid material support for palladium nanocatalyst. Langmuir. 2017. 33:7137–46. doi.10.1021/acs.langmuir.7b01247.
10. Modak A, Pramanik M, Inagaki S, Bhaumik A. Triazine functionalized porous organic polymer: Excellent CO_2 storage material and support for designing Pd nanocatalyst for C-C cross-coupling reactions. J Mater Chem A. 2014. 2:11642. doi.10.1039/C4TA02150A.
11. Hasanpour B, Jafarpour M, Eskandari A, Rezaeifard A. A Novel Star-Shaped Triazine-Based Vitamin B5 Copper (II) Nanocatalyst for Tandem Aerobic Synthesis of Bis(indolyl)methanes. Eur J Org Chem. 2020. 7:4122–. doi.10.1002/ejoc.202000270.

12. Shafiee M, Khosropour A, Mohammadpoor-Baltork I, Moghadam M, Tangestaninejad S, Mirkhani V. A new green catalyst: 1,3,5-triazine-functionalized bisimidazolium dichloride tethered SPION catalyzed Betti synthesis. Catal Sci Technol. 2012. 2:2440–4. doi.10.1039/C2CY20187A.

13. Sadeghzadeh S. Bis(4-pyridylamino)triazine-stabilized magnetite KCC-1: a chemoselective, efficient, green and reusable nanocatalyst for the synthesis of N-substituted 1,4-dihydropyridines. RSC Adv. 2016. 6: 99586–94. doi:10.1039/C6RA20488K.

14. Li Z, He T, Liu L, Chen W, Zhang M, Wu G. et al. Covalent triazine framework supported non-noble metal nanoparticles with superior activity for catalytic hydrolysis of ammonia borane: from mechanistic study to catalyst design Chem Sci.. 2017. 8:781–8. doi.10.1039/C6SC02456D.

15. Wang H, Wang Y, Guo Y, Ren X, Wu L, Liu L. et al. Pd nanoparticles confined within triazine-based carbon nitride NTs: an efficient catalyst for Knoevenagel condensation-reduction cascade reactions. Catal Today. 2019. 330:124–34. doi:10.1016/j.cattod.2018.04.020.

16. Sabuj Kanti D, Sauvik C, Sujan M, Asim B. A new triazine-thiophene based porous organic polymer as efficient catalyst for the synthesis of chromenes via multicomponent coupling and catalyst support for facile synthesis of HMF from carbohydrates. Mol. Catal. 2019. 475:110483. doi.10.1016/j.mcat.2019.110483.

17. Ozturk S, Xiao Y, Dietrich D, Giesen B, Barthel J, Ying J. et al. Nickel nanoparticles supported on a covalent triazine framework as electrocatalyst for oxygen evolution reaction and oxygen reduction reactions. Beilstein J. Nanotech. 2020. 11:770–81. doi: 10.3762/bjnano.11.62.

18. Vahedi NN, Heravi M, Alhampour A. Mohammad P. Ag nanoparticles immobilized on new mesoporous triazine based carbon (MTC) as green and recoverable catalyst for reduction of nitroaromaticin aqueous media. Scie Rep. 2020. 10:19322. doi:10.1038/s41598-021-96421-5.

19. Nouruzi N, Dinari M, Mokhtari N, Gholipour B, Rostamnia S, Khaksar S. et al. Porous triazine polymer: A novel catalyst for the three component reaction. Appl Organomet Chem. 2020. 34;8:e5677. doi.10.1002/aoc.5677.

20. Builla A, Vaquero J, Barluenga J, Jose. 2011. Modern Heterocyclic Chemistry. Wiley-VCH. Weinheim Verlag GmbH & Co. KGaA. 1821-1832. ISBN: 978-3-527-33201-4.

21. Jain S, Neumann K, Zhang Y, Valero E, Geng J, Bradley M. Tetrazine-Mediated Post polymerization Modification. Macromol. 2016. 49: 5438–43.doi.10.1021/acs.macromol.6b00867.

22. Aufaure R, Hardouin J, Millot N, Motte L, Lalatonne Y, Guenin E. Tetrazine click chemistry for the modification of 1-Hydroxy-1,1-methylenebisphosphonic acids: towards bio-orthogonal functionalization of gold nanoparticles. Chem Eur J. 2016. 22: 16022–7. doi:10.1002/chem.201602899.

23. Li Y, Louarn G, Aubert P, Alain-Rizzo V, Galmiche L, Audebert P. et al. Polypyrrole-modified graphene sheet nanocomposites as new efficient materials for supercapacitors. Carbon. 2019. 105: 510–520. doi.10.1016/j.carbon.2016.04.067.

24. Yao X, Wang X. Optimization of conditions for the reaction between β-lactam carbenes and 3, 6-di-(2-thienyl) tetrazine. ARKIVOC. 2016. 3:352–9. doi.10.3998/ark.5550190.p009.524.

25. Testa C, Gigot E, Genc S, Decreau R, Roger J, Hierso J. Ortho-Functionalized Aryltetrazines by Direct Palladium-Catalyzed C–H Halogenation: Application to Fast Electrophilic Fluorination Reactions. Angew Chem Int Ed. 2016. 55: 5555–9. doi:10.1002/anie.201601082.

26. Gross A, Haddad R, Travelet C, Reynaud E, Audebert P, Borsali R. et al. Redox-Active Carbohydrate-Coated Nanoparticles: Self-Assembly of a Cyclodextrin–Polystyrene Glycopolymer with Tetrazine–Naphthalimide. Langmuir. 2016. 32:11939–45. doi:10.1021/acs.langmuir.6b03512.

27. Fritea L, Gorgy K, Le Goff A, Audebert P, Galmiche L, Sandulescu R. Fluorescent and redox tetrazine films by host-guest immobilization of tetrazine derivatives within poly(pyrrole-β-cyclodextrin) films. J Electroanal Chem. 2016. 781:36–40. doi:10.1016/j.jelechem.2016.07.010.

28. Chung H, Reiner T, Budin G, Min C, Liong M, Issadore D. et al. Ubiquitous Detection of Gram-Positive Bacteria with Bioorthogonal Magnetofluorescent Nanoparticles. ACS Nano. 2011. 5:8834–41. doi:10.1021/nn2029692.

29. Haun J, Devaraj N, Hilderbrand S, Lee H, Weissleder R. Bioorthogonal chemistry amplifies nanoparticle binding and enhances the sensitivity of cell detection. Nature Nanotech. 2010. 5:660–5. doi:10.1038/nnano.2010.148.

30. Lai S, Mao W, Song H, Xia L, Xie H. A biocompatible inverse electron demand Diels–Alder reaction of aldehyde and tetrazine promoted by proline. New J Chem. 2016. 40:8194–7. doi.10.1039/ C6NJ01567K.

31. Samanta S, Das S, Biswas P. Synthesis of 3,6-di(pyridin-2-yl)-1,2,4,5-tetrazine (pytz) capped silvernanoparticles using 3,6-di(pyridin-2-yl)-1,4-dihydro-1,2,4,5-tetrazineas reducing agent: Application in naked eye sensing of Cu^{2+}, Ni^{2+} and Ag^+ ions in aqueous solution and paper platform. Sens Actuators B. 2014. 202:23–30. doi.10.1039/C6RA01509C.

32. Aufaure R, Hardouin J, Millot N, Motte L, Lalatonne Y, Guenin E. Tetrazine Click Chemistry for the Modification of 1-Hydroxy-1,1-methylenebisphosphonic Acids: Towards Bio-orthogonal Functionalization of Gold Nanoparticles. Chem. Eur. J. 2016. 22, 45: 16022-16027. doi.org/10.1002/ chem.201602899.

7 Synthesis of Quinolines, Isoquinolines, and Quinolones Using Various Nanocatalysts

Chetna Ameta,[1] Yogeshwari Vyas,[1] Purnima Chaubisa,[1] Dharmendra,[1] and Keshav Lalit Ameta[2]

[1] Department of Chemistry, University College of Science, M. L. Sukhadia University, Udaipur, Rajasthan, India
[2] Department of Chemistry, School of Liberal Arts and Sciences, Mody University of Science and Technology, Lakshmangarh, Rajasthan, India

7.1 INTRODUCTION

Nanocatalysts (NCs) have various features to work as a catalyst for the synthesis of organic compounds, such as greater reactivity, better selectivity, and higher stability. Nanoparticles (NPs) have vast applications in various fields including optronics, sensors, and. The catalytic efficiency of NPs can be changed by altering their size. Other than size, the surface plays a major role in the reactivity and selectivity of NPs. Their reactivity can be enhanced by doping and surface modification.

Heterocyclic compounds are the mainstay of medicinal chemistry research. Of all the heterocyclic moieties, quinoline (C_9H_7N), isoquinoline, and quinolones possess outstanding therapeutic effects and play eminent roles in medicinal, synthetic, and bi-organic chemistry. This chapter includes the synthesis of C_9H_7N, isoquinoline, and quinolones and their derivatives using various nanosized catalysts.

7.2 QUINOLINES

C_9H_7N is an N-heterocyclic aromatic compound. It has a strong smell and is a colorless hygroscopic liquid. C_9H_7N and its derivatives are important in medicine due to their unique biological and pharmacological uses.[1] Naturally, quinolines can be obtained from plants, such as check Fumariaceae, Rutaceae, Berberidaceae, and Papaveraceae.[2] Synthesis of quinolines is vital since they are widely used in drugs.[3,4] and biologically active materials, such as antibacterial,[5] antimalarial,[6] antiasthmatic,[7] anti-inflammatory,[8] and antihypertensive,[9] In general, quinolines are prepared by reactions, such as Friedlander,[10] Doebner,[11] Doebner-von Miller,[12] Combes,[13] Skraup,[14] and Pfitzinger,[15] Recently, various approaches have been utilized to synthesize quinolines with higher rates and greater yields. Quinolines and their derivatives help in the formation of polymers and conjugated molecules.[16] Their derivatives have useful applications in luminescence and polymerization.[17] They have been employed in the preparation of flavoring agents,[18] and used in refineries as antifoaming agents.[19]

DOI: 10.1201/9781003141488-7

147

7.3   SYNTHESIS OF QUINOLINE AND ITS DERIVATIVES

7.3.1   Using Salen catalyst

Ongoing research focuses on using NCs and provides an environmental-friendly way of synthesis. C_9H_7N was synthesized in a versatile and greenway using CoFe2O4@SiO2@Co(III Salen magnetic catalyst.[20]

C_9H_7N was synthesized in the presence of this catalyst by the treatment of a carbonyl compound with 2-amino benzophenone (Scheme 7.1). The yield was approximately 96% for the C_9H_7N derivatives when H_2O was utilized. Table 7.1 lists the use of various 1,3-dicarbonyl and 2-amino benzophenone compounds that were investigated using 10 mg of salen complex, 1 mmoL of both reactants in 2 cubic centimeters of H_2O at 80°C. In addition, this catalyst has distinctive merits, such as easy separation after use since it is highly magnetic. Therefore, the catalyst is inexpensive, with greater reusability and durability. Table 7.1 lists the yield that corresponds to the combination of various 1,3-dicarbonyl and 2-amino benzophenone compounds.

7.3.2   TiO2-Al2O3-ZrO2 nanocatalyst

A novel, convenient, highly versatile, and environmentally benign method for the synthesis of C_9H_7N was derived that used a TiO_2-Al_2O_3-ZrO_2 NC.[21] Synthesis involved the reaction between anilines and ethyl acetoacetate for an outstanding yield (Scheme 7.2). This method has greater merits, such as shorter reaction time, easy workup, and milder conditions.

Equal quantities of reactants were used and 5 mol% TiO_2-Al_2O_3-ZrO_2 were mixed and heated (60°C) with stirring. The effect of solvent, temperature, and concentration of catalyst was studied and optimized. Maximum yield (98%) was obtained when acetonitrile was used with 5 mol% catalysts at 60°C for 1 h.

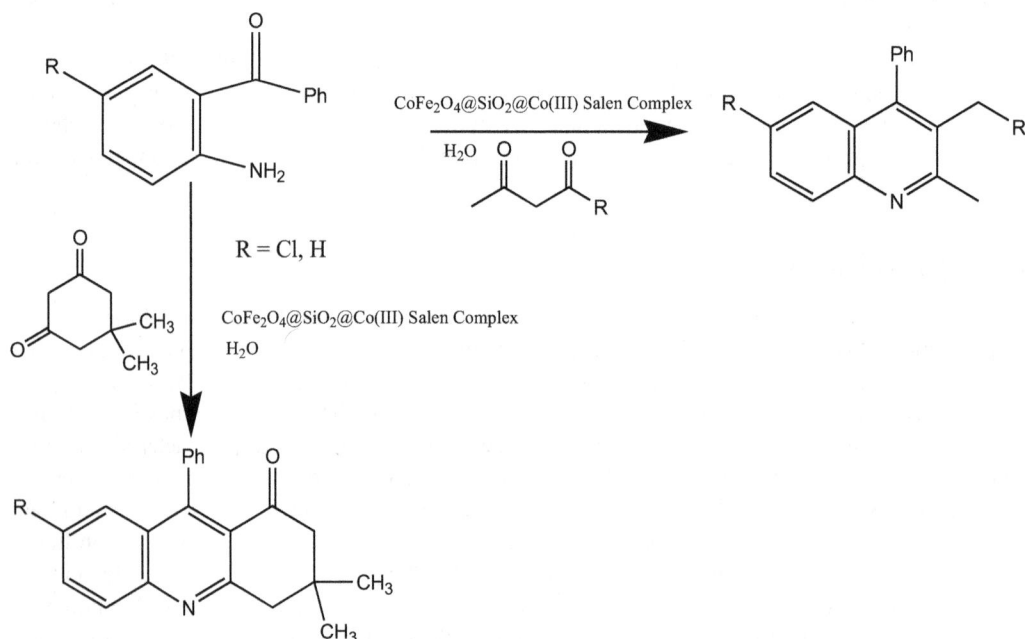

SCHEME 7.1   Synthesis of C_9H_7N by salen catalyst using H_2O.

TABLE 7.1
Yield Corresponding to Various Combinations

Number	Reactant 1	Reactant 2	Yield (%)	Time (min)
1	2-Aminobenzophenone	Dimedone	95	15
2	2-Aminobenzophenone	1,3-cyclohexadione	92	35
3	2-Aminobenzophenone	Acetophenone	86	40
4	5-chloro-2-aminobenzophenone	Methyl acetoacetate	87	20
5	5-chloro-2-aminobenzophenone	1,3-cyclohexadione	94	20
6	5-chloro-2-aminobenzophenone	Cyclohexanone	93	15
7	5-chloro-2-aminobenzophenone	Dimedone	96	10

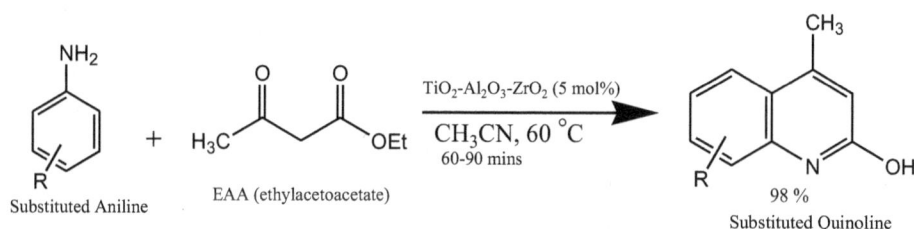

SCHEME 7.2   Synthesis of substituted C_9H_7N using TiO_2-Al_2O_3-ZrO_2 NC.

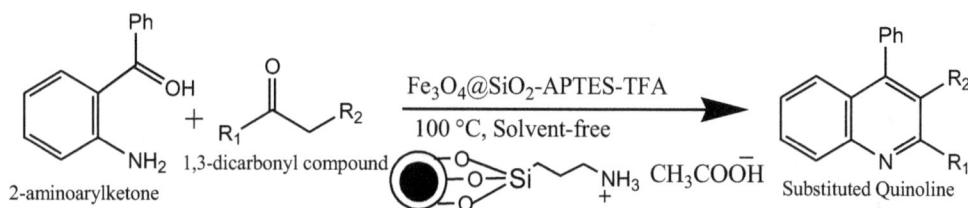

SCHEME 7.3   Procedure for production of quinolines.

7.3.3   Fe3O4@SiO2-APTES-TFA NANOCATALYST

2-aminoaryl carbonyls and alkynoates are suitable reactants, because their cyclization produced substituted quinolines. A cost-effective and non-toxic γ-aminopropyltriethoxysilanes (APTES)-trifluoroacetic acid (TFA) (Fe_3O_4@SiO_2-APTES-TFA) NC was prepared to synthesize C_9H_7N.[22] This catalyst gave the solvent-free synthesis of C_9H_7N via the Friedlander annulation reaction. 1,3-dicarbonyl compound and 2-aminoarylketone were used as precursors, and the catalyst was added under non-stop stirring for 5 h at 100°C. A typical procedure to produce quinolines is given in Scheme 7.3. This catalyst has high recyclability and could be reused numerous times because it was magnetically separable.

The method was further applied to several acyclic and cyclic β-dicarbonyl compounds as displayed in Table 7.2.

TABLE 7.2

Various Acid and Aminoaryl Ketones Used to Produce Quinolones

Number	CH acid	Aminoaryl ketones	Product	Yield
1.	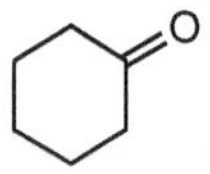	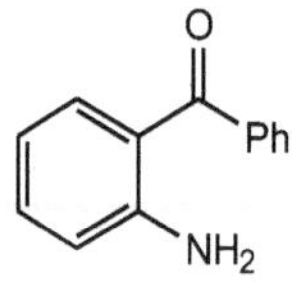	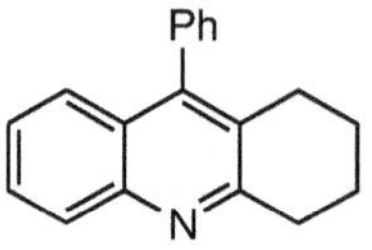	68 %
2.	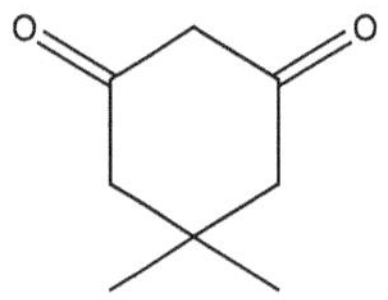	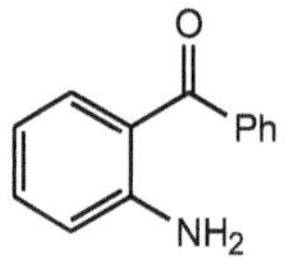	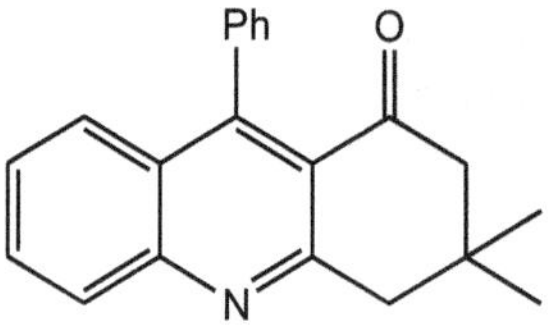	93%
3.	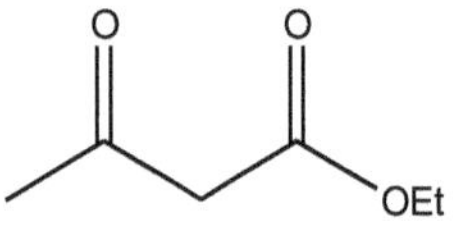	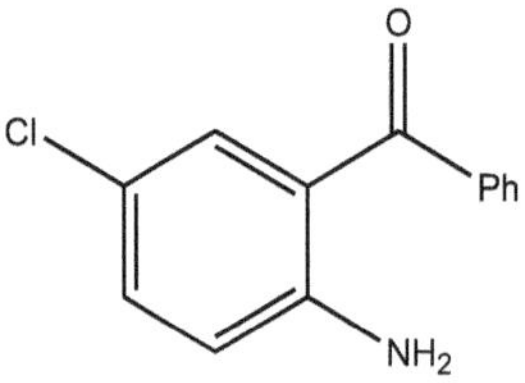	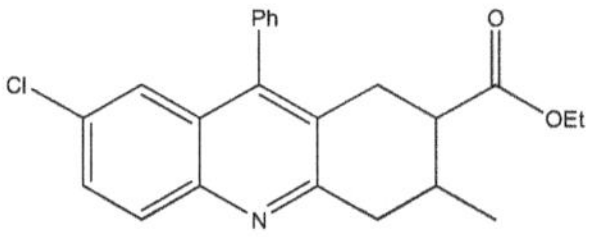	92%
4.	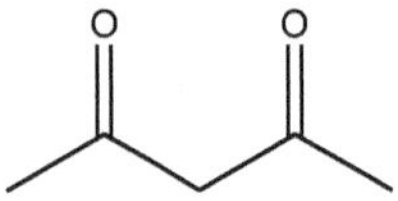	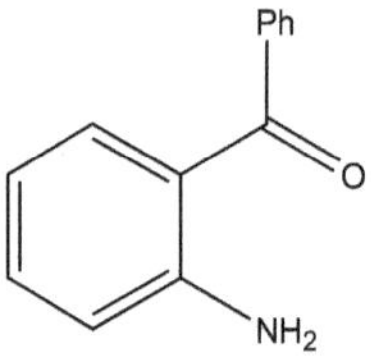	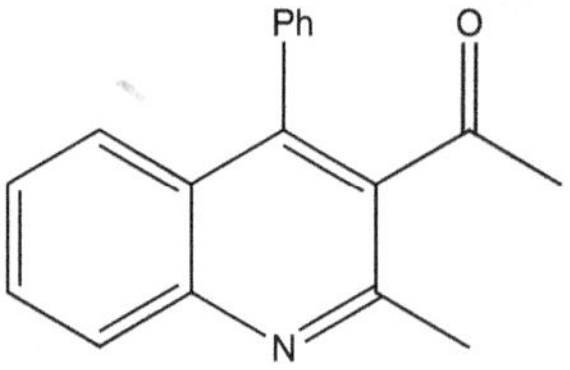	98%
5.	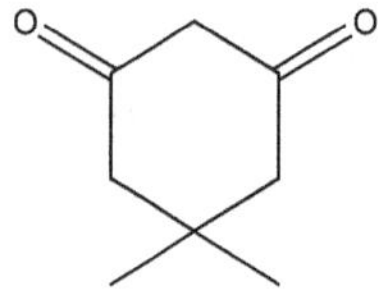	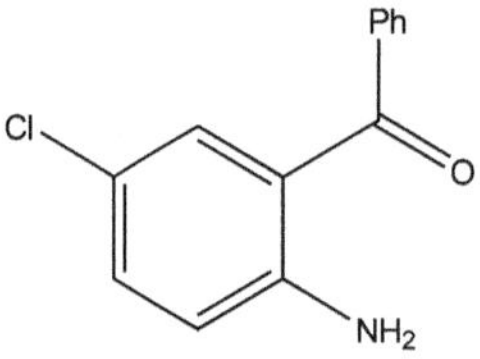	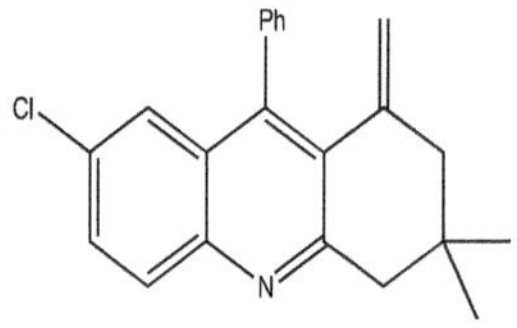	96%
6.	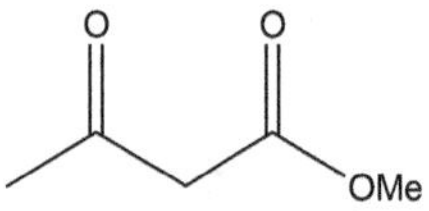	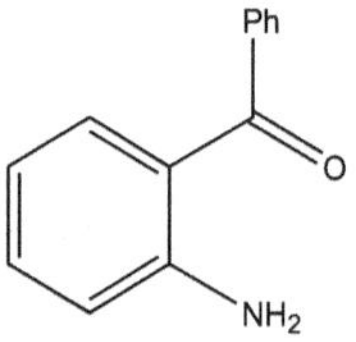	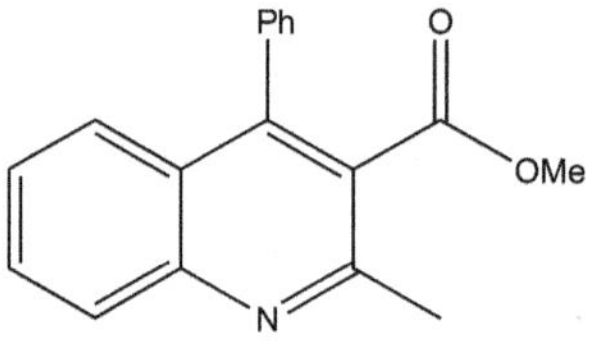	87%

5

7.3.4 COPPER-BASED NANOCATALYST

In recent studies, great attention has been given to copper-based (Cu) NCs since they are very selective and highly reactive in several multicomponent synthesis reactions, such as click and cross-coupling.[23,24] A one-pot production for C_9H_7N derivatives via a Cu(II) NC complex, which was obtained from 2-oxoquinoline-3-carbaldehyde Schiff base bonded on amino-functionalized silica (Cu@QCSSi) was reported under mild conditions.[25] The catalyst was recycled seven times without loss of activity. Scheme 7.4 represents the synthetic pathway for Cu@QCSSi. Synthesis of C_9H_7N derivatives involved refluxing with an NC (Scheme 7.5).

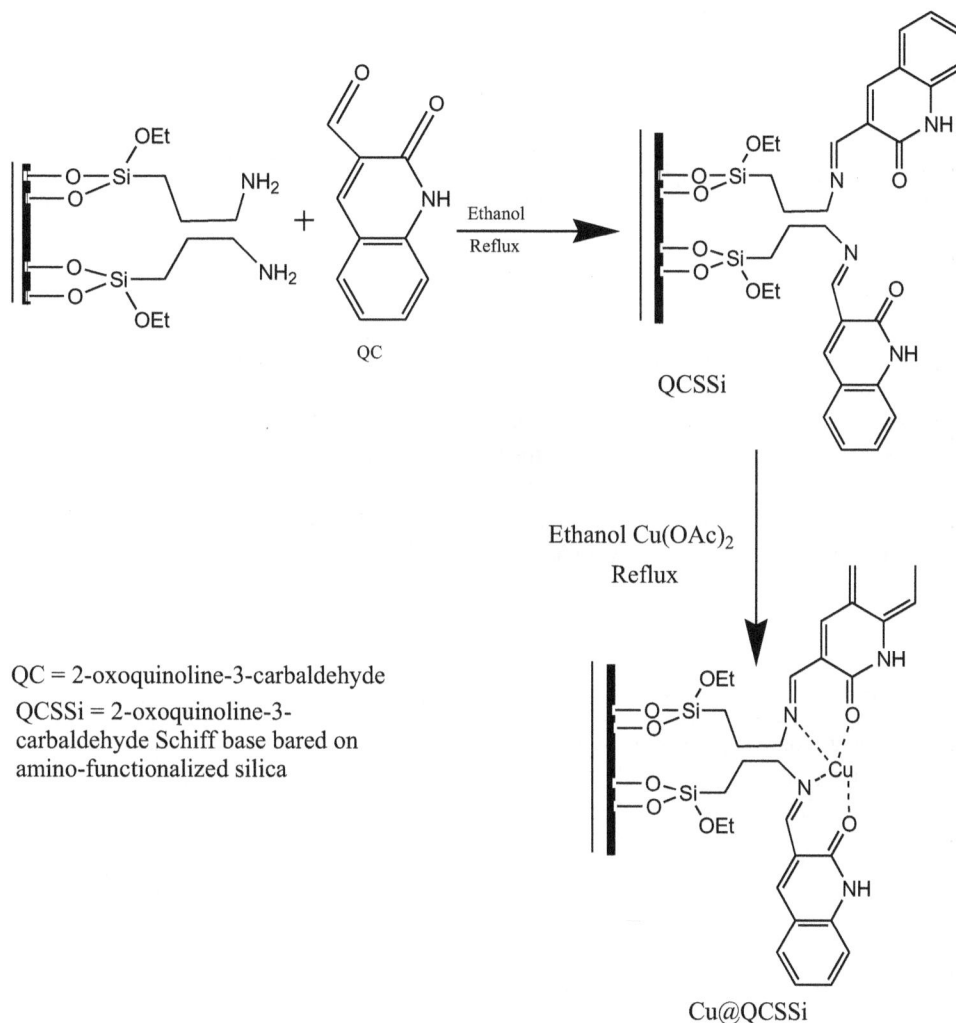

QC = 2-oxoquinoline-3-carbaldehyde

QCSSi = 2-oxoquinoline-3-carbaldehyde Schiff base bared on amino-functionalized silica

SCHEME 7.4 Synthetic pathway for Cu@QCSSi

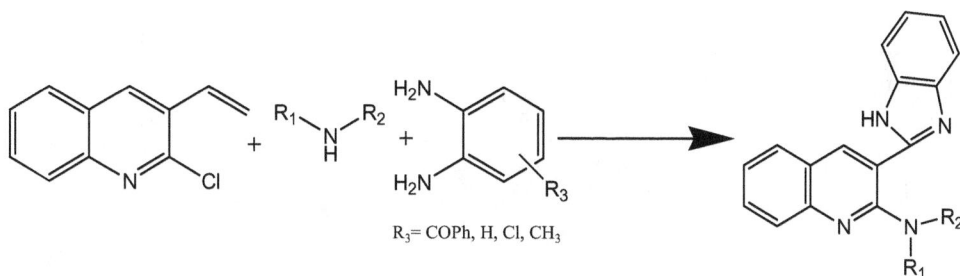

R_3= COPh, H, Cl, CH_3

SCHEME 7.5 Synthesis of C_9H_7N derivative using Cu@QCSSi

7.3.5 COBALT-BASED NANOCATALYST

Cobalt (Co) (Co/N-doped ZrO2@C) NC was made for reductive annulations of 2-nitroaryl carbonyls with alkynones and alkynoates to generate C_9H_7N.[26] This transformation synthesized various functionalized quinolines (Scheme 7.6).

Various functional groups were utilized in the synthetic protocol to determine the compatibility of Co NCs, such as methyl (–Me), dimethyl amine (–NMe$_2$), methoxy (–Ome), fluoro (–F), chloro (–Cl), nitro (–NO$_2$), and methoxy carbonyl (–COOMe). The results revealed that the yield was different for the different functional groups (Table 7.3). Reactants that had electron-withdrawing groups generated products with a higher yield compared with substrates that had electron-donating substituents. This might be because the electron-rich 2-nitrobenzaldehydes were less useful in the reduction of the –NO$_2$ group, and electron-withdrawing groups enhanced the reactivity of the carbonyl group and gave a better result.

7.3.6 IRON-BASED NANOCATALYST

Friedlander synthesis was applied that used a Fe3O4@SiO2/ZnCl2 catalyst for the generation of C_9H_7N.[27] This NC was prepared by a sol-gel method as illustrated in Scheme 7.7, where Fe_3O_4 acted as a shell and SiO_2 as a gel. α-methylene ketones and 2-aminoaryl ketones were mixed under solvent-free conditions and heated along with stirring (Scheme 7.8).

The catalytic activity of magnetic nanocrystal Fe3O4@SiO2/isoniazid/Cu(II) was explored in Friedlander synthesis.[28] It was utilized in the synthesis of C_9H_7N derivatives from 2-aminoaryl ketones and a-methylene ketones (Scheme 7.9; Table 7.4). This method was advantageous for a better yield and shorter reaction time. The catalyst could be easily detached using an external magnet and it could be recycled even after four cycles.

7.3.7 MANGANESE-BASED NANOCATALYST

Multicomponent reactions (MCRs) show their use in every field of organics, whether it is heterocyclic, medicinal, or pharmaceutical, since they have unique features, such as minimum time, a

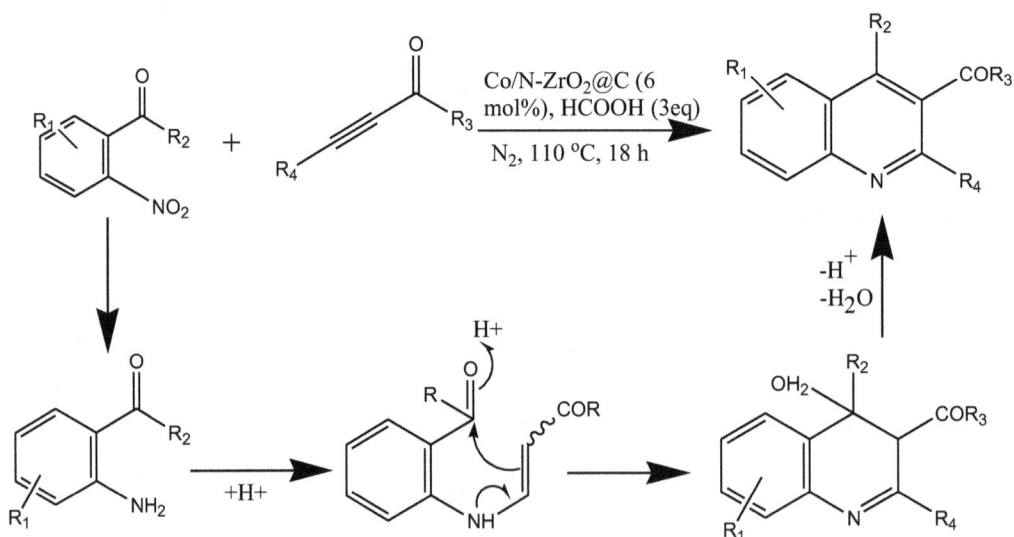

SCHEME 7.6 Synthesis route involving Co NC

TABLE 7.3
Effect of Various 2-nitobenzaldehyde on Yield of Product

Number	Variation in 2-nitrobenzaldehyde	Product	Yield (%)
1.			41
2.			48
3.			74
4.			78
6.			75
7.			65
8.			62

(*continued*)

TABLE 7.3 (Cont.)
Effect of Various 2-nitobenzaldehyde on Yield of Product

Number	Variation in 2-nitrobenzaldehyde	Product	Yield (%)
9.			38
10.			67
11.			71
12.			66
13.			76
14.			81

green approach, higher atom economy, and affordability. MCRs avoid a multistep reaction and produce superior yields and generate no by-products. A three-component reaction (condensation) of 1,3-cyclohexanedione, aromatic aldehydes, and 5-amino-3-methyl-1-phenylpyrazole was utilized in the presence of manganese (Mn) (2.5%) that was doped with multi-walled carbon nanotubes (MWCNT) NPs as a competent heterogeneous, recyclable, environmental benign catalyst, which yielded C_9H_7N derivatives (92%–98%) in 15 min[29] (Scheme 7.10). This catalyst has various qualities, such as easy synthesis, inexpensive, higher recyclability, even after eight the decrease in yield was negligible (5 %). The mechanism of the reaction is displayed in Scheme 7.11.

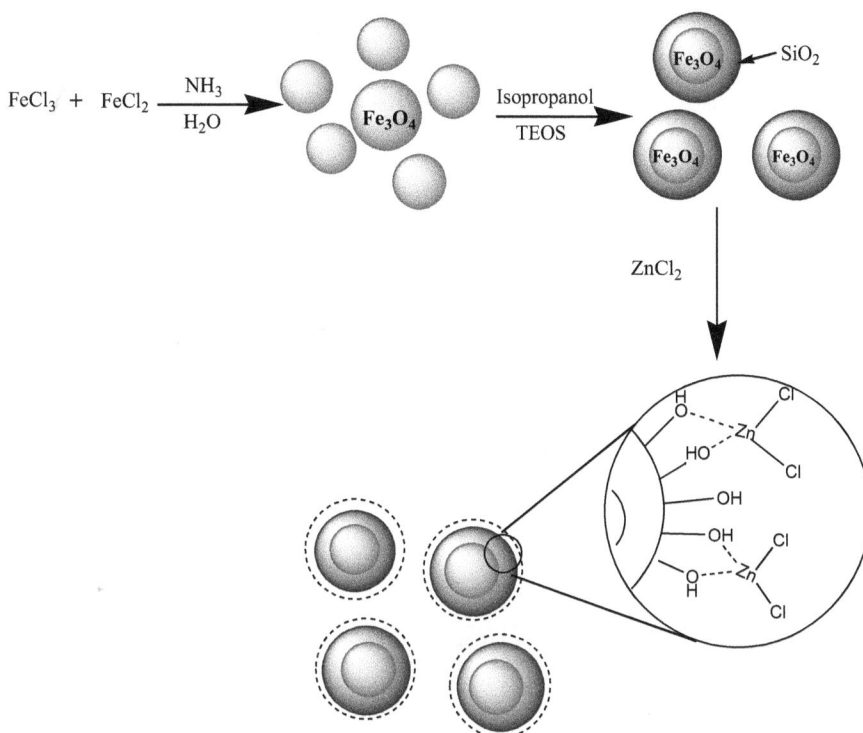

SCHEME 7.7   Systematic route for synthesis of Fe₃O4@SiO2/ZnCl2 core-shell NPs

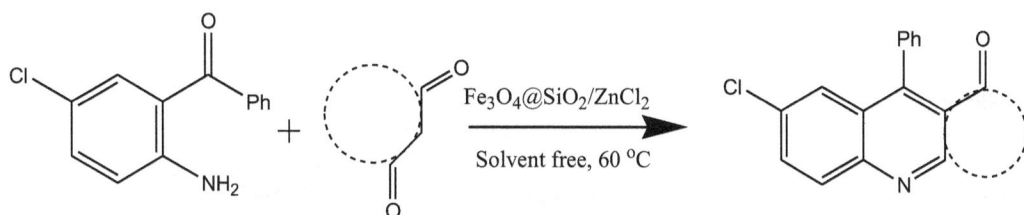

SCHEME 7.8   Synthesis of quinoline by Friedlander using core-shell NPs

7.3.8   KF/CPs NANOCATALYST

Green and proficient synthesis of quinolines was reported through the reaction of activated acetylenic compounds, alcohols, and isatin with potassium fluoride conductive polymers (KF/CPs) NCs[30] (Scheme 7.12). Optimization of the solvent, temperature, and amount was studied. The results showed that the highest yield was obtained under ambient conditions when H_2O was used as a solvent, and 10 % (w/w) of KF/CPs catalyst was utilized. The mechanism of the reaction is displayed in Scheme 7.13.

7.3.9   SILVER-BASED NANOCATALYST

A one-pot reaction was utilized for the generation of C_9H_7N derivatives that used a silver (Ag) NC.[31] Scheme 7.14 displays the model reaction for the generation of C_9H_7N derivatives. A potential mechanism is shown in Scheme 7.15.

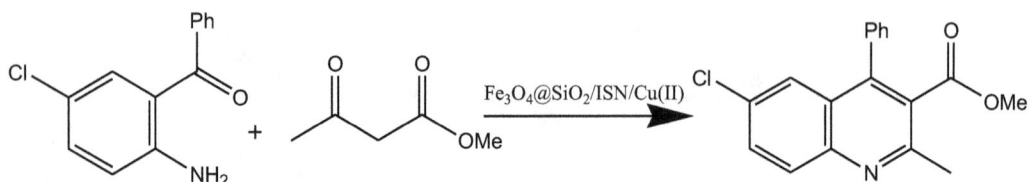

Catalyst (mg)	Yield	Time (h)	Temperature (°C)
0.05	69	2	60
0.07	95	2	60
0.1	95	2	60
0.07	70	2	Room Temperature

SCHEME 7.9   Synthesis of C_9H_7N derivatives

7.3.10   NICKEL-BASED NANOCATALYST

Nickel oxide (NiO) NPs were used in the synthesis of polysubstituted quinolines.[32] A condensation reaction took place between ketone and amino ketone without any solvent for 50–90 min. Scheme 7.16 shows a systematic synthesis procedure and a potential mechanism is shown in Scheme 7.17.

7.4   ISOQUINOLINES

Isoquinoline is a structural isomer of C_9H_7N. It is a benzopyridine constituted of a benzene ring attached to a pyridine ring. The isoquinoline configuration is present in a large number of alkaloids in isolated plant families. Isoquinoline derivatives show various biological activities, such as anti-bacterial, anti-inflammatory, antitumor, antifungal, analgesic, anticonvulsant, and antitubercular. In addition, isoquinoline derivatives are a novel group of cancer chemotherapeutic agents. Originally, isoquinoline was separated from coal tar by Hoogewerf and van Dorp in 1885.[33] Some methods for the synthesis of the isoquinoline ring could be improved to produce various isoquinoline derivatives. Potential methods for the formation of isoquinoline, such as Bischer–Napieralski, Pomeranz–Fritsch, and Pictet–Spengler reactions have the disadvantages of harsh reaction conditions, low yields, and partial substrate scope. Recently, NCs have received attention to synthesize isoquinoline derivatives. These compounds show enhanced catalytic activity that is associated with their bulk-sized forms due to their increased surface area.[34]

7.5   SYNTHESIS OF ISOQUINOLINE AND ITS DERIVATIVES

7.5.1   IRON-BASED NANOCATALYST

Green synthesis of pyrido[2,1-a]isoquinolines and pyrido[1,2-a]quinolins using Fe_3O_4– magnetic nanoparticles (MNPs) as an efficient NC was described and the antioxidant activity was studied. In this reaction, H_2O was used as a green solvent and Fe_3O_4-MNPs was as a green catalyst (Scheme 7.18).[35]

An MCR between isoquinoline, methyl malonyl chloride, alkyl bromides, and triphenylphosphine in the presence of a catalytic amount of Fe_3O_4-MNPs in H_2O at 80°C was investigated for the synthesis of pyrido[2,1-a]isoquinolines and pyrido[1,2-a]quinolines (Scheme 7.19). The magnetic iron

TABLE 7.4
Synthesis of Derivatives of Quinoline That Used Fe$_3$O$_4$@SiO$_2$/isoniazid/Cu(II) via Friedlander Synthesis

Number	Ketone	Aminoaryl ketone	Product	Yield (%)
1.				96
2.				92
3.				91
4.				95
5.				95
6.				87

oxide NP (Fe$_3$O$_4$-NPs) was formed by the reduction of ferric chloride solution with Clover Leaf water extract. These compounds have isoquinoline or C$_9$H$_7$N in their core; therefore, they have biological potential.[36]

The Fe$_3$O$_4$-MNPs is an easy, simple catalyst and is used in rapid and clean methods for the preparation of pyrrolo[2,1-a]isoquinoline derivatives (Scheme 7.20; Table 7.5). It is a novel, one-pot,

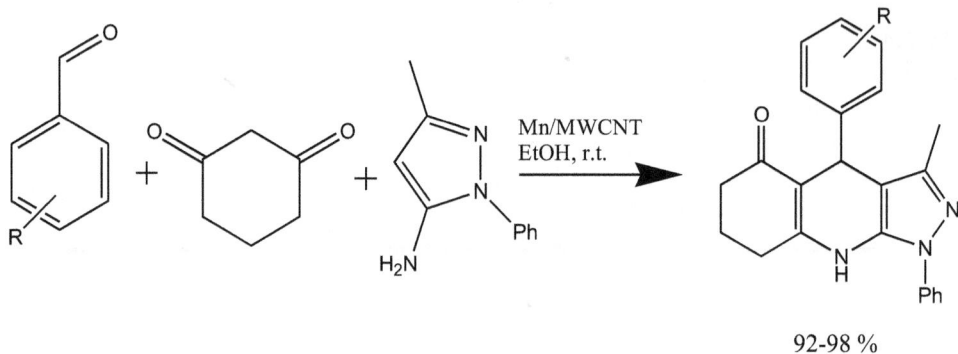

SCHEME 7.10   Three-component reaction for the synthesis of quinolone

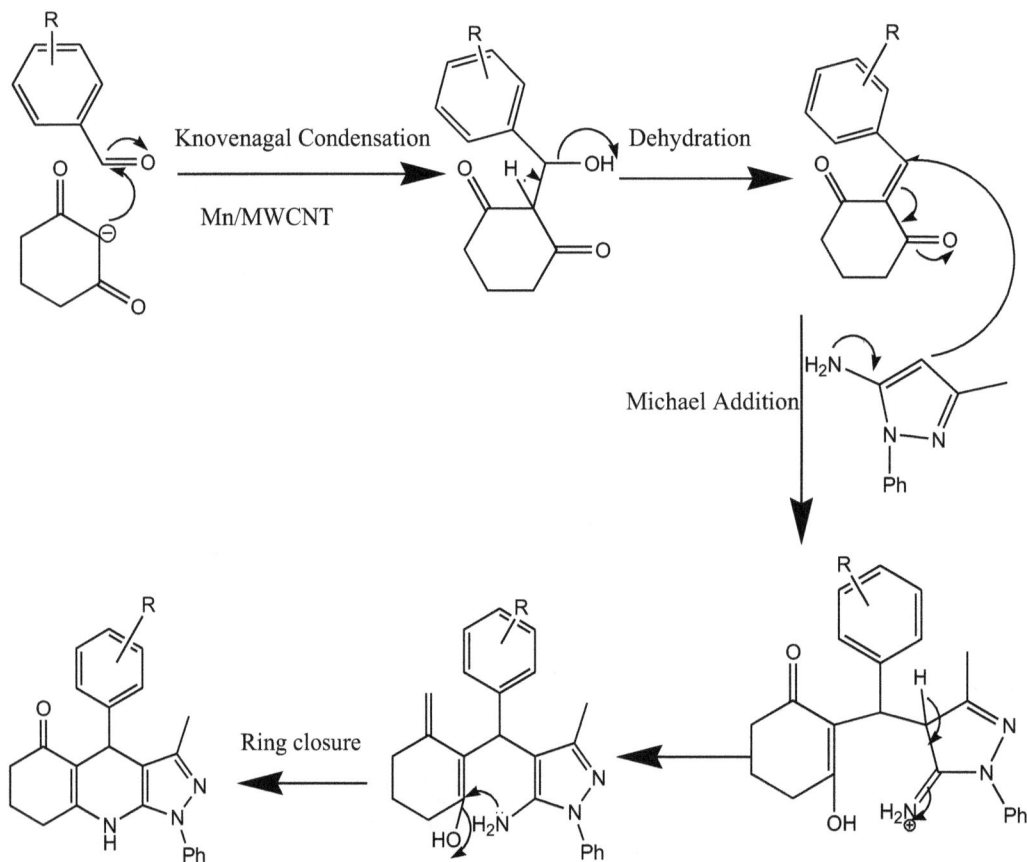

SCHEME 7.11   Mechanism of C_9H_7N production via three-component reaction using Mn NC

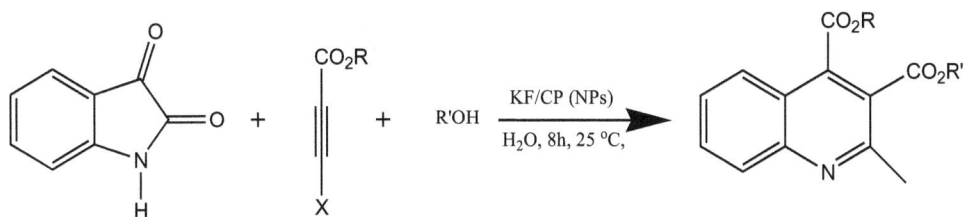

Sr. No.	R	R'	X	Yield
1.	Pr	Me	-CO$_2$Me	92
2.	Et	Et	-CO$_2$Me	93
3.	Me	Et	H	94
4.	Pr	Me	H	93
5.	Me	Me	H	92

SCHEME 7.12 Synthesis of quinolines via KF/CPs NC

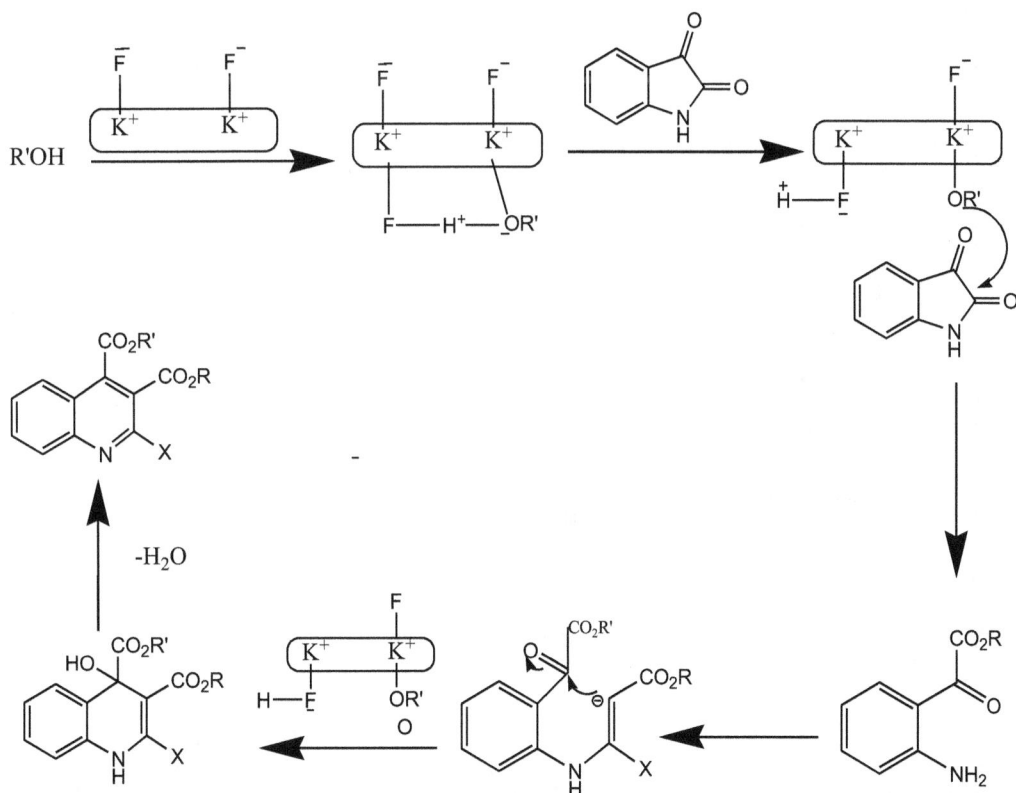

SCHEME 7.13 Mechanism of synthesis of C$_9$H$_7$N via KF/CPs catalyst

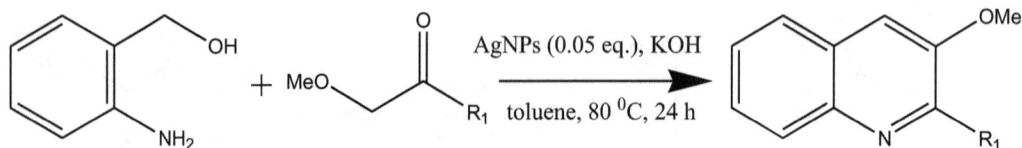

R_1 = Alkyl, Heteroaryl, Aryl

SCHEME 7.14 Synthesis of C_9H_7N derivatives using Ag NC

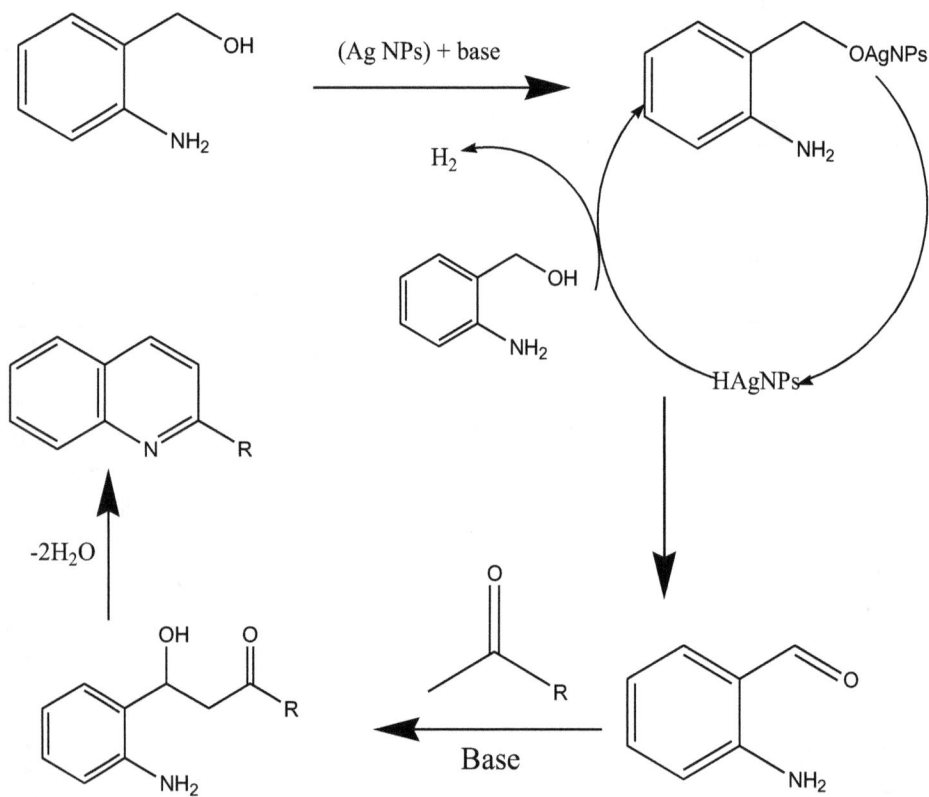

SCHEME 7.15 Proposed mechanism for synthesis of C_9H_7N using Ag NC

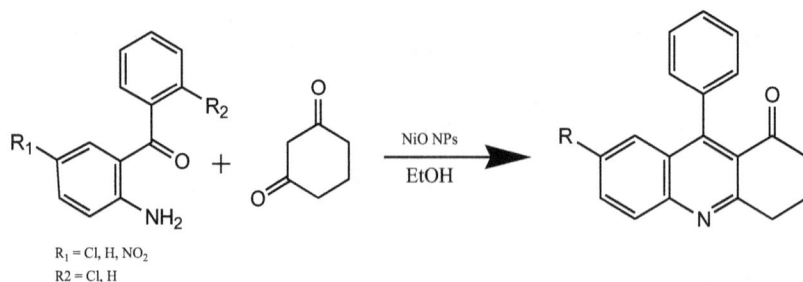

R_1 = Cl, H, NO$_2$
R2 = Cl, H

SCHEME 7.16 Synthesis procedure of C_9H_7N using NiO NPs

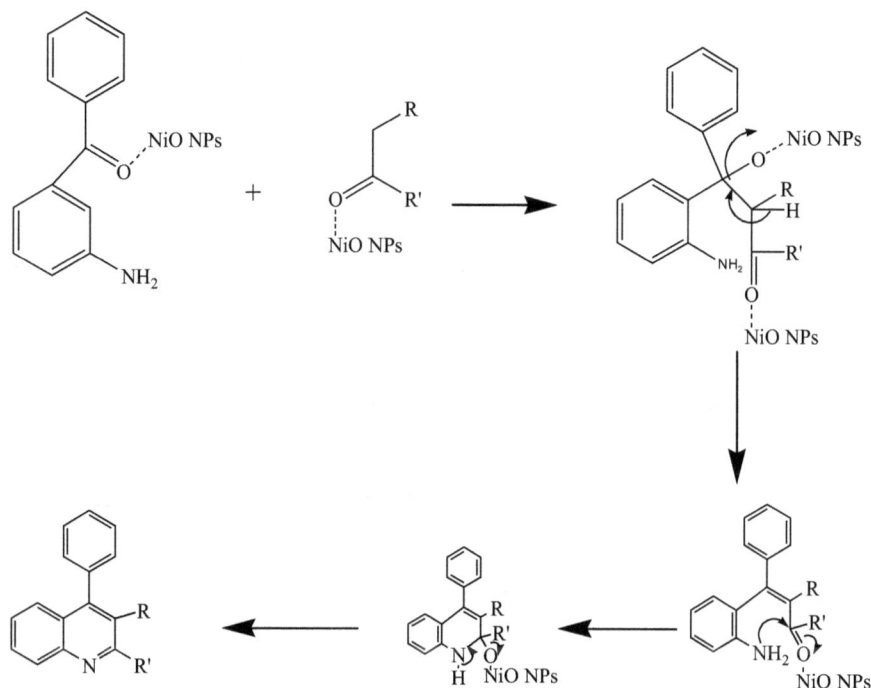

SCHEME 7.17 Potential mechanism for synthesis using NiO NPs

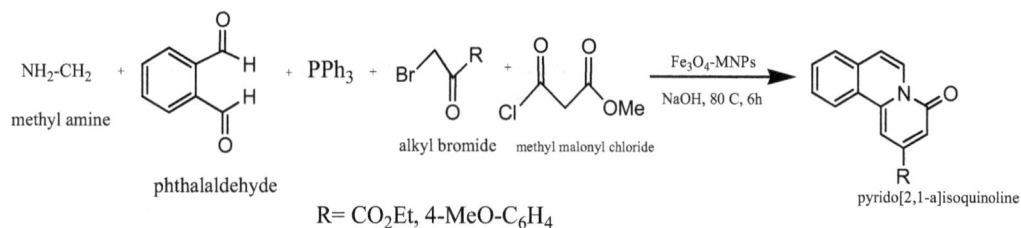

R= CO$_2$Et, 4-MeO-C$_6$H$_4$

SCHEME 7.18 Synthesis of pyrido[2,1-α]isoquinolines

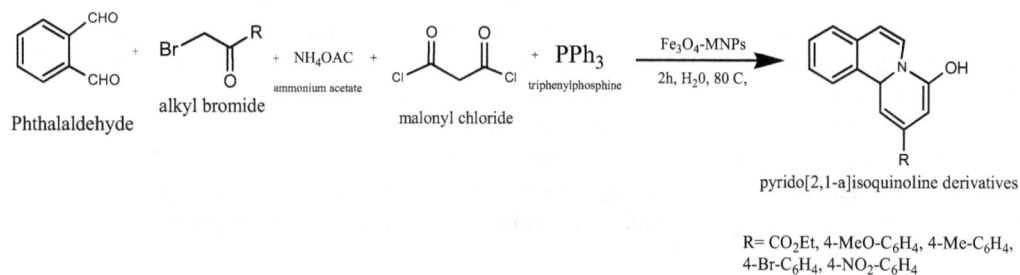

R= CO$_2$Et, 4-MeO-C$_6$H$_4$, 4-Me-C$_6$H$_4$,
4-Br-C$_6$H$_4$, 4-NO$_2$-C$_6$H$_4$

SCHEME 7.19 Synthesis of pyrido[2,1-a]isoquinolines derivatives

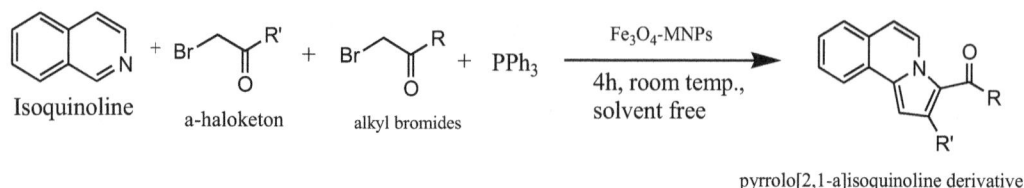

SCHEME 7.20 Synthesis of pyrrolo[2,1-α]isoquinoline derivative ethyl 3-(2-ethoxy-2-oxoacetyl)pyrrolo[2,1-a]isoquinoline-2- carboxylate

TABLE 7.5
Effect of Temperature and Catalyst on Yield of Ethyl
3-(2-ethoxy-2-oxoacetyl) Pyrrolo [2, 1-a]isoquinoline-2-carboxylate

Number	Catalyst	Temperature (°C)	Yield (%)
1	CM ZnO	RT	36
2	CM ZnO	90	38
3	Pyridine	RT	55
4	Pyridine	90	58
5	CuO NPs	RT	60
6	CuO NPs	90	62
7	ZnO NPs	RT	80
8	TiO$_2$ NPs	RT	45

efficient process with a high yield for the synthesis of pyrrolo[2,1-a]isoquinoline derivatives. It employed an MCR of isoquinoline, alkyl bromides, and triphenylphosphine in the presence of Fe$_3$O$_4$-MNPs as the catalyst under solvent-free conditions at room temperature (RT). The Fe$_3$O$_4$-MNPs were obtained by the reduction of ferric chloride solution with pomegranate peel water extract.[37]

7.5.2 Zinc-based nanocatalyst

Pyrido[2,1-a]isoquinoline and pyrido[1,2-a]quinoline derivatives were formed with good yields by the reaction of isoquinoline or C$_9$H$_7$N, activated acetylenic compounds, α-halo ketones, and triphenylphosphine in the presence of zinc oxide (ZnO) NPs as an efficient catalyst under solvent-free conditions at RT.[38] The reaction workup was easy, and the products could be readily separated from the reaction mixture. ZnO NPs markedly improved the yield of the product. The catalyst showed significant reusable activity. In the solvent-free conditions, primed the pyrido[2,1- a]isoquinoline derivatives a-e were obtained in excellent yields, as shown in Scheme 7.21 (Table 7.6).

1-hydrazino-3-(4-chlorophenyl)isoquinoline and chalcone were dissolved in dry acetic acid in the presence of Fe$_3$O$_4$ NPs for several hours to produce pyrazolo derivatives of isoquinoline. (Scheme 7.22). The benefits of this catalyst are the mild reaction state condition, non-toxicity, easy removal from the reaction mixture, and easy removal by auto-oxidation of the preferred pyrazolines to consistent pyrazoles.[39]

The reaction of isoquinoline, formamide, and dimethyl acetylene dicarboxylate in the presence of ZnO nanorod particles (ZnO NRs) as a catalyst in a solvent-free environment at RT was described to produce methyl 1-formyl-2-oxo-1,11 b-dihydro-2H-pyrimido[2,1-a] isoquinoline-4-carboxylate (Scheme 7.23). ZnO NRs displayed a significant improvement in the product yield and had considerable reusability.[40]

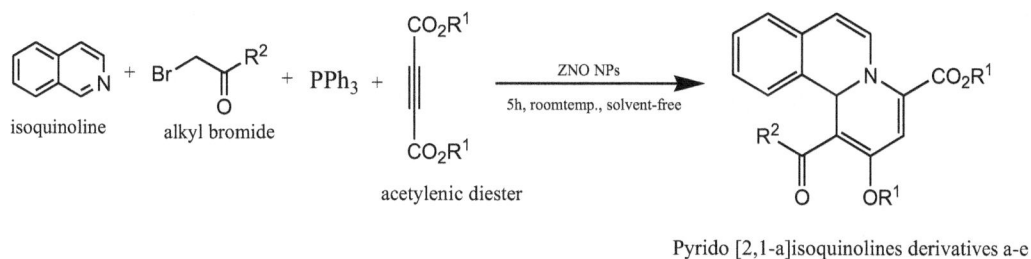

SCHEME 7.21   Synthesis of pyrido [2,1-a]isoquinolines

TABLE 7.6
Excellent Yield of Pyrido[2,1- a]isoquinoline Derivatives a–e

Product	R1 (substituents)	R2 (substituents)	Yield (%)
a	Methyl	CO_2Et	95
b	Methyl	4-Tol	90
c	Methyl	4-MeOC_6H_4	87
d	Ethyl	CO_2Et	93
e	Ethyl	4-MeOC_6H_4	85

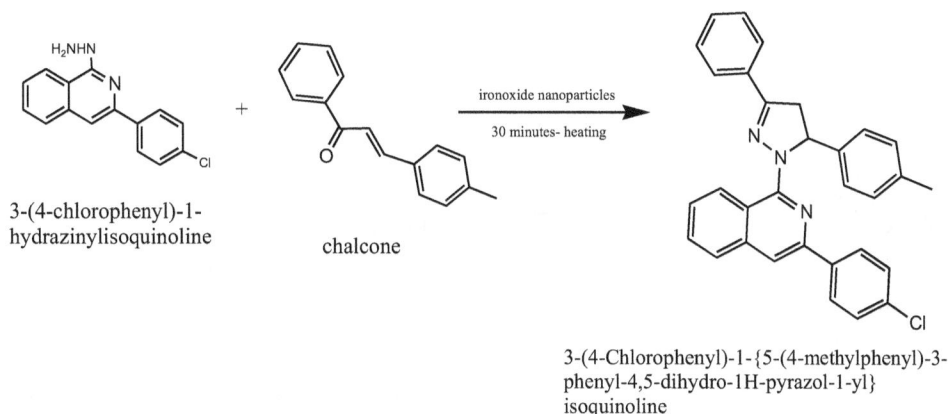

3-(4-Chlorophenyl)-1-{5-(4-methylphenyl)-3-
phenyl-4,5-dihydro-1H-pyrazol-1-yl}
isoquinoline

SCHEME 7.22   Synthesis of 3-(4-Chlorophenyl)-1-{5-(4-methylphenyl)-3-phenyl-4,5-dihydro-1H-pyrazol-1- yl} isoquinoline

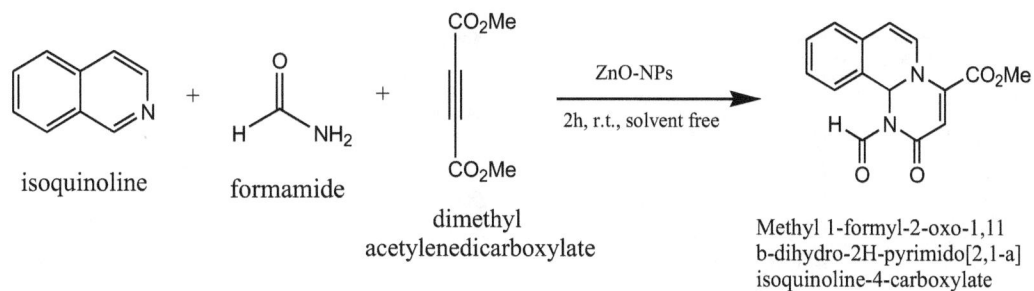

Methyl 1-formyl-2-oxo-1,11
b-dihydro-2H-pyrimido[2,1-a]
isoquinoline-4-carboxylate

SCHEME 7.23   Synthesis of pyrimido[2,1-a] isoquinoline derivative

7.5.3 KF/CLINOPTILOLITE NANOCATALYSTS

Punica granatum peel water extract was used as the green media for the synthesis of PG-KF/clinoptilolite NPs with a high yield. Thus obtained PG-KF/clinoptilolite NPs showed a significant basic catalytic activity when preparing the product with a high yield and were used several times. The synthesis of pyrrolo isoquinoline derivatives was performed using the MCR of isoquinoline, alkyl bromides, 2-hydroxyacetophenone, and dimethyl carbonate as a green reagent and KF/clinoptinolite NPs as a catalyst in an aqueous media at 80°C. The antioxidant capacity of some of the synthesized compounds was investigated using diphenyl-picrylhydrazine (DPPH) radical trapping. The short time of the reaction, high yields of the product, easy separation of the catalyst and products are some of the advantages of this procedure[41] (Scheme 7.24). Solvent effect on pyrazine containing pyrrolo[2,1-α]isoquinoline derivatives shown in Table 7.7 (Mousavi et al. 2020).

A four-component reaction is used for the synthesis of pyrrolo[2,1-a]isoquinoline derivatives. Phthalaldehyde or its derivatives, primary amines, alkyl bromides, activated acetylenic compounds and potassium fluoride/Clinoptilolite nanoparticles (KF/CP NPs) was reacted under solvent-free conditions at RT. It involved Diels-Alder reaction between synthesized pyrrolo[2,1-a]isoquinoline derivatives, activated acetylenic compounds and triphenylphosphine in the presence of KF/CP NPs under solvent-free conditions at RT (Scheme 7.26). In addition, the antioxidation property was investigated using DPPH radical. This eco-friendly procedure has a few advantages, such as a faster rate of reaction with high efficiency and easy removal of the catalyst.[42] The recommended mechanism for the reaction is shown in Scheme 7.27.

A novel four-component reaction of isocyanides for the green synthesis of pyrimidoisoquinolines in H_2O was studied using KF/clinoptilolite@MWCNTs nanocomposites (Scheme 7.28).[43]

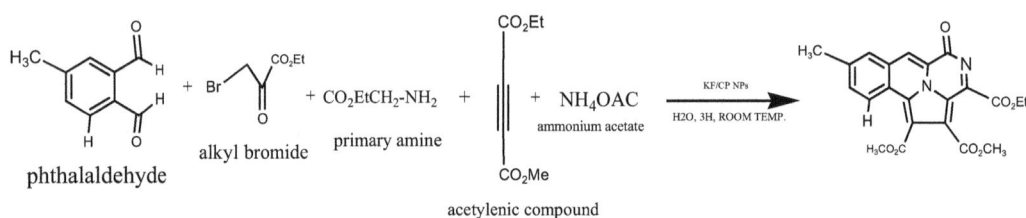

SCHEME 7.24 Synthesis of pyrazine containing pyrrolo[2,1-α]isoquinoline

TABLE 7.7
Best Temperature and Solvent for the Preparation of Pyrrolo[2,1-α]isoquinoline

Number	Solvent	Time (h)	Temperature (°C)	Yield%
1	EtOH	8	RT	-
2	EtOH	8	90	5
3	H_2O	3	RT	95
4	H_2O	3	80	97
5	H_2O	3	90	97
6	CH_2Cl_2	5	RT	75
7	CH_2Cl_2	5	40	75
8	Solvent-free	3	RT	85

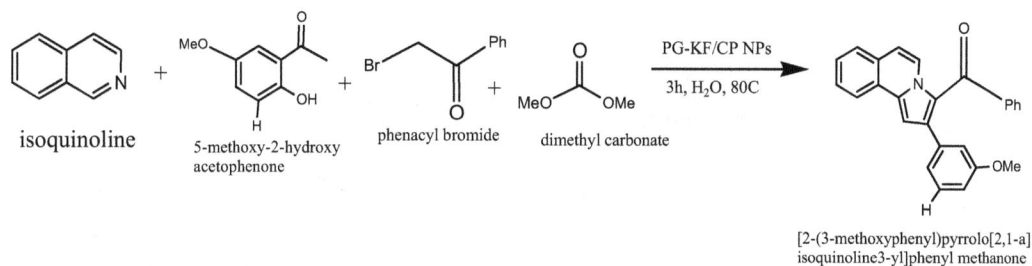

SCHEME 7.25   Synthesis of [2-3-methoxyphenyl)pyrrolo[2,1-a]isoquinoline 3-yl]phenyl methanone

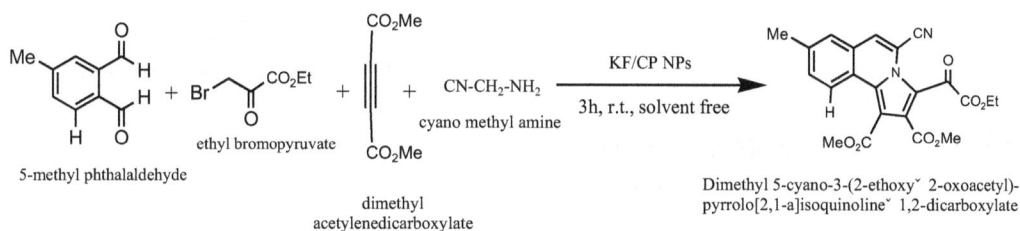

SCHEME 7.26   Synthesis of Dimethyl 5-cyano-3-(2-ethoxy2-oxoacetyl)-pyrrolo [2, 1-a]isoquinoline 1,2-dicarboxylate

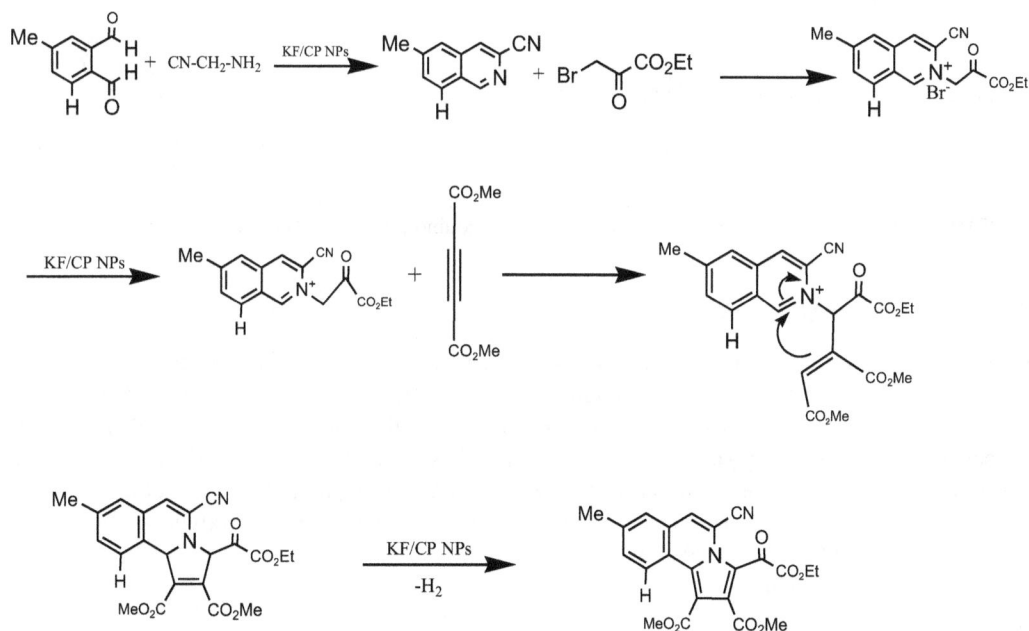

SCHEME 7.27   Mechanism for the generation of Dimethyl 5-cyano-3-(2-ethoxy2-oxoacetyl)-pyrrolo [2,1-a] isoquinoline1,2-dicarboxylate

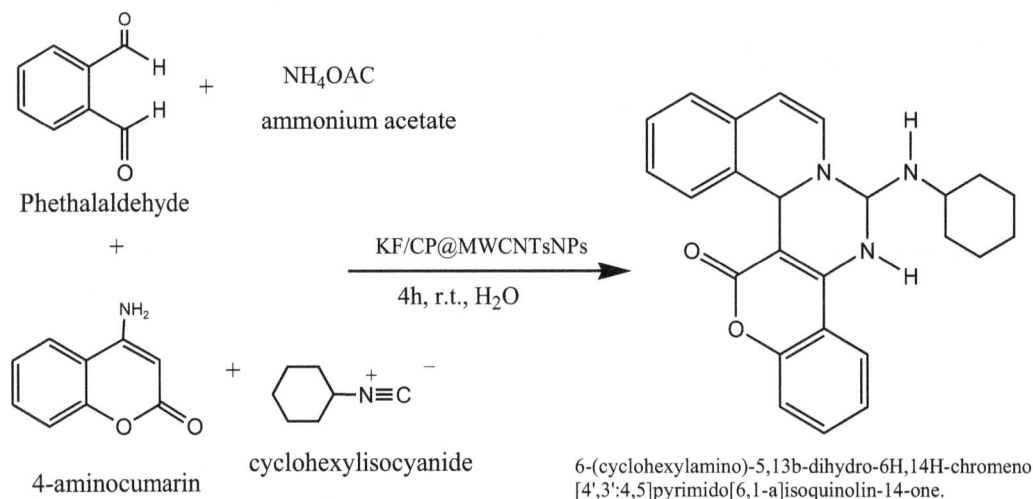

Phethalaldehyde

+

NH4OAC

ammonium acetate

+

NH2

4-aminocumarin

+

cyclohexylisocyanide

KF/CP@MWCNTsNPs

4h, r.t., H2O

6-(cyclohexylamino)-5,13b-dihydro-6H,14H-chromeno
[4',3':4,5]pyrimido[6,1-a]isoquinolin-14-one.

SCHEME 7.28 6-(cyclohexylamino)-5,13b-dihydro-6H,14H-chromeno [4',3':4,5] pyrimido [6,1-a] isoquinoline-14- one

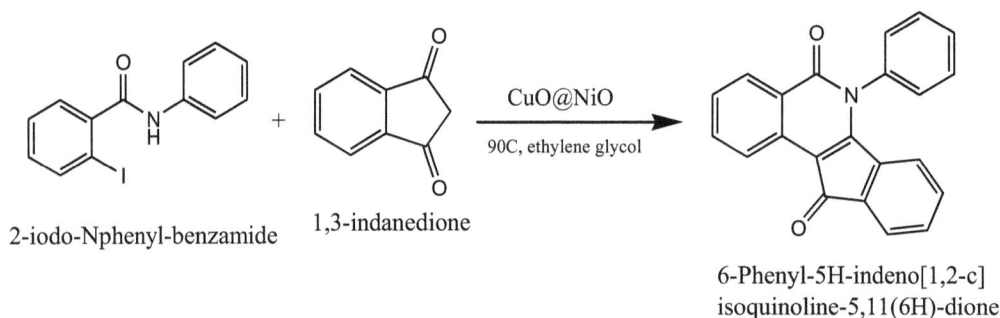

2-iodo-Nphenyl-benzamide   1,3-indanedione

CuO@NiO

90C, ethylene glycol

6-Phenyl-5H-indeno[1,2-c]
isoquinoline-5,11(6H)-dione

SCHEME 7.29 Synthesis of 6-phenyl-5H-indeno[1,2-c]isoquinoline-5,11(6H)-dione

7.5.4 COPPER-BASED NANOCATALYST

Indenoisoquinolines are synthetic compounds that have a wide range of biological activities, and some of the compounds have shown potent anticancer activity. An environmentally benign synthetic method was developed for the synthesis of indenoisoquinolines that used a novel CuO@NiO nanocatalyst and ethylene glycol as a green solvent. This method has several advantages, such as extensive substrate choice, exceptional yield, shorter reaction time, no need for an additive or base, and the catalyst was recycled up to six times without a major loss in its catalytic activity.[44] The method is shown in Schemes 7.29 and 7.30.

7.6 QUINOLONE

A wide range of synthetic approaches can be used for the synthesis of quinolones and their analogs. These are an important class of organic compounds that have several applications including suppressing tumor growth, promoting apoptosis DNA repair, and combating malarial infection. In the treatment of patients with human immunodeficiency virus infection, quinolone-based drugs can be used alone or in combination with existing antiretroviral drugs. Despite all the advantages, it has

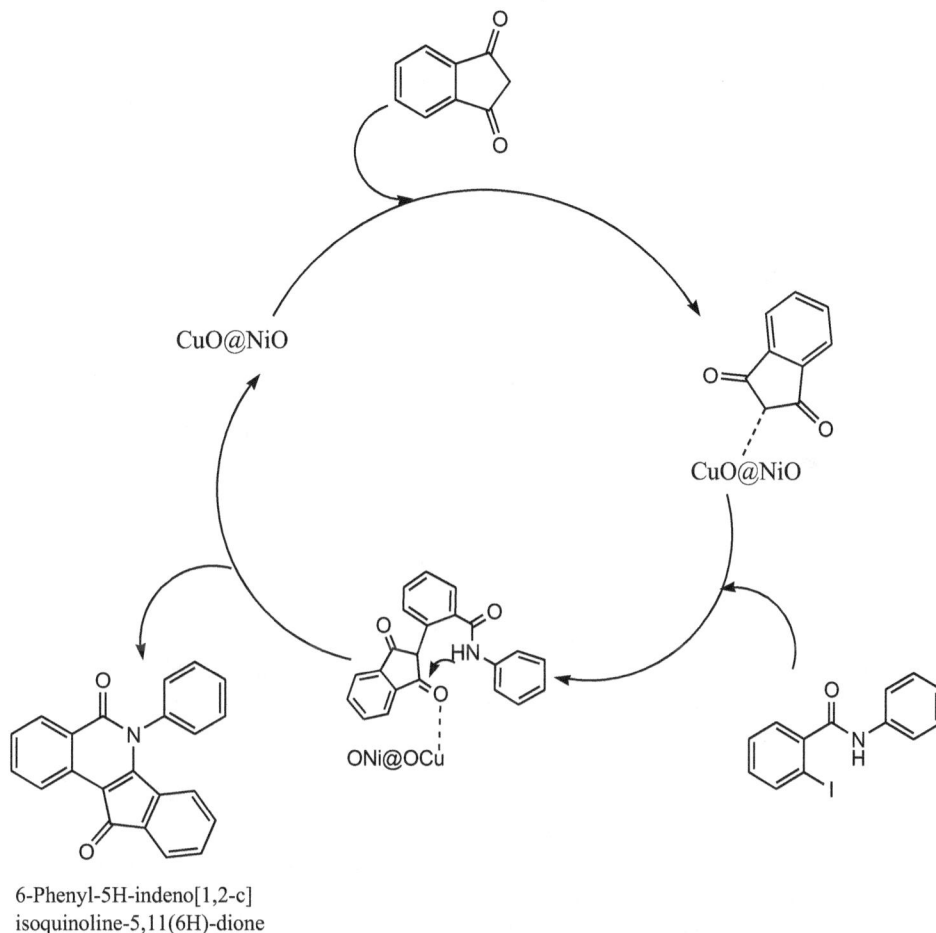

SCHEME 7.30 Mechanism of 6-phenyl-5H-indeno[1,2-c]isoquinoline-5,11(6H)-dione synthesis by CuO@ NiO NPs

been difficult to substitute the quinolone framework with various chemical functionalities with a short-step reaction under mild reaction conditions. Catalytic transformations could be used, which is attractive from environmental and industrial perspectives in agreement with the principle of green chemistry. Some of the recent developments in the preparation of quinolones and their derivatives that use NCs are discussed in the following sections.

7.7   SYNTHESIS OF QUINOLONE AND ITS DERIVATIVES

7.7.1   POLYSTYRENE-SUPPORTED PALLADIUM NANOCATALYST

Substituted 2-quinolones were synthesized from 2-iodoanilines and alkynes using oxalic acid as the carbon monoxide (CO) source under microwave exposure. Polystyrene-supported palladium (Pd@ PS) NPs were used as a catalyst. The use of a heterogeneous Pd catalyst was discovered for the first time for 2-quinolone synthesis that involved a carbonylation reaction employing $(CO_2H)_2 \cdot 2H_2O$ as a solid and bench stable CO source. The reaction revealed good substrate generalization for 2- iodoanilines and alkynes with wide functional group acceptance and good regioselectivity. The ligand-free operation, recyclability of the heterogeneous Pd@PS catalyst, and use of a bench stable carbon (C1) source are t helpful advantages of the procedure.[45]

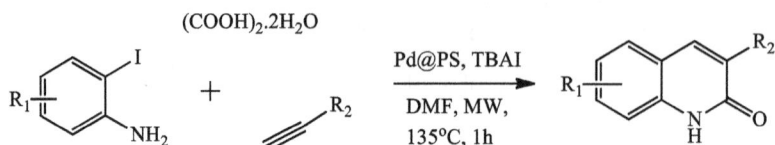

R_1 = H, Cl, CH$_3$, 6-Cl, 6-Br, 6-CH$_3$, 6-CN, 7-Cl, 6-COOMe etc.

SCHEME 7.31 Synthesis of quinolone derivative using MW by Pd@PS catalyst

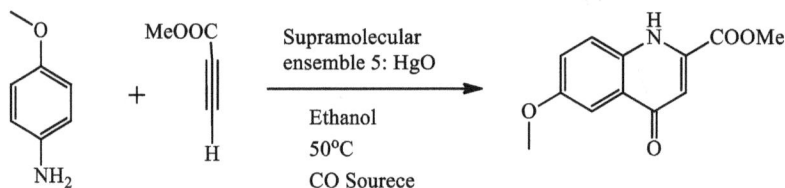

SCHEME 7.32 Synthesis of quinolone derivative catalyzed by supramolecular ensemble 5: HgO

Carbon dioxide (CO_2) is a benign source of CO. Currently, abundantly available CO_2 has been used as a CO replacement for quinolone synthesis that employs transition metals, such as Pd, Ag, and Cu. For the last few years $(CO_2H)_2 \cdot 2H_2O$ has been explored as in situ CO, CO_2, and hydrogen (H_2) sources and their applications in the diverse and exciting area of organic synthesis under-supported catalytic conditions. The best compatibility of the support (PS) was shown to hold the $(CO_2H)_2 \cdot 2H_2O$ over the surface, which made the blend effective for better interactions with a closely associated catalyst for productive reactions.

To optimize the reaction conditions, synthesis was performed with various catalysts, solvents, and bases at different temperatures. The study established $(CO_2H)_2 \cdot 2H_2O$ as the most efficient C1 source in the presence of a heterogeneous Pd@PS catalyst for the synthesis of 3-substituted-2-quinolones. The role of CO and CO_2 as CO sources in the reaction were recognized through mechanistic evaluations. The major highlights of the procedure are the use of recyclable heterogeneous NC, oxalic acid as a bench stable CO substitute, microwave irradiation, easy handling of the reaction, and regioselectivity of products.

7.7.2 SUPRAMOLECULAR ASSEMBLIES AND MERCURY NANOCATALYSTS

A one-pot approach for the synthesis of C_9H_7N and quinolone derivatives was studied.[46] A single catalytic system based on supramolecular assemblies and metal NPs for the preparation of 2,3-disubstituted quinoline and 4- quinolone derivatives were used. In this approach, fluorescent aggregates in aqueous media were formed via aggregation-induced emission enhancement that used electron-deficient tetraphenylcyclopentadienone. These aggregates served as reactors for the generation of mercury oxide (HgO) NPs. These in situ generated assemblies and HgO nanomaterials were used in the synthesis of N-heterocyclic derivatives with high catalytic efficiency through ortho C–H functionalization of less reactive anilines. Supramolecular ensemble 5: HgO NPs exhibited better catalytic efficiency than HgO NPs.

7.7.3 TITANIUM-BASED NANOCATALYST

A high-power sonicator for the synthesis of 8-aryl-7,8-dihydro-[1,3]-dioxolo[4,5-g]quinolin-6(5H)-ones from the MCR of Meldrum's acid, 3,4-methylenedioxy aniline, and various aromatic aldehydes

Proved by IR studies

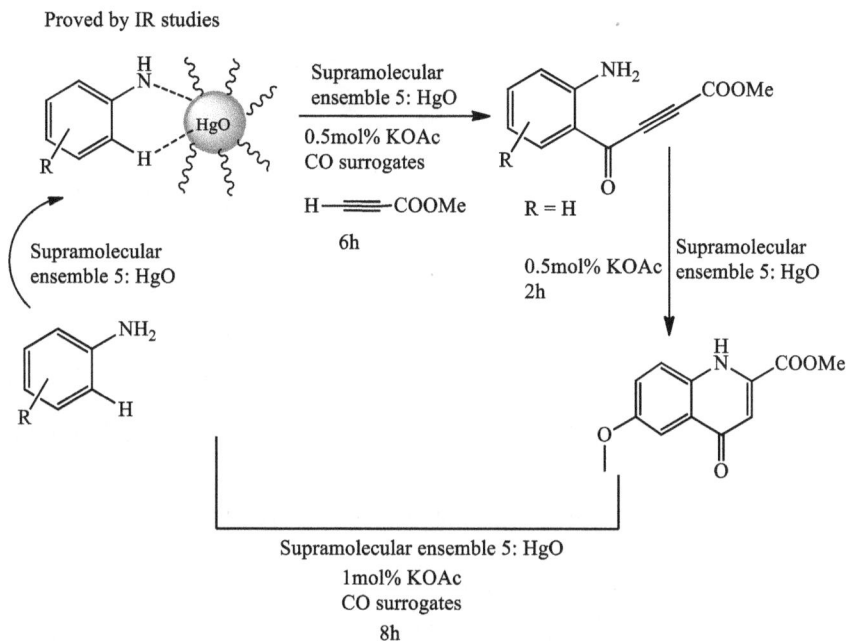

SCHEME 7.33 Potential mechanism for the synthesis of quinolone derivatives catalyzed by supramolecular ensemble 5: HgO

TABLE 7.8
Optimization of Reaction Conditions under Ultrasound Irradiation

Number	Solvent	Time (min)	Catalyst (mol %)	Yield (%)
1	H_2O	35	Boric acid (10 mol %)	60
2	H_2O	35	ZnO NPs (10 mol %)	72
3	H_2O	15	Commercial TiO_2 (10 mol %)	79
4	H_2O	40	Catalyst-free	Traces
5	H_2O	15	TiO_2 NPs (10 mol %)	90
6	Acetonitrile	30	TiO_2 NPs (10 mol %)	72
7	H_2O	15	TiO_2 NPs (5 mol %)	70

in the presence of a catalytic amount of titanium dioxide (TiO_2) NPs was proposed.[47] H_2O was used as a medium. First, TiO_2 NPs were synthesized by the biochemical method that used a leaf extract of the *Origanum majorana* plant as a reducing and capping agent under ultrasound. This was based on the decomposition of the precursor and its reduction and stabilization by appropriate agents present in the reaction mixture. TiO_2 NPs can also be synthesized conventionally; however, ultrasound offered the advantage of reducing the reaction time to 20 min from 5 h. This was due to the formation of scattered NPs with high yields. Therefore, it proved to be an excellent catalyst with operational ease and high yield under benign conditions without any environmental concerns.

Table 7.8 shows that TiO_2 NPs (10 mol %) in an aqueous medium gave better yields in 15 min compared with other conditions. This might be due to the largest surface area and presence of the most reactive acidic sites due to its nanosized TiO_2 NPs. After the completion of the reaction, the prepared TiO_2 NPs were easily recovered and the catalytic activity of the catalyst remained unchanged after use.

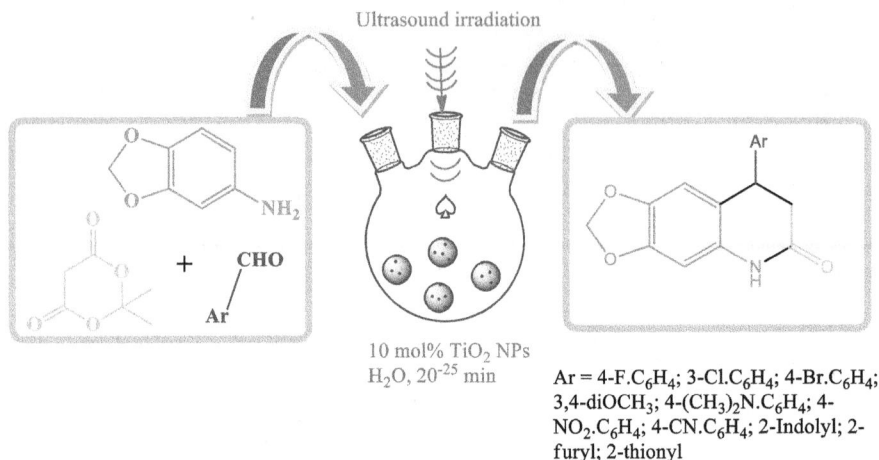

SCHEME 7.34 Proposed mechanism for synthesis of 8-aryl-7,8-dihydro-[1,3]-dioxolo[4,5-g]quinolin-6 (5H)-ones

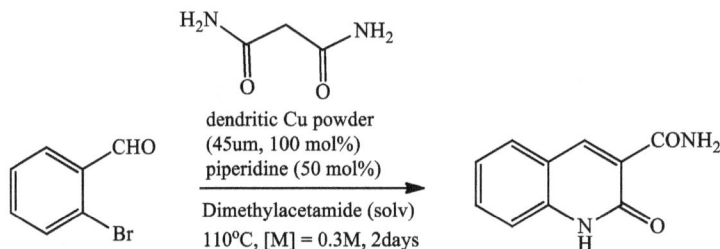

SCHEME 7.35 One-pot protocols for the synthesis of 3-substituted 2-quinolones

7.7.4 SBA-15/PrN(CH2PO3H)2 AS NANOCATALYST

pyrido[2,3-d]pyrimidines and pyrimido[4,5-b]quinolones were synthesized in the presence of Santa Barbara Amorphous-15 (SBA-15)/PrN(CH$_2$PO$_3$H)$_2$ under dry conditions.[48] SBA-15/ PrN(CH$_2$PO$_3$H)$_2$ is a novel and heterogeneous catalyst that contains phosphorous acid groups. The major advantages of this method are high yields, short reaction times, and reusability of the catalyst. The reaction of 4-nitro benzaldehyde (1 mmoL), malononitrile (1 mmoL), and 6-amino-1,3-dimethylpyrimidine-2,4(1H,3H)-dione (1 mmoL) was performed at 100°C. The reaction mixture was allowed to cool at RT and the obtained solid mixture was dissolved in ethanol (EtOH). The progress of the reaction is monitored by thin layer chromatography (TLC). The removed catalyst from the solution was washed with hot ethyl acetate (10 mL) and dried for use in the next run. The catalytic activity of the catalyst was restored within the limits of the experimental errors for three successive recycling runs.

7.7.5 COPPER-BASED NANOCATALYST

The step-economical synthesis of 3-amido-2-quinolones by dendritic Cu powder-mediated one-pot reaction has been described.[49] This reaction's setup is easy, compatible with moisture, and has many functional groups under mild conditions. This method is very useful for the synthesis of the key intermediates of biologically relevant 3-amido-2-quinolones.

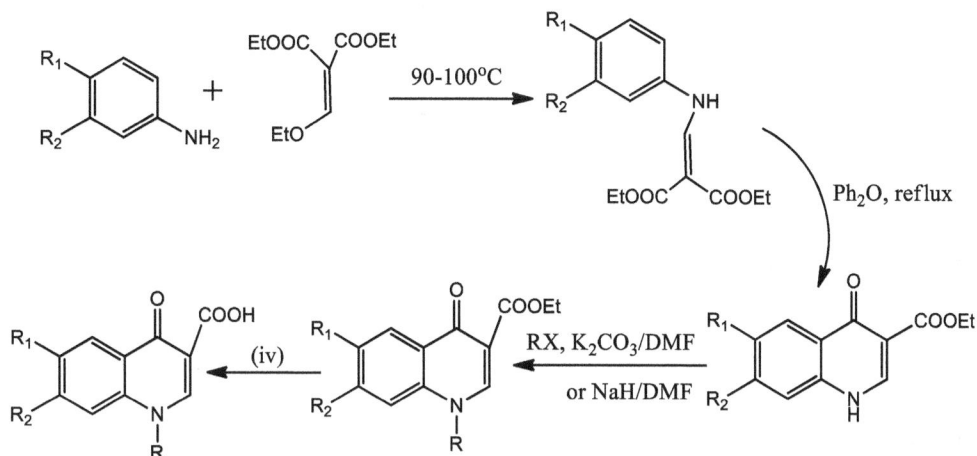

SCHEME 7.36   Synthetic route for the synthesis of 4-quinolone-3-carboxylic acids by chit-Cu-NP and NO_2BF_4

Replacing dendritic Cu powder with Cu NPs (e.g., 25 and 60–80 nm) gave 60%–62% product yields. Dendritic Cu powder has two roles, promoting the Knoevenagel condensation and assisting C–N bond formation without the help of a base, although with reduced efficacy. Many functional groups are resistant to reacting in mild reaction conditions. In addition, this method is user-friendly because it has a one-pot easy setup with moisture tolerance, and it is cost-effective and uses low-cost Cu powder. Chitosan-supported Cu NPs have been synthesized and utilized for the synthesis of 3-nitro-4-quinolones from 3-carboxy-4-quinolones via IPSO nitration. The synthesized 3-nitro derivatives of 4-quinolones were successfully converted into their 3-tetrazolyl bioisosteres, which showed increased antibacterial activity compared with the standard ciprofloxacin.[50]

Chitosan has the bifunctionality of hydroxyl and amine groups in its molecular structure; therefore, it has outstanding stabilization strength for metal NPs. It works as a potential catalyst for the synthesis of various heterocyclic compounds. A mild, cost-effective, and environmentally benign method for the synthesis of 3-nitroquinolones was developed that used chitosan-Cu-NP, and its efficiency was further compared with cellulose-Cu-NP and starch-Cu-NP.

The recyclability of the catalyst was tested before and after five uses in the reaction and showed no remarkable change in the morphology and catalytic activity after recycling five times. The size of the NPs was approximately 266 nm. Initially, in the presence of atmospheric O_2, the Cu oxidized to Cu^{2+}. These Cu^{2+} formed a chelate with both carbonyl groups of the quinolones through O_2 with Cu^{2+}. A concerted mechanism takes place via decarboxylative nitration, in which NO^{2+} from nitronium tetrafluoroborate attacks at the charge developed on the C-3 carbon, and decarboxylation occurred simultaneously to form the product.

7.7.6   ZIRCONIUM-BASED NANOCATALYST

The direct amination of 7-halo-6-fluoroquinolone-3-carboxylic acids with a variety of piperazine derivatives and (4aR, 7aR)-octahydro-1H-pyrrolo[3,4-b] pyridine that used zirconia sulfuric acid (ZrSA) NPS was used for the synthesis of various antibacterial fluoroquinolone compounds. H_2O was used as a medium. ZrSA exhibited high catalytic activity, with high yields of the desired product. In addition, the catalyst was recyclable and could be reused at least three times without any noticeable loss in its catalytic activity. This catalytic method has a simple workup procedure and avoids the use of harmful organic solvents and results in the rapid synthesis of fluoroquinolone

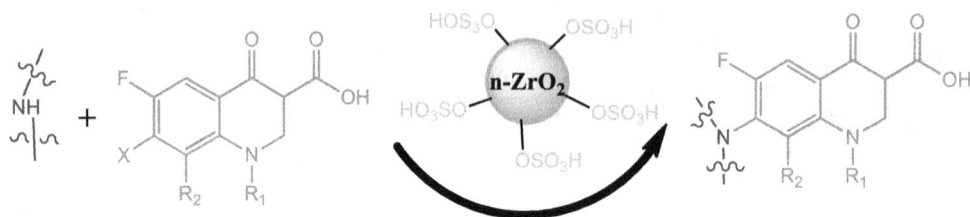

SCHEME 7.37 Synthesis of fluoroquinolone derivatives

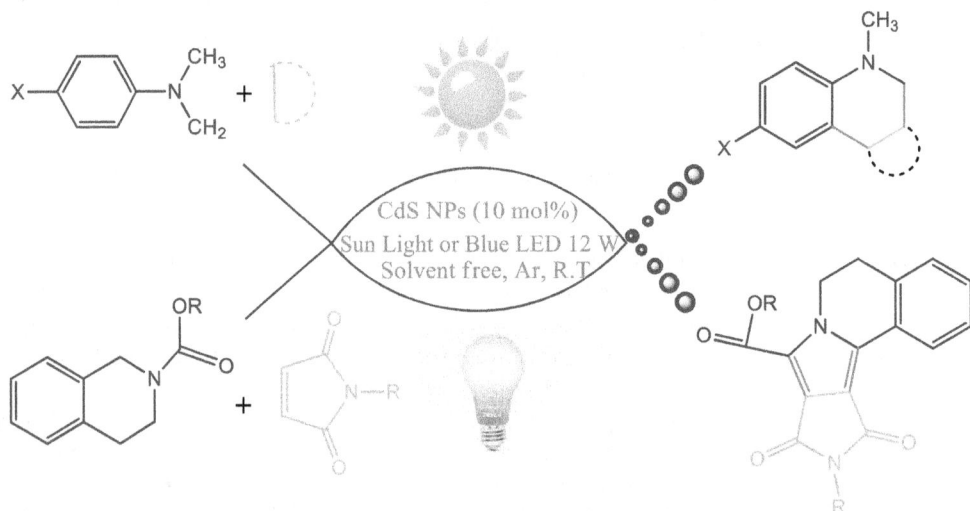

SCHEME 7.38 Solvent-free and RT visible-light-induced C–H activation

derivatives in refluxing water. Therefore, this method represents a considerable enhancement over the conventional methods.[51]

7.7.7 Iron-based Nanocatalyst

Propylsilan and arginine were used for the functionalization of Fe_3O_4 magnetic NPs.[52] The synthesized Fe3O4@PS-arginine (Arg) magnetic NPs were altered to obtain Fe_3O_4@PS-Arg[HSO_4]. These NPs were used as eco-friendly solid acid magnetic NCs for the synthesis of 2-amino-4-arylbenzo[h]quinoline-3-carbonitrile and 10,10-dimethyl-7-aryl-9,10,11,12-tetrahydrobenzo[c] acridin-8(7H)-one derivative via a one-pot reaction of α-naphthilamine and aromatic aldehydes with malononitrile or dimedone. Simple operation, high reaction yields, reusability of catalyst several times, short reaction time, and easy separation from the reaction mixture are the significant benefits of using this catalyst.

7.7.8 Cadmium-based Nanocatalyst

The solvent-free, RT, visible-light-induced C–H activation was studied. [53] Nanosized cadmium sulfide (CdS) were synthesized and applied as a highly efficient reusable photocatalyst. This catalyst was used for the synthesis of pyrrolo[3,4-c]quinolone and pyrrolo[2,1-a]isoquinoline-8-carboxylate derivatives via a condensation reaction. It involved the reaction between N, N-dimethylanilines, or alkyl 2-(3,4-dihydroisoquinolin-2(1H)-yl)acetates with maleimides. This reaction was proceeded through a C–H activation approach under benign and eco-friendly conditions at RT without using any solvent and oxidant under visible light irradiation. Using this method, all favorable products were obtained with good yields with relatively short reaction times under benign conditions with the application of visible light irradiation, which is a renewable energy source. The catalyst was easily recovered and reused several times without any loss of activity.

7.8 CONCLUSION

Quinolines, isoquinolines, and quinolones are important organic compounds because they have greater potential in medicinal and biological fields. Quinolines and isoquinoline derivatives function as antibacterial, antimalarial, antifungal, analgesic, and antihypertensive agents. Isoquinoline is used in the treatment of solid tumors. Quinolone-based drugs are used in many serious diseases. They are obtained naturally from plants and can be synthesized by various named reactions. A variety of synthetic approaches are used for the synthesis of quinolines, isoquinolines, and quinolones and their analogs. The Friedlander and Pfitzinger reactions are commonly used for the synthesis of quinolines. Bischler–Napieralski, Pictet–Spengler, and Pomeranz–Fritsch are employed for the preparation of isoquinolines. However, these reactions have major drawbacks including harsh conditions and lower yields. The use of NCs in the synthesis of quinolines, isoquinolines, and quinolones has gained attention since they offer better reaction conditions, such as mild conditions, are environmentally friendly, with fewer steps. These catalytic transformations are useful in the green synthesis of compounds.

REFERENCES

1. Joule JA, Mills K. Heterocyclic chemistry. 4th ed. Oxford: Blackwell; 2000.
2. Gerd C, Hartmut H. Quinoline and Isoquinoline, Ullmann's Encyclopedia of Industrial a Chemistry. Weinheim: Wiley-VCH: 2005.
3. Hu W, Zhang Y, Zhu H, Ye D, Wang D. Unsymmetrical triazolylnaphthyridinyl-pyridine bridged high active copper complexes supported on reduced graphene oxide and their application in water. Green Chem. 2019. 21:5345–51. doi.10.1039/C9GC02086A.
4. Yang Q, Zhang YL, Zeng W, Duan ZC, Sang X, Wang D. Merrifield resin supported quinone as an efficient biomimetic catalyst for metal-free, base free, chemoselective synthesis of 2,4,6-trisubstituted pyridines. Green Chem. 2019. 21:5683–90. doi./10.1039/C9GC02409C.
5. Bouzian Y, Karrouchi K, Sert Y, Lai CH, Mahi L, Ahabchane NH, Talbaoui A, Mague JT, Essassi EM. Synthesis, spectroscopic characterization, crystal structure, DFT, molecular docking and in vitro antibacterial potential of novel quinoline derivatives. J Mol Struct 2020. 1209:127940–50. doi.10.1016/j.molstruc.2020.127940
6. Ozyanik M, Demirci S, Bektas H, Dem N, Demirbas A, Alpay Karaoglu S. 2012. Preparation and antimicrobial activity evaluation of some quinoline derivatives containing an azole nucleus. Turk J Chem. 2017. 36:233–46. doi.10.3906/kim-1109-9.
7. Graves PR, Kwiek JJ, Fadden P, Ray R, Hardeman K, Coley AM, Foley M, Haystead TAJ. Discovery of novel targets of quinoline drugs in the human purine binding proteome. Mol Pharmacol 2002. 62:1364–72. doi.10.1124/mol.62.6.1364
8. Chen YL, Fang KC, Sheu JY, Chen YL, Fang KC, Sheu JY, Hsu SL, Tzeng CC. Synthesis and antibacterial evaluation of certain quinolone derivatives. J Med Chem. 2001. 44:2374–7. doi.10.1021/jm0100335
9. Pradhan S, Roy S, Ghosh S, Chatterjee I. Regiodivergent aromatic electrophilic substitution using nitrosoarenes in hexafluoroisopropanol: a gateway for diarylamines and p-iminoquinones synthesis, Adv Synth Catal. 2019. 361:4294–401. doi.10.1002/adsc.201900788.
10 Nitidandhaprabhas O. Doebner's reaction with 6-methyl-2-amino pyridine. Nature. 1966. 212:504–5. doi.10.1038/212504b0.

11. Bergstrom FW. Heterocyclic nitrogen compounds. Part IIA. Hexacyclic compounds: pyridine, quinoline, and isoquinoline. Chem Rev. 1944. 35:77–277. doi.10.1021/CR60111A001

12. Born JL. Mechanism of formation of benzo[g]quinolones via the Combes reaction. J Org Chem. (1972) 37:3952–3. doi.10.1021/jo00797a045

13. Theoclitou ME, Robinson LA. Novel facile synthesis of 2, 2, 4 substituted 1, 2-dihydroquinolines via a modified Skraup reaction. Tetrahedron Lett. 2002. 43:3907–10. doi.10.1016/S0040-4039(02)00614-7.

14. Chen SM, Cheng JY, Ma LT, Zhou S, Xu X, Zhi C, Zhang W, Zhi L, Zapien JA. Light-weight 3D Co–N-doped hollow carbon spheres as efficient electro catalysts for rechargeable zinc–air batteries. Nanoscale. 2018, 10:10412–19. doi.10.1039/C8NR01140K

15. Calaway PK, Henze HR. Utilization of aryloxy ketones in the synthesis of quinolines by the pfitzinger reaction. J Am Chem Soc. 1939. 61:1355–8.

16. Tumambac GE, Rosencrance CM, Wolf C. Selective metal ion recognition using a fluorescent 1, 8-diquinolylnaphthalene-derived sensor in aqueous solution. Tetrahedron. 2004. 60:11293–7. doi.10.1016/j.tet.2004.07.053.

17. Calus S, Gondek E, Danel A, Jarosz B, Pokładko M, Kityk AV. Electroluminescence of 6-R-1, 3-diphenyl-1H-pyrazolo [3, 4-b] quinoline-based organic light-emitting diodes (R= F, Br, Cl, CH$_3$, C$_2$H$_3$ and N (C$_6$H$_5$)$_2$ Mater Lett. 2007. 61:3292–5. doi.10.1016/j.matlet.2006.11.055

18. Jones G. In: Katritzky, CW Rees KT, editors. Comprehensive Heterocyclic Chemistry II, Vol. 5, Six-membered rings with one nitrogen atom. AR Potts, Oxford: Pergamon; 1984. p. 167.

19. Caeiro G, Lopes JM, Magnoux P, Caeiro G, Lopes J, Magnoux P, Ayrault P, Ramoaribeiro F. A FT-IR study of deactivation phenomena during methylcyclohexane transformation on H-USY zeolites: Nitrogen poisoning, coke formation, and acidity–activity correlations. J Catal. 2007. 249:234–43. doi.10.1016/j.jcat.2007.04.005

20. Hemmat K, Nasseri MA, Allahresani A. CoFe$_2$O$_4$@SiO$_2$@Co(III) Salen Complex: A Magnetically Recyclable Heterogeneous Catalyst for the Synthesis of Quinoline Derivatives in Water. Chemistry Select. 2019. 4:4339–46. doi.10.1002/slct.201900696.

21. Agasar M, Patil MR, Keri RS. Titanium-based nanoparticles: A novel, facile and efficient catalytic system for one-pot synthesis of quinoline derivatives. Chem Data Collect. 2018. 17:178–86. doi.10.1016/j.cdc.2018.08.001

22. Jafarzadeh M, Soleimani E, Norouzi P, Adnan R, Sepahvand H. Preparation of trifluoroacetic acid-immobilized Fe$_3$O$_4$@ SiO$_2$–APTES nanocatalyst for synthesis of quinolines. J Fluor Chem. 2015. 178:219–24. doi.10.1016/j.jfluchem.2015.08.007.

23. Ojha NK, Zyryanov GV, Majee A, Charushin VN, Chupakhin ON, Santra S. Copper nanoparticles as inexpensive and efficient catalyst: A valuable contribution in organic synthesis. Coord Chem Rev. 2017. 353:1–57. doi.10.1016/j.ccr.2017.10.004.

24. Bihani M, Pasupuleti BG, Bora PP, Bez G, Lal RA. Copper (II) Nitrate Catalyzed Azide–Alkyne Cycloaddition Reaction: Study the Effect of Counter Ion, Role of Ligands and Catalyst Structure. Catal Lett. 2018.148:1315–23. doi.10.1007/s10562-018-2357-9

25. Sharghi H, Aberi M, Shiri P. Silica-supported Cu(II)–quinoline complex: Efficient and recyclable nanocatalyst for one-pot synthesis of benzimidazolquinoline derivatives and 2 H -indazoles. Appl. Organomet. Chem. 2019. 33:e4974. doi:10.1002/aoc.4974

26. Xie R, Lu GP, Jiang HF, Zhang M. Selective reductive annulation reaction for direct synthesis of functionalized quinolines by a cobalt nanocatalyst. J Catal. 2020. 383:239–43. doi.10.1016/j.jcat.2020.01.034.

27. Soleimani E, Naderi Namivandi M, Sepahvand H. ZnCl$_2$ supported on Fe$_3$O$_4$@ SiO$_2$ core–shell nanocatalyst for the synthesis of quinolines via Friedländer synthesis under solvent-free condition. Appl Organomet Chem. 2017. 31:e3566–e74. doi.10.1002/aoc.3566.

28. Lotfi S, Nikseresht A, Rahimi N. Synthesis of Fe$_3$O$_4$@ SiO$_2$/isoniazid/Cu (II) magnetic nanocatalyst as a recyclable catalyst for a highly efficient preparation of quinolines in moderate conditions. Polyhedron. 2019. 173:114148–55. doi.10.1016/j.poly.2019.114148

29. Harikrishna S, Robert AR, Ganja H, Maddila S, Jonnalagadda SB. A green, facile and recyclable Mn3O4/MWCNT nano-catalyst for the synthesis of quinolines via one-pot multicomponent reactions. Sustain Chem Pharm. 2020. 16:100265–71. doi.10.1016/j.scp.2020.100265.

30. Sajjadi-Ghotbabadi H, Javanshir S, Rostami-Charati F. Nano KF/clinoptilolite: an effective heterogeneous base nanocatalyst for synthesis of substituted quinolines in water. Catal Lett. 2016. 146:338–44. doi.10.1007/s10562-015-1652-y.

31. Mahajan A, Arya A, Chundawat TS. Green synthesis of silver nanoparticles using green alga (*Chlorella vulgaris*) and its application for synthesis of quinolines derivatives. Synth Commun. 2019. 49:1926–37. doi.10.1080/00397911.2019.1610776.

32. Kumar NS, Reddy MS, Bheeram VR, Mukkamala SB, Raju Chowhan L, Chandrasekhara Rao L. Zinc oxide nanoparticles as efficient catalyst for the synthesis of novel dispiroindolizidine bisoxindoles in aqueous medium. Environ Chem Lett. 2019. 17:455–64. doi.10.1007/s10311-018-0772-1.

33. Hoogewerf S, van Dorp WA. Sur quelques dérivés de l'isoquinoléine. Recueil des Travaux Chemiques des Pays-Bas. 1886. 5:305–312.

34. Rostamizadeh S, Nojavan M, Aryan R Isapoor E, Azad M. Amino acid-based ionic liquid immobilized on α-Fe$_2$O$_3$-MCM-41: An efficient magnetic nanocatalyst and recyclable reaction media for the synthesis of quinazolin-4(3H)-one derivatives. J Mol Catal A: Chem. 2013. 374:102–10. doi.10.1016/j.molcata.2013.04.002

35. Hamedani NF, Ghazvini M, Azad L, Noushin A. Green synthesis of pyrido[2,1-a]isoquinolines and pyrido[1,2-a]quinolins using Fe3O4-MNPs as efficient nanocatalyst: Study of antioxidant activity. J Heterocyclic Chem. 2019. 57:1–9. doi.10.1002/jhet.3782

36. Ezzatzadeh E, Hargalani FZ, Shafaei F, Ezzatzadeh E, Hargalani FZ, Shafaei F. Bio-Fe3O4-MNPs Promoted Green Synthesis of Pyrido[2,1-a]isoquinolines and Pyrido[1,2-a]quinolines: Study of Antioxidant and Antimicrobial Activity. Polycycl Aromat Compnd. 2021. doi.10.1080/10406638.2021.1879882

37. Abbasi M, Hargalani FZ, Afrashteh S, Rostamian R. Bio-Fe3O4-MNPs catalyzed green synthesis of pyrrolo[2,1-a]isoquinoline derivatives using isoquinolium bromide salts: study of antioxidant activity. Can J Chem. 2019. 00: 1–8.doi.10.1139/cjc-2019-0167

38. Ghazvini M, Farahani FS, Amiri SS, Sheikholeslami-Farahani F, Ghazvini M, Soleimani-Amiri S, Salimifard M, Rostamian R. Green Synthesis of Pyrido[2,1-a]isoquinolines and Pyrido[1,2-a]quinolines by Using ZnO Nanoparticles. Syn Lett. 2018. 29:493–96. doi.10.1055/s-0036-1591509.

39. Khan FN, Manivel P, Prabakaran K. Jin JS, Jeong ED, Kim HG, Maiyalagan T. Iron-oxide nanoparticles mediated cyclization of 3-(4-chlorophenyl)-1-hydrazinylisoquinoline to 1-(4,5-dihydropyrazol-1-yl)isoquinolines. Res Chem Intermed. 2012. 38:571–82.

40. Amiri SS, Hossaini Z, Arabkhazaeli M, Karami H, Afshari Sharif Abad S. Green synthesis of pyrimido-isoquinolines and pyrimidoquinoline using ZnO nanorods as an efficient catalyst: Study of antioxidant activity. J Chin Chem Soc. 2018. 1–8. www.jccs.wiley-vch.de/

41. Mousavi SF, Hossaini Z, Zareyee D. Green synthesis of pyrrolo isoquinolines using in situ synthesis of 4-hydroxycumarines: Study of antioxidant activity. J Heterocyclic Chem. 2020. 57(11):3856–67. doi.10.1002/jhet.4091.

42. Amiri SS. Green production and antioxidant activity study of new pyrrolo[2,1-a]isoquinolines. J Heterocyclic Chem. 2020. 1–13. doi.10.1002/jhet.4115

43. Amiri SS, Ghazvini M, Khandan S, Afrashteh S. KF/Clinoptilolite@MWCNTs Nanocomposites Promoted a Novel Four-Component Reaction of Isocyanides for the Green Synthesis of Pyrimidoisoquinolines in Water. Polycycl Aromat Compd. 2021. doi.10.1080/10406638.2021.1912122

44. Rawat M, Rawat DS. CuO@NiO Nanocomposite Catalyzed Synthesis of Biologically Active Indenoisoquinoline Derivatives. ACS Sustainable Chem Eng. 2020. 8: 13701–12. doi.10.1021/acssuschemeng.0c03898.

45. Thakur V, Sharma A, Yamini, Sharma N, Das P. Supported Palladium Nanoparticles-Catalyzed Synthesis of 3- Substituted 2-Quinolones from 2-Iodoanilines and Alkynes Using Oxalic Acid as C1 Source. Adv Synth Catal. 2019. 361:426–31.

46. Kataria M, Kumar M, Bhalla V. Supramolecular Ensemble of Tetraphenylcyclopentadienone Derivative and HgO nanoparticles: A One-Pot Approach for the Synthesis of Quinoline and Quinolone Derivatives. Chemistry Select. 2017. 2:3018–27.

47. Bhardwaj D, Singh A, Singh R. Eco-compatible sonochemical synthesis of 8-aryl-7,8-dihydro-[1,3]-dioxolo[4,5-g]quinolin-6(5H)-ones using green TiO$_2$. Heliyon 5. 2019. e01256.doi:10.1016/j.heliyon.2019.e01256

48. Jalili F, Zarei M, Zolfigol MA, Rostamnia S, Moosavi-Zare AR. SBA-15/PrN(CH$_2$PO$_3$H$_2$)$_2$ as a novel and efficient mesoporous solid acid catalyst with phosphorous acid tags and its application on the synthesis of new pyrimido[4,5-b]quinolones and pyrido[2,3-d]pyrimidines via anomeric based oxidation. Microporous Mesoporous Mater. 2019. doi.10.1016/j.micromeso.2019.109865.

49. Ahn BH, Lee Y, Lim HM. Step-economical synthesis of 3-amido-2-quinolones by dendritic copper powder-mediated one-pot reaction. Org Biomol Chem. 2018. 16:7851–60.

50. Azad CS, Narula Ak. An operational transformation of 3-carboxy-4-quinolones into 3-nitro-4-quinolones via ipso nitration using polysaccharide supported copper nanoparticles: synthesis of 3-tetrazolyl bioisosteresm of 3-carboxy-4-quinolones as antibacterial agents. RSC Adv. 2016. 6:19052–9.

51. Nakhaei A, Davoodnia A, Yadegarian S. Application of ZrO$_2$–SO$_3$H as highly efficient recyclable nanocatalyst for the green synthesis of fluoroquinolones as potential antibacterial. QJICC. 2019. 7:230–306.

52. Karkhah MK, Kefayati H, Shariati S. Synthesis of benzo[*h*]quinolone and benzo[*c*]acridinone derivatives by Fe$_3$O$_4$@PS-Arginine[HSO$_4$] as an efficient magnetic nanocatalyst. J of Heterocycl Chem. 2020. 57: 4181–91.

53. Firoozi S, Hosseini-Sarvari M, Koohgard M. Solvent-free and room temperature visible light-induced C–H activation: CdS as a highly efficient photo-induced reusable nano-catalyst for the C–H functionalization cyclization of *t*-amines and C–C double and triple bonds. Green Chem. 2018. 20: 5540–9.

8 Recent Advances in Nanocatalyzed Synthesis of Triazoles and Tetrazoles and Their Biological Studies

Popat M. Jadhav,[1] A. B. Kanagare,[1] Anand B. Dhirbassi,[1]
Atam B. Tekale,[2] R. M. Borade,[3] S. U. Tekale,[1]
Keshav Lalit Ameta,[4] and R. P. Pawar[5]

[1] Department of Chemistry, Deogiri College, Aurangabad, Maharashtra, India

[2] Department of Chemistry, Shri Shivaji College, Parbhani, Maharashtra, India

[3] Department of Chemistry, Government Institute of Forensic Science, Aurangabad, Maharashtra, India

[4] Department of Chemistry, School of Liberal Arts and Sciences, Mody University of Science and Technology, Lakshmangarh, Rajasthan, India

[5] Department of Chemistry, Shiv Chattrapati College, Aurangabad, Maharashtra, India

8.1 INTRODUCTION

Triazole is a five-membered heterocyclic compound that has three nitrogen (N) and two carbon (C) atoms. It exists in two isomeric forms: -1,2,3-triazole (**1**), and 1,2,4-triazole(**2**). The 1,2,3 isomer contains three N atoms adjacent to one another, and the 1,2,4 isomer has two N atoms adjacent to each other, and the third N is present between both C atoms.

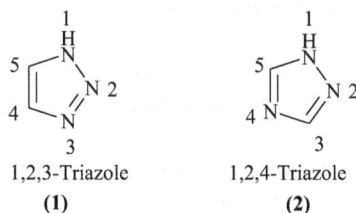

1,2,3-Triazole   1,2,4-Triazole
(1)   (2)

1,2,3-triazole and its derivatives are well documented for various biological activities, such as antimicrobial, analgesic, anti-HIV, anti-inflammatory, anti-allergic, anticancer, antimalarial, and antitubercular.[1,2] The 1, 2, 4-triazoles play an important role in medicinal chemistry and have various biological activities, such as antimicrobial, antimalarial, anticancer, antioxidant, and antimycotic.[3] The triazole ring has proved to be a medicinally important scaffold for various commercially marketed drugs, such as alprazolam, rizatriptan, trazodone, and hexaconazole. Therefore, the small triazole nucleus has several biological activities and is a privileged scaffold for medicinal chemists.

DOI: 10.1201/9781003141488-8

Tetrazoles are the heterocyclic compounds that have a five-membered ring composed of four N atoms and one C atom and exists in three different isomeric forms (**3**), (**4**), (**5**):

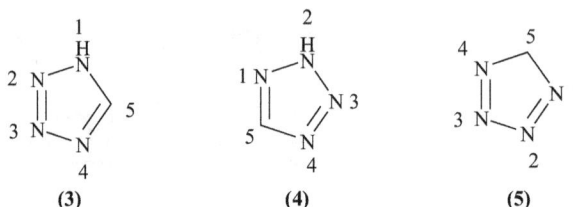

| (3) | (4) | (5) |

The heterocyclic compounds that have a tetrazole moiety have attracted the attention of medicinal and organic chemists due to their unique structures in various antihypertensive, anti-allergic, anti-biotic, and anticonvulsant agents.[4–5] These tetrazoles have extensive applications in photography, recording systems, and the biological sciences.[6–7]

Structural modifications of the triazole and tetrazole rings can lead to improved biological activities with improved potency and lower toxicity. This chapter provides an overview of recent updates on the biological potential and various methods for the synthesis of triazole and tetrazole based heterocycles that use nanomaterials as catalysts.

8.2   BIOLOGICAL SIGNIFICANCE OF TRIAZOLES AND TETRAZOLES:

The Schiff bases of 4-amino-1, 2, 4-triazoles (**6**) were synthesized by the condensation of 4-amino-1,2,4-triazol-3-ones with aromatic aldehydes under ultrasound irradiation and documented for antioxidant activity using the 2,2-diphenyl-1-picrylhydrazyl (DPPH) method. The DPPH inhibition values of the compounds were from 71.2% to 96.4% at 1.20 μM. Molecular docking of the synthesized compounds with the active site of angiotensin I-converting enzyme (ACE) revealed good inhibitory effects of the triazole Schiff's bases.[8]

The glycosyl 1, 2, 3-triazoles (**7**) were synthesized by reactions of the corresponding azides with vinyl acetate under microwave irradiation. The unprotected glucosyl and galactosyl triazoles did not display inhibitory activity at 1 mM. Among the screened samples, the GlcNAc-triazole was hydrolyzed by *Talaromyces flavus* CCF 2686 β-N-acetyl hexosaminidase. Furthermore, the β-GlcNActriazole acted as a strong ligand for rat and human natural killer cell-activating receptors.[9]

The 1, 2, 4-triazoles (**8**) were evaluated for antimicrobial activity by Stingaci et al. The compounds were highly active against *Xanthomonas campestris*. The antifungal activity of these compounds was better than the reference drugs.[10]

1,2,4-triazole-spirodienone (**9**) was a promising pharmacophore for anticancer activity. It showed remarkable in vitro cytotoxic activity by arresting the cell cycle and showed induction of apoptosis in MDA-MB-231 cells.[11]

The 1, 2, 4-triazoles (**10**) were evaluated for tyrosinase inhibition potential by Akin et al. The inhibition mechanism of these compounds was reversible and uncompetitive on tyrosinase activity. The most promising compound was bound weakly with the receptor via interactions with His244, His263, Phe264, and Val283.[12]

The Schiff bases that contained 1, 2, 4-triazole-3(4H)-thione (**11**) were documented for antifungal activity. These compounds were more effective against *Wheat gibberellic* compared with the fluconazole standard. The more active compounds were evaluated for enzyme inhibition efficacy against the receptor CYP51 by docking.[13]

The 1H-1,2,3-triazol-4-ylindoline-2,3-diones (**12**), (**13**) were highly active against *Staphylococcus epidermidis*, *Bacillus subtilis*, *Escherichia coli*, and *Pseudomonas aeruginosa*. Some of them exhibited better antifungal potential than the standard fluconazole against *Aspergillus niger* and

Candida albicans. The results demonstrated the key role of the triazole unit in these compounds for high antimicrobial activities.[14]

The 3-amino-1, 2, 4-triazole scaffolds that contained compounds (**14**) and (**15**) were evaluated for anticancer activity against cancer cell lines using a (3-(4,5-dimethylthiazol-2-yl)-2,5-diphenyltetrazolium bromide (MTT) assay. In addition, these compounds exhibited good anti-angiogenic activity that indicated their highly promising dual anticancer activity.[15]

The 1,2,3-triazoles (**16**) were synthesized via an azide–alkyne click chemistry approach and evaluated for anti-leishmanial activity against the promastigote form of *Leishmania donovani.* Three of these compounds were identified for a promising anti-leishmanial activity and were non-cytotoxic towards macrophage cells. The molecular docking study supported good interactions with the key residues in the catalytic site of trypanothione reductase.[16]

The 1,4-disubstituted triazole or a-ketotriazole (**17**) derivatives synthesized by the copper-catalyzed (Cu)[3+2] cycloaddition of alkynes with different azides that had a lipophilic chain mimicking the substrate were able to inhibit InhA. One of the compounds exhibited a minimum inhibitory concentration <2 mg/mL against *Mycobacterium tuberculosis* H37Rv.[17]

The disubstituted-1,2,3-triazole-thiosemicarbazone hybrid molecules (**18**) exhibited an excellent potency result for *B. subtilis* and *P. aeruginosa* compared with the reference drug ciprofloxacin. Antibacterial activity results were supported by molecular docking and density-functional theory (DFT) studies.[18]

The triazoles (**19**) were reported for an inhibitory potential of cyclin-dependent kinase 5 enzyme.[19]

The fluorine and piperazine moiety that had 1,2,4-triazole thione derivatives (**20**) synthesized by the Mannich reaction of triazole intermediates, substituted piperazines, and formaldehyde was documented for significant fungicidal activity against *Cercospora arachidicola*, *Physalospora piricola*, and *Rhizoctonia cerealis* at 50 mg/mL.[20]

The Schiff bases of 1, 2, 4-triazole derivatives (**21**) synthesized by the condensation of N-[(4-amino-5-sulfanyl-4H-1, 2, 4-triazol-3-yl)methyl]-4-substituted-benzamides with various aldehydes exhibited good antibacterial and antifungal activity.[21]

The 1, 2, 4-triazole-3(4H)-thiones (**22**) were screened for antibacterial and antifungal activity by Spoor et al. Some of the compounds exhibited significant antimicrobial activity.[22]

Khan et al developed the triazole heterocyclic derivatives (**23**) for analgesic, ulcerogenic, and anti-inflammatory activity.[23]

Penjarla et al. documented tetrazoles (**24**) that had C-nucleoside analogs for antitumor activity.[24]

The newly synthesized drug candidate (**25**) was shown to have in vitro anticancer potential by Dhiman et al.[25]

Maheshwari et al. documented a series of 1H-tetrazole derivatives (**26**) for protein tyrosine phosphatase 1B (PTP1B) inhibitory activity. Among the series, the 5-Cl substituted benzothiazole analogs revealed considerable PTP1B inhibition with an IC_{50} of 1.88 μM aligned with the reference standard suramin ($IC_{50} \geq 10$ μM). In addition, excellent in vivo antidiabetic activity of these compounds was observed compared with the standard drugs glimepiride and metformin. Studies revealed the necessity of the presence of a tetrazole moiety for the enhancement of non-carboxylic inhibitors of PTP1B through antidiabetic potential.[26]

Inspired by the chemical structure of cilostazol, a selective phosphodiesterase 3A (PDE3A) inhibitor, which are the new hybrids of nucleobases and tetrazoles (**27**) were synthesized and studied for inhibitory activity on PDE3A and their cytotoxicity on HeLa and MCF-7 cancerous cell lines by Shekouhy et al. The obtained results showed a linear correlation between the inhibitory effect of the synthesized compounds and their cytotoxicity. In some cases, the PDE3A inhibitory effects of synthesized compounds were higher than cilostazol. Some of the synthesized compounds revealed higher cytotoxicity against the HeLa and MCF-7 cancerous cell lines.[27]

Zhang et al. documented 31 ursolic acids that had a tetrazole moiety (**28**) for potential antitumor activities as a HIF-1α transcriptional inhibitor. The structure–activity relationships of these

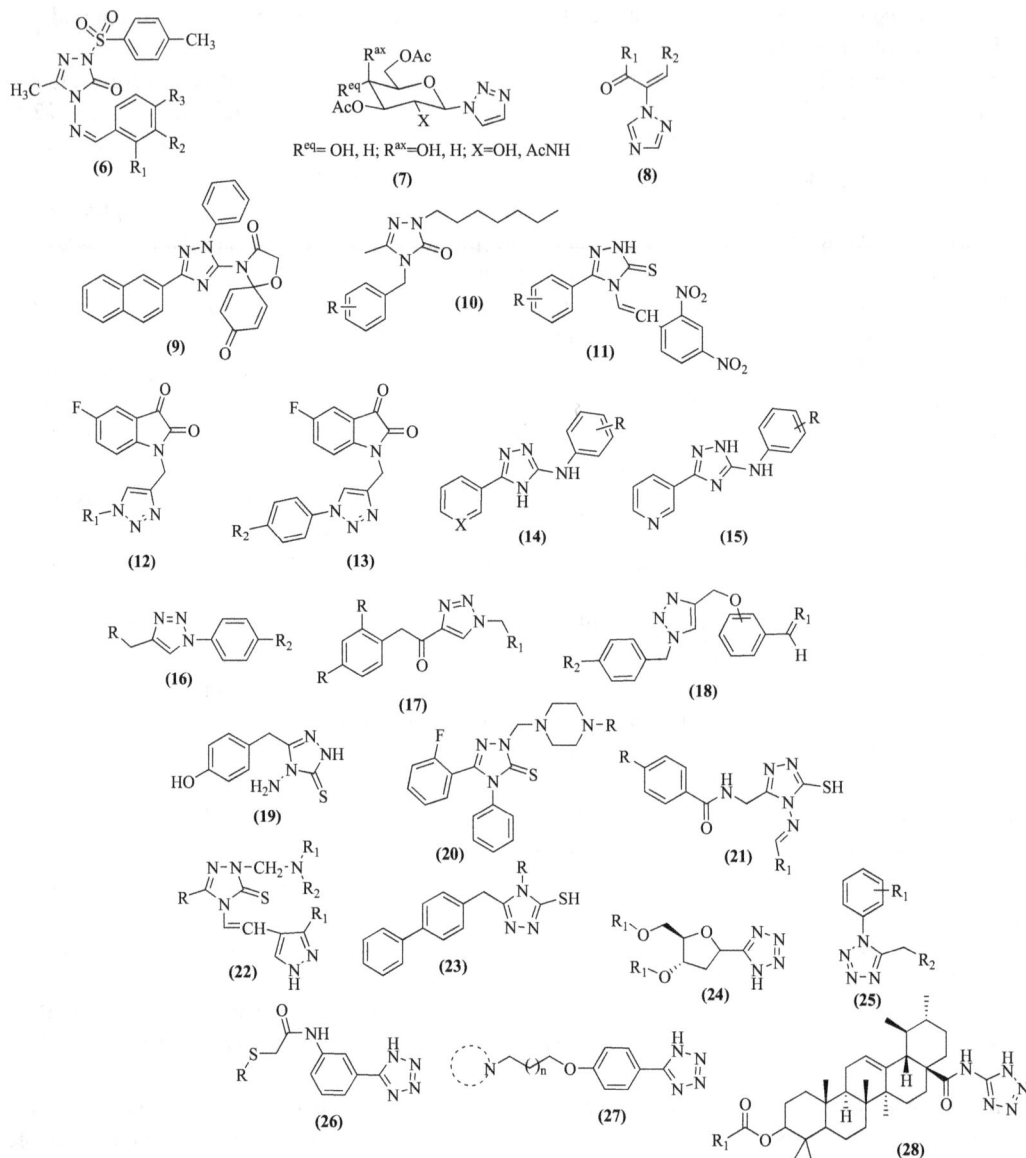

FIGURE 8.1 Structures biologically active compounds containing triazoles and tetrazoles

compounds through HIF-1α highlighted the existence of a tetrazole group at C-28 to enhance their inhibitory activities.[28]

The structures of some biologically active heterocyclic compounds that have triazoles and tetrazole moieties are shown in Figure 8.1.

8.3 RECENT DEVELOPMENTS IN THE NANOMATERIAL CATALYZED SYNTHESIS OF TRIAZOLES AND TETRAZOLES

A literature survey revealed various developments in the synthesis of triazoles and tetrazoles that used nanomaterials as efficient heterogeneous catalysts. This section will discuss the recent developments in this field.

Bahadorikhalili et al. introduced β-cyclodextrin functionalized polyethylene glycol (PEG)ylated mesoporous silica nanoparticles–graphene oxide hybrid (Si NP–GO) as heterogeneous support for the immobilization of a copper (Cu) catalyst (Cu@βCD-PEG-mesoGO). The mesoporous Si NP–GO hybrid (mesoGO) was synthesized and functionalized using PEG_{600} ended β-cyclodextrin. Then, the Cu was immobilized onto the modified NPs and Cu@βCD-PEG-mesoGO was evaluated for the synthesis of 1, 2, 3-triazoles via the three-component click reaction using benzyl bromides, alkynes, and sodium azide (Scheme 8.1). This catalyst has excellent properties, such as easy workup process, high efficiency, and turnover frequency (TOF), mild reaction conditions, use of water (H_2O) as a green solvent, and easy catalyst recovery.[29]

Basu et al. developed silver (Ag) NPs supported on an Al2O3@Fe2O3 core-shell nanostructured material that used the aqueous phase reduction method. The material exhibited a large scope in heterogeneous catalysis due to the fine dispersion of the reactive NPs on the increased surface area of the material. This core-shell mesoporous NC exhibited high catalytic efficiency during the acylation of benzyl alcohol under solvent-free conditions and the synthesis of 1, 4-disubstituted 1, 2, 3-triazoles in an aqueous medium (Scheme 8.2). The catalyst was heterogeneous, and therefore, could be easily recovered and reused without a significant decrease in catalytic activity.[30]

Sarma et al. synthesized Cu NPS using hydrotalcite as solid support for the azide–alkyne cycloaddition reaction for the development of a facile route to the synthesis of 1, 4-disubstituted-1, 2, 3-triazoles (Scheme 8.3). The catalyst was heterogeneous and could be easily reused and recycled. The reaction was carried out at room temperature (RT) and the use of ethylene glycol as a solvent made it an environmentally friendly system for the synthesis of 1,4-disubstituted-1,2,3-triazoles.[31]

Elayadi et al. developed a method for the synthesis of nanowire copper oxide (CuO) as a catalyst for the 1, 3-dipolar cycloaddition of organic azides to terminal alkynes under mild reaction conditions to give 1, 4-disubstituted 1, 2, 3-triazole as a single regioisomer with excellent yields with the reusability of the catalyst (Scheme 8.4).[32]

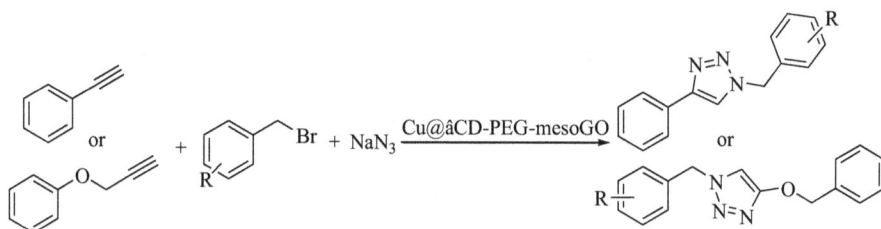

SCHEME 8.1

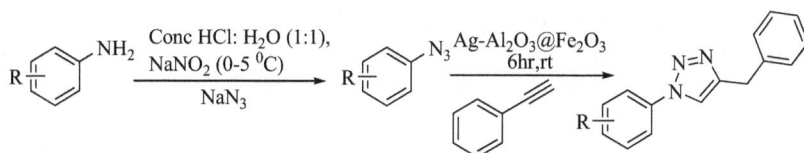

SCHEME 8.2

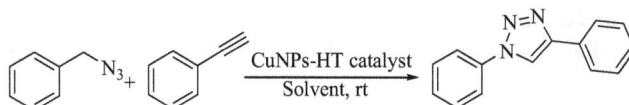

SCHEME 8.3

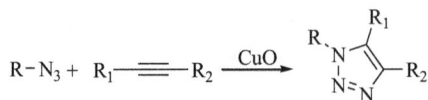

SCHEME 8.4

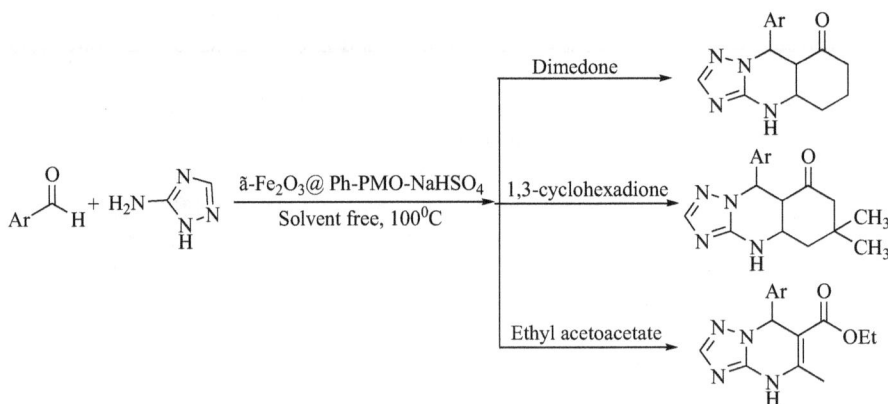

SCHEME 8.5

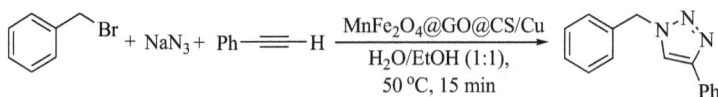

SCHEME 8.6

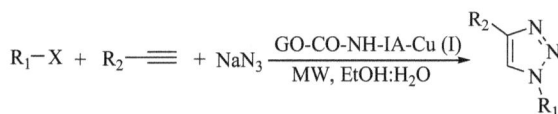

SCHEME 8.7

Haghighat et al. developed core-shell phenylene bridged mesoporous periodic magnetic organosilica NPs immobilized on $NaHSO_4$ (γ-Fe2O3@Ph-PMO-NaHSO4) as a novel magnetically separable acidic nanocatalyst (Scheme 8.5). This protocol offered several advantages, such as high yields, easy and quick isolation of the products, short reaction time, and good reusability of the catalyst.[33]

Mahdavinasab et al. reported a magnetic chitosan-based biocomposite, MnFe2O4@GO@chitosan/Cu, and used it as a competent heterogeneous catalyst for the synthesis of triazoles (Scheme 8.6). The easy separation, reusability, recovery, and high yields of the products made this protocol cheap and gave an environmentally friendly material for the synthesis of triazoles.[34]

Naeimi et al. developed functionalized Go–Cu(I) complex as a catalyst for the synthesis of 1, 2, 3-triazoles by the reaction of alkynes, alkyl halides, and sodium azide under microwave irradiation with excellent yields (Scheme 8.7).[35]

Oxidized Cu NPs supported on titanium dioxide (TiO_2) were shown to catalyze the multicomponent synthesis of 1,2,3-triazoles via [3+2] Huisgen's 1, 3-dipolar cyclo-addition in

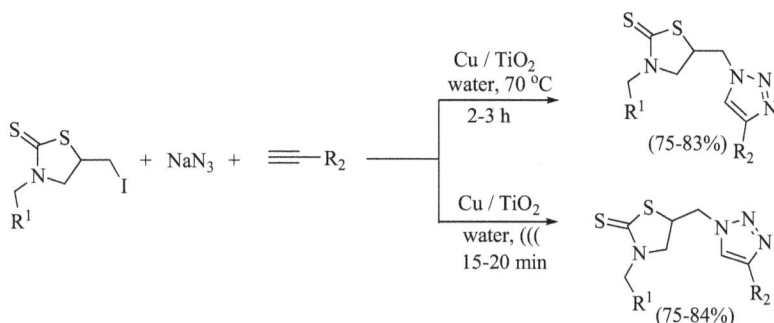

SCHEME 8.8

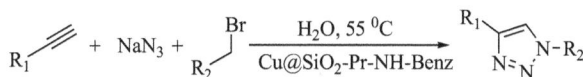

SCHEME 8.9

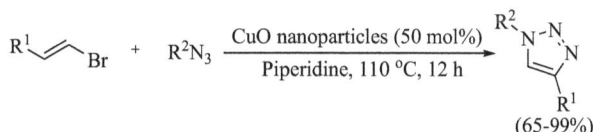

SCHEME 8.10

an aqueous medium under conventional heating and ultrasonic irradiation conditions (Scheme 8.8). The catalyst was easily synthesized by copper nitrate in deionized water via the ultrasound-enhanced impregnation (UIM) method. These compounds exhibited good antibacterial activity against *Staphylococcus aureus* and *E. coli*.[36]

Shadjou et al. synthesized an innovative NC (Cu/SiO$_2$-Pr-NH-Benz) and utilized it for coupling and click reactions in an aqueous medium. They reported a resourceful and simple approach for synthesizing a variety of 1, 2, 3-triazole, and propargylamine derivatives with excellent yields within a short reaction time (Scheme 8.9). The most significant advantage of this catalyst was enhanced catalytic activity with competent recycling in the one-pot synthesis of propargyl amine derivatives and 1, 4-disubstituted triazoles under green conditions.[37]

Commercially available CuO nanoparticles (CNP) were used as a heterogeneous catalyst for the synthesis of 1, 2, 3-triazoles with good to excellent yields. The synthesis of triazoles was achieved by the azide–olefin cycloaddition on bromoalkenes and organic azides (Scheme 8.10).[38]

The CNPs on activated carbon (AC) were shown to be an efficient catalyst for the multicomponent synthesis of β-hydroxy-1,2,3-triazoles from variously substituted epoxides and alkynes in an aqueous medium (Scheme 8.11). Mechanistic aspects of the reaction were studied by researchers to understand the participation of Cu(I) acetylides during the reactions.[39]

CNPs on AC were used as a catalytic material for the multicomponent synthesis of 1, 2, 3-triazoles from different azide precursors in an aqueous medium. The contents were heated at 70°C and the products were obtained in high purity without the need for further purification (Scheme 8.12).[40]

Sharghi documented CNPs supported on C (Cu/C) as a heterogeneous catalyst for the one-pot three-component regioselective [3+2] Huisgen cycloaddition of alkyl or benzyl halides, terminal

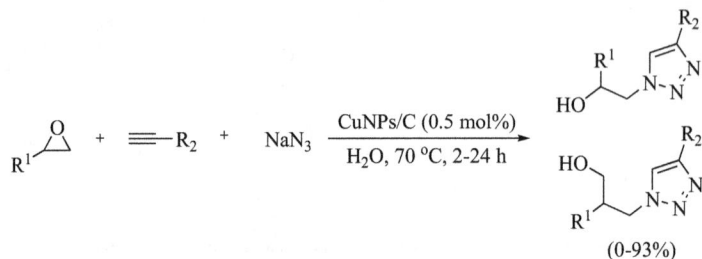

SCHEME 8.11

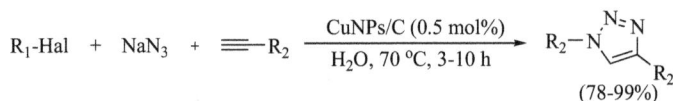

SCHEME 8.12

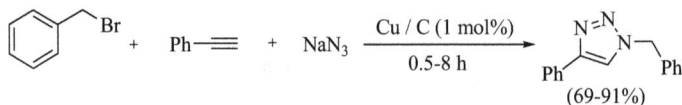

SCHEME 8.13

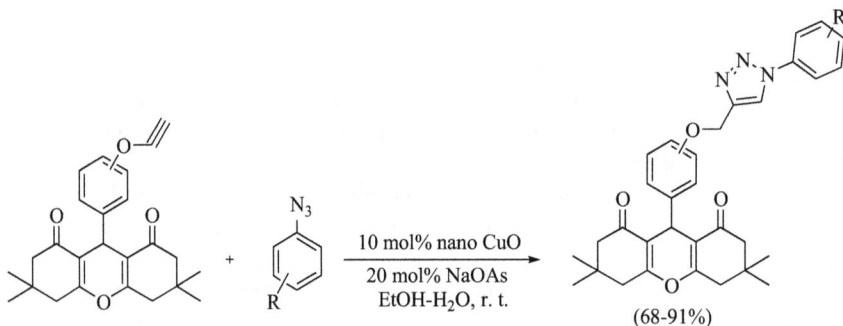

SCHEME 8.14

alkynes, and sodium azide in H_2O as a green solvent that gave the corresponding 1, 2, 3-triazoles in excellent yields. The inductively coupled plasma (ICP) analysis study revealed the presence of Cu in the heterogeneous catalyst as 9.97% (w/w) (Scheme 8.13).[41]

Iniyavan et al. studied the 1, 3-dipolar cycloaddition (CuAAC) of aromatic azides and acetylenic xanthenes that used Cu (II) oxide (CuO) NPs that gave the corresponding xanthene substituted triazoles with excellent yields. The protocol produced the products under mild reaction conditions (RT), within a short reaction time (Scheme 8.14).[42]

Rajabi-Moghaddam developed Cu(II)-coated magnetic core-shell NPs Fe3O4@ SiO_2-2-aminobenzohydrazide as an efficient catalyst for the synthesis of 1,2,3-triazoles by the reaction of benzyl bromides, sodium azide, and terminal alkynes via click chemistry (Scheme 8.15). The catalyst had high efficiency along with good reusability for up to six consecutive runs.[43]

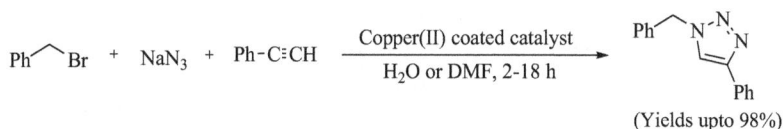

SCHEME 8.15

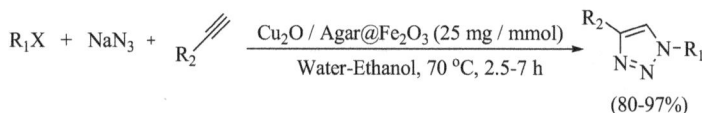

SCHEME 8.16

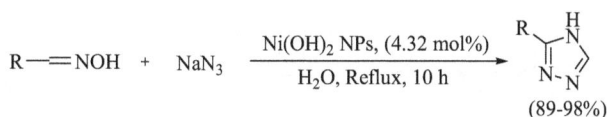

SCHEME 8.17

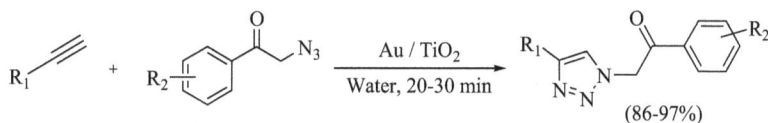

SCHEME 8.18

Copper (I) oxide nanoparticles (CNPs) supported on magnetic agar (Cu₂O/Agar@ Fe₃O₄) were used as a green and cost-effective heterogeneous NC for the synthesis of 1, 4-disubstituted 1, 2, 3-triazoles in high yields in H₂O: ethanol (EtOH) as the reaction medium (Scheme 8.16). Separation of the catalyst was successfully carried out by an external magnet, which could be reused for at least five subsequent runs without significant activity loss.[44]

Halder et al. documented the synthesis of β-nickel hydroxide NPs, which were used as an efficient catalyst for the synthesis of variously substituted tetrazoles by the reaction of oximes with sodium azide under mild reaction conditions (Scheme 8.17). This method had several advantages, such as high efficiency, broad substrate scope, easy handling, higher efficiency, low cost, and reusability of the heterogeneous catalytic system. The catalyst exhibited excellent catalytic activity due to its nanocrystalline nature, small particle size, large surface area, and good thermal stability.[45]

Nanoporous TiO₂ supported gold (Au) NPs were synthesized by the deposition–precipitation method and the synthesized NPs were reported for the green synthesis of 1,4-disubstituted-1,2,3-triazole derivatives via the 1,3-dipolar cycloaddition of organic azides with a variety of terminal alkynes in an aqueous medium. The method gave good to excellent yields with high selectivity for the regioselective synthesis of 1, 2, 3-triazoles involving the Huisgen [3+2] cycloaddition reaction (Schemes 8.18 and 8.19).[46]

A green and efficient method was developed for the synthesis of 1,2,3-triazoles using CNPs supported on nanocellulose (CuNPs/NC) as a reusable catalyst for the synthesis of 1,2,3-triazoles via the azide–alkyne cycloaddition reaction in glycerol as the environmentally benign solvent at an ambient temperature (Scheme 8.20).[47]

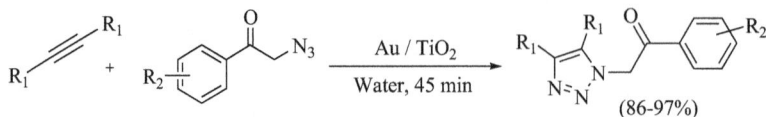

SCHEME 8.19

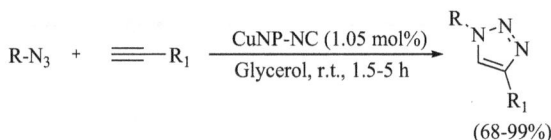

SCHEME 8.20

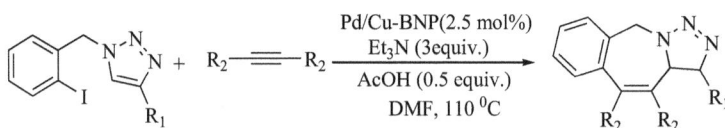

SCHEME 8.21

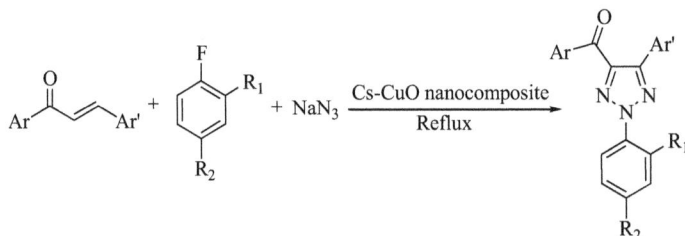

SCHEME 8.22

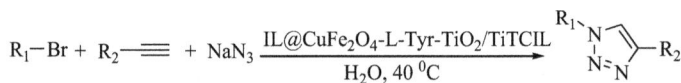

SCHEME 8.23

Saha et al. synthesized metal–C bond stabilized alloy structured palladium (Pd/Cu) bimetallic NPs with binaphthyl moiety as a stabilizer (Pd/Cu-BNP). The Pd/Cu-BNP was used as a capable and recyclable catalyst for the synthesis of polycyclic triazoles through domino alkyne insertion and C–hydrogen (C–H) bond functionalization reaction sequence (Scheme 8.21).[48]

Khalil et al. developed a chitosan Cu(II) oxide nanocomposite, which was developed for the synthesis of [1, 2, 3] triazoles. The nanocomposite showed a powerful catalytic activity to catalyze the multicomponent regioselective cycloaddition of chalones, aryl halides, and sodium azide to give N-2-aryl[1,2,3]triazoles (80%–95% yield) (Scheme 8.22).[49]

Sharma et al. reported the synthesis of novel heterogeneous magnetic NC (IL@CuFe2O4-L-Tyr-TiO2/TiTCIL), which provided an eco-friendly procedure with several advantages, such as aqueous medium as the solvent, operational simplicity, easy workup, short reaction time, and excellent

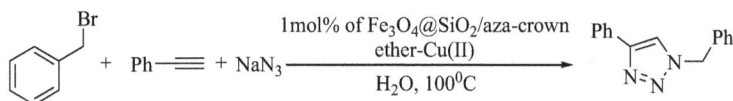

SCHEME 8.24

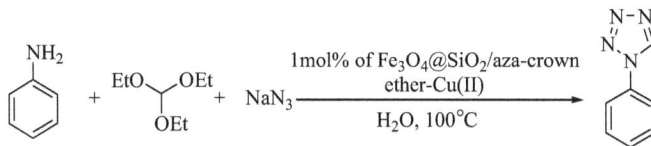

SCHEME 8.25

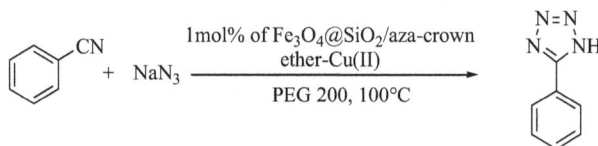

SCHEME 8.26

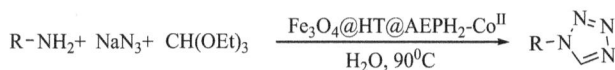

SCHEME 8.27

yields during the synthesis of 1,4-disubstituted-1,2,3-triazoles (Scheme 8.23) via click reaction. Furthermore, IL@CuFe$_2$O$_4$-L-Tyr-TiO$_2$/TiTCIL showed good photocatalytic activity in the degradation of methylene blue dye in visible light.[50]

Rezaei et al. reported a novel and efficient magnetic NC using covalent grafting of Si-coated aza crown ether Cu(II) complex on an iron oxide (FeO) support. The newly developed catalyst was studied for the synthesis of tetrazole and triazole derivatives (Schemes 8.24–26). This method had several important features, such as short reaction time, high yields, simple synthesis, magnetic separation, and favorable recoverability of the catalyst.[51]

Salimi et al. developed a novel NC Fe3O4@HT@AEPH2-CoII using Co(II) immobilized onto aminated ferrite NPs. The resultant NC showed large catalytic activity for the synthesis of 1-substituted-1-H-tetrazole in an aqueous medium (Scheme 8.27). The developed method acted as a green protocol that offered an excellent yield of the products along with an easy operational procedure, minimum chemical waste, mild reaction conditions, short reaction time, easy catalyst synthesis, and up to four cycles of recyclability of the catalyst.[52]

Tamoradi et al. synthesized three novel and nanoscale green magnetic solid base catalysts (CoFe2O4@glycine-M (where M = Pr, Tb, or Yb)) and used them as reusable heterogeneous NCs for the synthesis of 5-substituted 1H–tetrazoles under green reaction conditions (Scheme 8.28). This method had excellent advantages, such as operational simplicity, easy isolation of the products, high activity, and reusability for several consecutive runs without major loss of their catalytic efficiency.[53]

Zarchi et al. developed a novel method for the one-pot synthesis of 5-substituted 1H tetrazole from aryl halide including in situ cyanide group (-CN) insertion from an inorganic salt in the presence of a novel magnetic catalyst, Pd on a surface-modified Schiff Base complex (Scheme 8.29). The NC

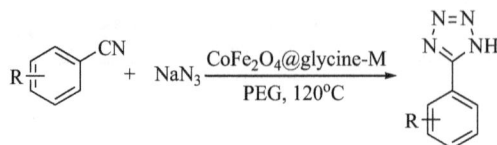

SCHEME 8.28

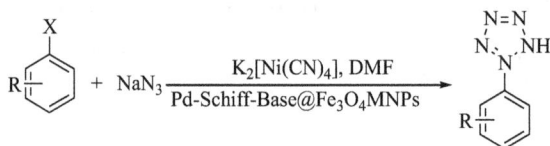

SCHEME 8.29

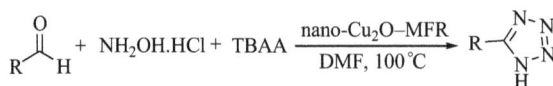

SCHEME 8.30

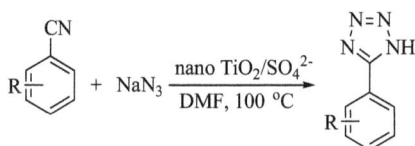

SCHEME 8.31

was simply recovered by an outer magnetic field and reused several times without significant loss of its catalytic activity.[54]

Behrouz developed a protocol for an easy and facile one-pot three-component synthesis of 5-substituted 1H-tetrazole derivatives from aldehydes using doped nanosized Cu_2O on a melamine–formaldehyde resin (nano-Cu_2O-MFR) as a catalyst with good to excellent yields (Scheme 8.30). The major advantages of nano-Cu_2O-MFR were its inexpensive nature, high stability, and recycling ability for several consecutive reactions runs without any appreciable decrease in its activity.[55]

Hosseini-Sarvari demonstrated an efficient and cheap protocol for the synthesis of 5-substituted-1H-tetrazoles from different sodium azides and nitriles using nano $TiO_2/SO_4{}^{2-}$ as an effective heterogeneous catalyst (Scheme 8.31). Broad varieties of aryl nitriles undergo [3+2] cycloaddition to give tetrazoles with good to excellent yields.[56]

Kritchenkov et al. synthesized a tetrazole bearing chitosan with moderate and low degrees of substitution using a novel metal-catalyzed 1,3-dipolar cycloaddition of an azide ion to cyano ethyl chitosan in an aqueous medium (Scheme 8.32).[57]

Mani et al. synthesized Ag NPs which were used as efficient and reusable heterogeneous catalysts for the synthesis of 5-substituted 1H-tetrazoles from different nitriles that had a diverse functional group and sodium azide in N,N-dimethyl formamide (DMF) at 120°C with excellent yields (Scheme 8.33).[58]

Moradi et al. documented the synthesis of biochar NPs from the pyrolysis of chicken manure, which was used as an environmentally friendly and reusable biocatalyst for the synthesis of tetrazole

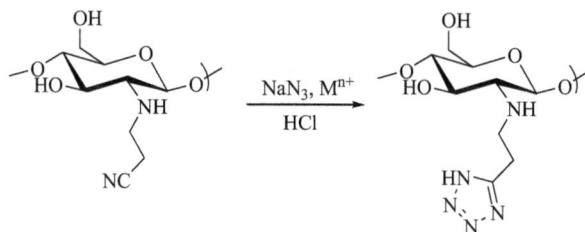

SCHEME 8.32

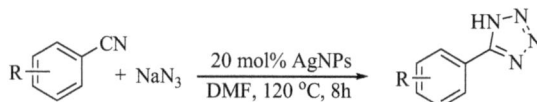

SCHEME 8.33

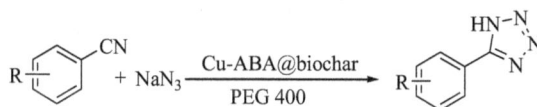

SCHEME 8.34

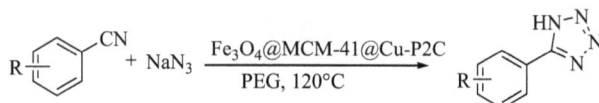

SCHEME 8.35

derivatives (Scheme 8.34). The tetrazoles were achieved in high turnover number (TON) and TOF values in the presence of copper nanoparticles supported on biochar, which showed the high efficiency of this catalyst. The catalyst was reused for several runs without Cu leaching or decreased catalytic activity.[59]

Nikoorazm et al. reported Fe_3O_4 magnetic NPs as a core for Cu(II) Schiff base complex functionalized mesoporous MCM-41 shell to offer a core-shell nanostructure (Fe_3O_4@MCM-41@ Cu-P2C). This material was employed as a simple, inexpensive, environmentally friendly catalyst using PEG as the reaction medium for the synthesis of 5-substituted 1H-tetrazoles (Scheme 8.35). Fe_3O_4@MCM-41@Cu-P2C is cost-effective, stable, heterogeneous, easy to handle, and recoverable NC and can be reused for several consecutive runs without any considerable loss of catalytic activity.[60]

Padmaja et al. successfully employed recyclable CNPs to catalyze the microwave-assisted (3+2) cycloaddition reaction of nitriles with sodium azide (NaN_3) to give the corresponding 5-substituted 1H-tetrazoles with excellent yields (Scheme 8.36). The features associated with this protocol include rapid synthesis, cost-effectiveness, reusability, stability, mild reaction conditions, no need for additives, high tolerance to various functional groups, and excellent yields under microwave irradiation and as an alternative to conventional protocols that involved Lewis's acid catalysts and operational simplicity.[61]

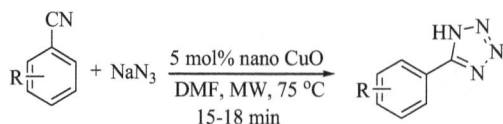

SCHEME 8.36

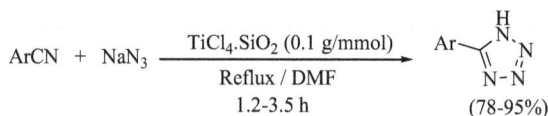

SCHEME 8.37

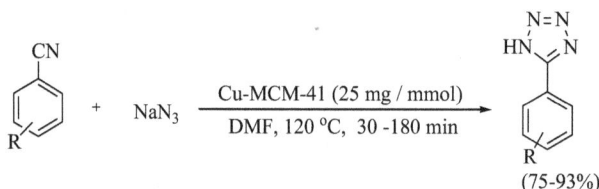

SCHEME 8.38

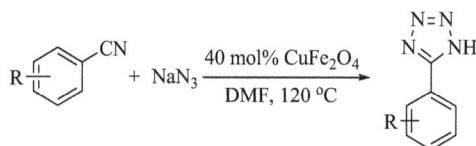

SCHEME 8.39

Nanoparticulate $TiCl_4.SiO_2$ was employed as an efficient solid Lewis acid catalyst for the synthesis of 5-substituted 1H-tetrazole derivatives (Scheme 8.37). The catalyst could be conveniently recovered and was reused at least three times without significant loss of activity.[62]

Nano sized Cu-MCM-41 mesoporous molecular sieves with various Si: Cu molar ratios were synthesized and used as an efficient heterogeneous catalyst for the synthesis of 5-substituted 1H-tetrazoles by the [3+2] cycloaddition reaction of nitriles and sodium azide (Scheme 8.38). Among the ratios, the Cu-MCM-41 with Si: Cu molar ratio was better for catalyzing the [3+2] cycloaddition reaction.[63]

Sreedhar et al. developed a competent and cheap protocol for the synthesis of 5-substituted 1H-tetrazoles by the reaction of various nitriles and sodium azide using magnetically reusable and recoverable $CuFe_2O_4$ NPs (Scheme 8.39). A large variety of aryl nitriles underwent the [2+3] cycloaddition under mild reaction conditions to give tetrazoles with good to excellent yields. The catalyst was magnetically separated and reused five times without significant loss of catalytic activity.[64]

Magnetic $CoFe_2O_4$ centered asparagine functionalized noble metal (where M = Cu or Ni) anchored nanocomposite ($CoFe_2O_4$@Lasparagine anchored Cu, Ni) NC proved an efficient heterogeneous catalyst for the synthesis of 5-substituted 1H-tetrazoles by the azide–alkyne cycloaddition reaction in PEG as the green reaction medium (Scheme 8.40). The developed protocol had an operationally simple procedure, short reaction time, high yield of the corresponding products that gave the corresponding products along with good reusability of the catalyst.[65]

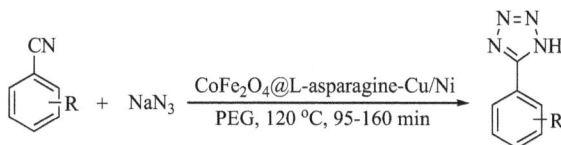

SCHEME 8.40

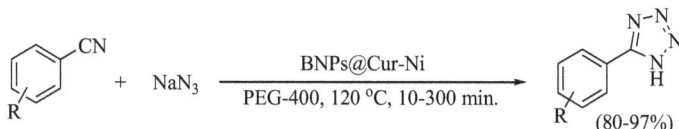

SCHEME 8.41

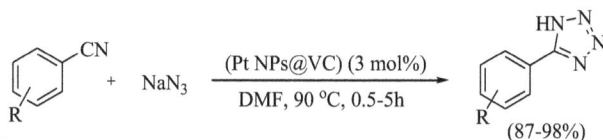

SCHEME 8.42

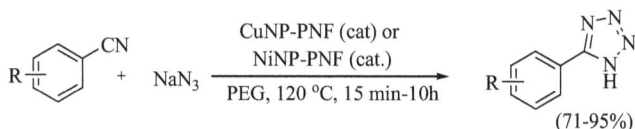

SCHEME 8.43

Nickel-anchored curcumin-functionalized boehmite NPs (BNPs@Cur-Ni) were developed as a versatile and robust NC for the synthesis of 5-substituted 1H-tetrazoles along with excellent TON and TOF outcomes (Scheme 8.41). The use of curcumin and boehmite as the natural source and poly(ethylene glycol) (PEG) as a solvent made the protocol a good tool for green chemistry.[66]

Baskaya et al. developed a facile and highly efficient protocol for the synthesis of new 5-substituted 1H-tetrazoles by the reaction of nitriles with sodium azide catalyzed by monodisperse carbon black decorated NPs as heterogeneous NCs (Scheme 8.42). The catalyst showed good recycling ability and excellent catalytic performance for the synthesis of tetrazoles.[67]

Ghorbani-Choghamarani and Taherinia develop peptide nanofibers decorated with Cu and Ni NPs as a catalyst for the synthesis of 5-substituted 1H-tetrazoles (Scheme 8.43). The developed Cu and Ni materials were cost-effective and non-toxic when immobilized on woven peptide nanofibres.[68]

CuO/aluminosilicate was developed as an efficient heterogeneous NC for the sequential one-pot synthesis of various 5-substituted-1H-tetrazoles by Movaheditabar et al. The synthetic strategy involved [3+2] cycloaddition reaction of aliphatic and aromatic nitriles with sodium azide in refluxing DMF. The tetrazoles were obtained with good to excellent yields along with good reusability and high catalytic performance (Scheme 8.44).[69]

The tandem synthesis of 5-substituted 1H tetrazoles can be accomplished by the reactions of aryl halides with $K_4[Fe(CN)_6]$ and sodium azide catalyzed by cross-linked poly(4-vinyl pyridine)-stabilized Pd(0) NPs, [P4-VP]-PdNPs in the presence of potassium carbonate as the base (Scheme 8.45). Only a slight decrease in catalytic activity was associated with this protocol.[70]

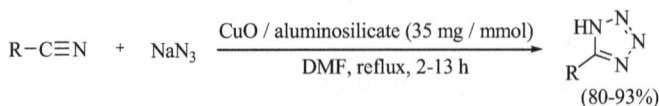

(80-93%)

SCHEME 8.44

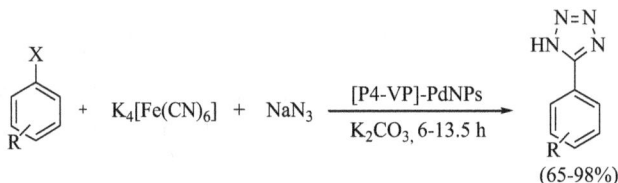

(65-98%)

SCHEME 8.45

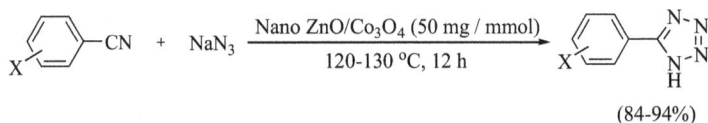

(84-94%)

SCHEME 8.46

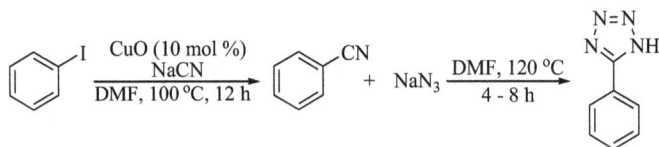

SCHEME 8.47

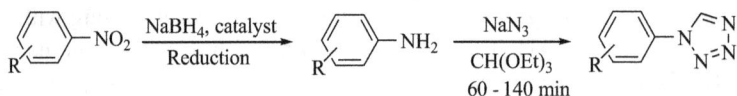

SCHEME 8.48

Nano ZnO/Co$_3$O$_4$ was used as an effective catalyst for the synthesis of substituted 1H-tetrazoles via the reaction of nitriles and sodium azide. Under the optimized reaction conditions, all nitriles reacted efficiently with sodium azide and afforded good to excellent yields of the desired products (Scheme 8.46). The nature of substituents present on the nitriles did not play a significant role in the yield of the corresponding products. The nanosized ZnO/Co$_3$O$_4$ heterogeneous material exhibited better catalytic activity than ZnO or Co$_3$O$_4$ under the optimized reaction conditions.[71]

Yapuri et al. synthesized a sequential and expedient one-pot synthesis of 5-substituted tetrazoles via the [2+3] cycloaddition of aryl nitriles with sodium azide (Scheme 8.47). The essential aryl nitriles were synthesized by using the nano-CuO supported cyanation of aryl iodides generated in situ.[72]

A green and versatile protocol was developed for the synthesis of 1-substituted-1H-1, 2, 3, 4-tetrazoles by Pd(II)-polysalophen coated magnetite NPs as a robust versatile nanocomposite by Xu et al. (Scheme 8.48).[73]

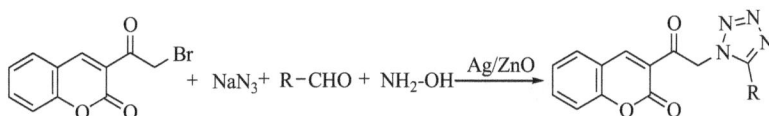

SCHEME 8.49

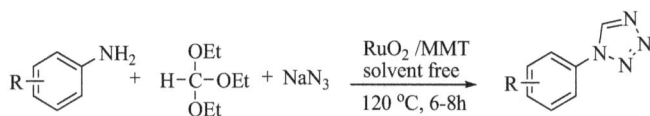

SCHEME 8.50

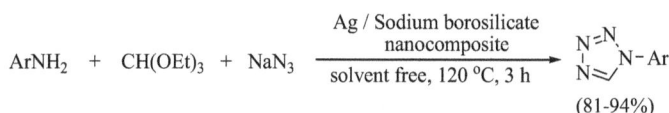

SCHEME 8.51

Attia et al. synthesized 1,5-disubstituted tetrazole (1,5-DST) based chromone derivatives by the one-pot multicomponent reaction between sodium azide, aldehyde derivatives, and chromenocyl bromide in the presence of triethylamine using Ag-doped ZnO nanocomposites and ZnO nanorods (NRs) as a photocatalyst (Scheme 8.49). Optimization of the reaction was developed under ambient conditions at room temperature in the dark and in the presence of visible light irradiation, which showed that Ag/ZnO NCs had proficient catalytic activity for the synthesis of novel 1, 5-DST during photocatalytic [3 +2] cycloaddition reaction. The synthesized tetrazole derivatives were studied for cytotoxic assessment toward HepG2, MCF-7, A549, and Wi38 cancer cell lines.[74]

Pawar et al. developed a facile, one-pot three-component catalytic method for the synthesis of N-substituted tetrazole using a RuO_2 nanocomposite (Scheme 8.50). This strategy resulted in good to excellent yields (84%–97%), moderate reaction time, and excellent reusability for up to five cycles. The useful catalytic activity of the bifunctional nanocomposite was credited to the uniformly dispersed RuO_2 NPs on the surface of the MMT and the RuO_2 site was responsible for the coordination of isocyanide intermediate and the strong acidic character of MMT induced the cyclization steps and condensation synergistically.[75]

Nasrollahzadeh et al. reported a suitable protocol for 1-substituted 1H-1,2,3,4-tetrazoles that used sodium borosilicate glass-supported Ag NPs as a novel heterogeneous catalyst under solvent-free reaction conditions (Scheme 8.51). The Ag/sodium borosilicate nanocomposite (ASBN) catalyst was developed using *Aleurites moluccana* leaf extract as a stabilizing and reducing agent. The method produced the corresponding 1-substituted tetrazoles with good to high yields under environmentally friendly and solvent-free conditions.[76]

Naeimi et al. documented an ultrasound-assisted rapid synthesis of 1-substituted tetrazoles by the cyclization of diversely substituted primary amines, sodium azide, and triethyl orthoformate catalyzed by ZnS NPs (Scheme 8.52). The ZnS NPs were efficient, recoverable, and reusable catalysts that highlighted their use as an excellent substitute for Bronsted acids for the preparation of 1-substituted tetrazoles.[77]

Khorramabadi et al. developed the synthesis of tetrazoles by the three-component condensation of amines, triethyl orthoformate, and sodium azide catalyzed by a novel Cu NC coated with Fe_3O_4 magnetic NPs (Scheme 8.53). Under the optimized reaction conditions, a wide range of

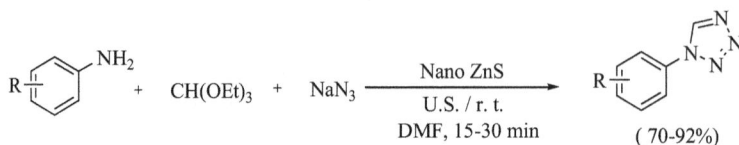

SCHEME 8.52

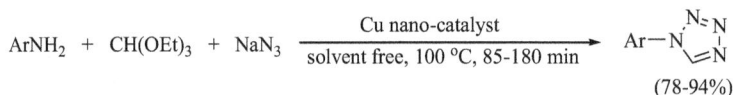

SCHEME 8.53

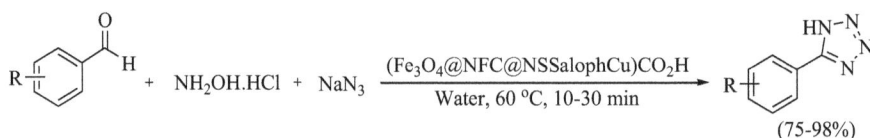

SCHEME 8.54

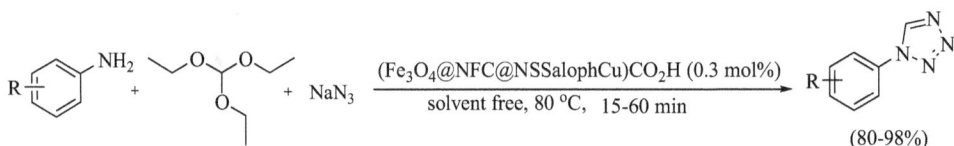

SCHEME 8.55

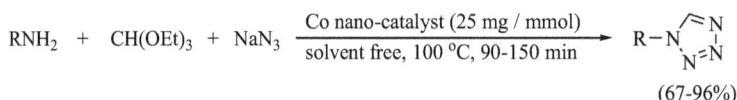

SCHEME 8.56

tetrazoles were synthesized by the reaction of various aromatic amines with sodium azide and tri-ethyl orthoformate under the solvent-free condition at 100°C.[78]

Cu(II)-salophen complex anchored on magnetic mesoporous cellulose nanofibers ((Fe3O4@NFC@NSalophCu)CO2H) was used as an NC for the synthesis of 5-substituted-1H-tetrazole and 1-substituted-1H-tetrazole derivatives via the one-pot multicomponent reactions. The synthesis was achieved by the $(Fe_3O_4@NFC@NSalophCu)CO_2H$ catalyzed cyclo condensation of aldehydes, hydroxylamine hydrochloride, sodium azide or amines, triethyl orthoformate, and sodium azide (Schemes 8.54 and 55). The NC served as a safe, easily available, cheap, and recyclable catalyst in an aqueous medium as a green solvent within a short reaction time.[79]

Magnetic Co NPs were synthesized by coating Fe_3O_4 magnetic NPs on tetraethyl orthosilicate functionalized with (3-chloropropyl)trimethoxysilane and 2-amino-5-mercapto-1,3,4-thiadiazole ligands followed by complexation with $Co(OAc)_4$[Fe3O4@SiO2@CPTMS@AMTDA@Co]. This material was used as a catalyst for the synthesis of various tetrazoles (Scheme 8.56). The

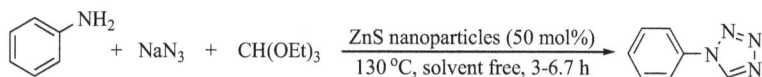

SCHEME 8.57

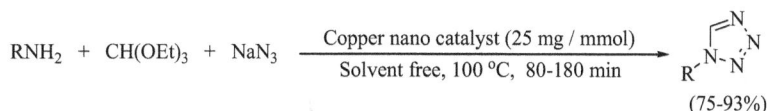

SCHEME 8.58

transformation was achieved by the condensation of aromatic amines, sodium azide, and triethyl orthoformate (TEOF) under solvent-free conditions at 100°C.[80]

The synthesis of 1-substituted-1H tetrazoles can be carried out by the cyclization reaction of various primary amines, sodium azide, and triethyl orthoformate under solvent-free conditions in the presence of ZnS NPs as an efficient and reusable heterogeneous catalyst (Scheme 8.57). This is an attractive protocol for the synthesis of tetrazoles due to the clean reaction conditions, nonacidic and solvent-free conditions using a solid recyclable catalyst. The ZnS NPs were synthesized under microwave irradiation and had a high surface area, and fine monodisperse particles. The catalyst showed good reusability results.[81]

Ariannezhad et al.developed a Cu NC by coating Fe_3O_4 magnetic NPs with tetraethylorthosilicate (TEOS), followed by functionalization with 3-chloropropyl(trimethoxy)silane and 4H-1,2,4-triazol-4-amine and complexation with Cu(II) chloride. This new material was used successfully used for the synthesis of 1-aryl-1H-tetrazoles by the reaction of aromatic amines with sodium azide and triethyl orthoformate under solvent-free conditions at 100°C (Scheme 8.58).[82]

8.4 CONCLUSION

In summary, triazoles and tetrazoles are biologically significant five-membered heterocyclic compounds that are the core structures of several commercially marketed drugs and other heterocyclic compounds of great biological significance. This chapter summarized various biological activities of triazole and tetrazole-based heterocyclic compounds along with the recent developments in heterocyclic compounds that used nanomaterials as efficient and reusable heterogeneous catalysts.

REFERENCES

1. Sahu A, Sahu P, Agrawal R. A Recent Review on Drug Modification Using 1, 2, 3-Triazole. Curr Chem Bio. 2020. 14:71–87. doi.10.2174/2212796814999200807214519.
2. Zhang B. Comprehensive Review on the Anti-Bacterial Activity of 1, 2, 3-Triazole Hybrids. Eur J Med Chem. 2019. 168:357–72.doi:10.1016/j.ejmech.2019.02.055.
3. Sharma V, Shrivastava B, Bhatia R, Bechwati M, Khandelwal R, Ameta J. Exploring Potential of 1, 2, 4-Triazole: A Brief Review. Pharm. 2011. 1:1192–222.
4. Sarvary A, Maleki A. A Review of Syntheses of 1, 5-Disubstituted Tetrazole Derivatives. Mol Div. 2015. 19:189–212. doi:10.1007/s11030-014-9553-3.
5. Aljamali NM, Mahmood RM, Baqi RA. Review on Preparation and Application Fields of Triazole & Tetrazole Derivatives. Int J Anal Appl Chem. 2020. 6:50–60.
6. Durr CJ, Lederhose P, Hlalele L, Abt D, Kaiser A, Brandau S. et al. Photo-Induced Ligation of Acrylonitrile-Butadiene Rubber: Selective Tetrazole-Ene Coupling of Chain-End-Functionalized Copolymers of 1, 3-Butadiene. Macromolecules. 2013. 46:5915–23. doi.10.1021/ma401154k.

7. Li Z, Qian L, Li L, Bernhammer JC, Huynh HV. et al. Tetrazole Photo Click Chemistry: Reinvestigating its Suitability as a Bioorthogonal Reaction and Potential Applications. Ang Chemie Int Ed. 2016. 55:2002–6. doi.10.1002/anie.201508104.

8. Saadaoui I, Krichen F, Salah BB, Mansour RB, Miled N, Bougatef A. et al. Design, Synthesis and Biological Evaluation of Schiff Bases of 4-Amino-1,2,4-Triazole Derivatives as Potent Angiotensin-Converting Enzyme Inhibitors and Antioxidant Activities. J Mol Stru. 2019. 1180: 344–54. doi.10.1016/j.molstruc.2018.12.008.

9. Slamova K, Marhol P, Bezouska K, Lindkvist L, Hansen SG, Kren V. et al. Synthesis and Biological activity of Glycosyl-1H-1,2,3-Triazoles. Bioorg Med Chem Lett. 2010. 20:4263–5. doi.10.1016/j.bmcl.2010.04.151.

10. Stingaci E, Zveaghinteva M, Pogrebnoi S, Lupascu L, Valica V, Uncu L et al. New Vinyl-1, 2, 4-Triazole Derivatives as Antimicrobial Agents: Synthesis, Biological Evaluation, and Molecular Docking Studies. Bioorg Med Chem Lett. 2020. 30(17): 127368. doi:10.1016/j.bmcl.2020.127368.

11. Luo L, Jia JJ, Zhong Q, Zhong X, Zheng S, Wang G. et al. Synthesis and Anticancer Activity Evaluation of Naphthalene-Substituted Triazole Spirodienones. Eur J Med Chem. 2021. 213: 113039: doi.10.1016/j.ejmech.2020.113039.

12. Akin S, Demir EA, Colak A, Kolcuoglu Y, Yildirim N, Bekircan O. Synthesis, Biological Activities and Molecular Docking Studies of Some Novel 2,4,5-Trisubstituted-1,2,4-Triazole-3-One Derivatives as Potent Tyrosinase Inhibitors. J Mol Stru. 2019. 1175: 280–6. doi.10.1016/j.molstruc.2018.07.065.

13. Wu S, Zhang W, Qi L, Ren Y, Ma H. Investigation on 4-Amino-5-Substituent-1, 2, 4-Triazole-3-Thione Schiff Bases an Antifungal Drug by Characterization (Spectroscopic, XRD), Biological Activities, Molecular Docking Studies, and Electrostatic Potential (ESP). J Mol Stru. 2019. 1197:171–82. doi:10.1016/j.molstruc.2019.07.013

14. Deswal S, Naveen, Tittal RK, Vikas DG, Lal K, Kumar A. 5-Fluoro-1H-indole-2, 3-dione-triazoles-Synthesis, Biological Activity, Molecular Docking, and DFT Study. J Mol Stru. 2020. 1209:127982. doi.10.1016/j.molstruc.2020.127982.

15. Grytsai O, Valiashko O, Penco-Campillo M, Dufies M, Hagege A, Demange L. et al. Synthesis and Biological Evaluation of 3-Amino-1,2,4-Triazole Derivatives as Potential Anticancer Compounds. Bioorg Chem. 2020. 104:104271. doi.10.1016/j.bioorg.2020.104271.

16. Masood MM, Hasan P, Tabrez S, Ahmad BB, Yadava U, Daniliuc CG et al. Anti-leishmanial and Cytotoxic Activities of Amino Acid-Triazole Hybrids: Synthesis, Biological Evaluation, Molecular Docking and In Silico Physicochemical Properties. *Bioorg Med Chem Lett.* 2017. 27(9):1886–91. doi.10.1016/j.bmcl.2017.03.049.

17. Menendez C, Gau S, Lherbet C, Rodriguez F, Inard C, Pasca MR et al. Synthesis and Biological Activities of Triazole Derivatives as Inhibitors of InhA and Antituberculosis Agents. Eur J Med Chem. 2011. 46:5524–31. doi.10.1016/j.ejmech.2011.09.013.

18. Naveen, RK Tittal, Ghule VD, Kumar N, Kumar L, Lal K et al. Design, Synthesis, Biological Activity, Molecular Docking and Computational Studies on Novel 1,4-Disubstituted-1,2,3-Triazole-Thiosemicarbazone Hybrid Molecules. J Mol Stru. 2020. 1209:127951. doi.10.1016/j.molstruc.2020.127951.

19. Srivastava AK, Kumar A, Misra N, Manjula PS, Sarojini BK, Narayana B. Synthesis, Spectral (FT-IR, UV-visible, NMR) Features, Biological Activity Prediction and Theoretical Studies of 4-Amino-3-(4-hydroxybenzyl)-1*H*-1,2,4-triazole-5(4*H*)-thione and its Tautomer. J Mol Stru. 2016. 1107:13744. doi.10.1016/j.molstruc.2015.11.042.

20. Zhang L-Y, Wang B-L, Zhan Y-Z, Zhang Y, Zhang X, Li Z-M. Synthesis and Biological Activities of Some Fluorine- and Piperazine-Containing 1, 2, 4-Triazole Thione Derivatives. Chin Chem Lett. 2016. 27:163–7. doi.10.1016/j.cclet.2015.09.015.

21. Mange YJ, Isloor AM, Malladi S, Isloor S, Fun H-K. Synthesis and Antimicrobial Activities of Some Novel 1, 2, 4-Triazole Derivatives. Arabian J Chem. 2013. 6: 177–81. doi.10.1016/j.arabjc.2011.01.033

22. Isloor AM, Kalluraya B, Shetty P. Regioselective Reaction: Synthesis, Characterization and Pharmacological Studies of Some New Mannich Bases Derived From 1, 2, 4-Triazoles. Eur J Med Chem. 2009. 44: 3784–7. doi.10.1016/j.ejmech.2009.04.038

23. Khan SA, Imam SM, Ahmad A, Basha SH, Husain A. Synthesis, Molecular Docking with COX 1& II Enzyme, ADMET Screening and In Vivo Anti-Inflammatory Activity of Oxadiazole, Thiadiazole

and Triazole Analogues of Felbinac. J Saudi Chem Soc. 2017. 1319(6103):30064–9. doi.10.1016/
j.jscs.2017.05.006.

24. Penjarla S, Sabui SK, Reddy DS, Banerjee S, Reddy PY, Penta S. et al. An Efficient Synthesis Tetrazole
and Oxadiazole Analogs of Novel 2'-Deoxy-Nucleosides and Their Antitumor Activity. Bioorg Med
Chem Lett. 2020. 30(24): 127612. doi.10.1016/j.bmcl.2020.127612.

25. Dhiman N, Kaur K, Jaitak V. Tetrazoles as Anticancer Agents: A Review on Synthetic Strategies,
Mechanism of Action and SAR Studies. Bioorg Med Chem. 2020. 28(15): 115599. doi:10.1016/
j.bmc.2020.115599

26. Maheshwari N, Karthikeyan C, Bhadada SV, Verma AK, Sahi C, Moorthy NSHN. et al. Design, Synthesis
and Biological Evaluation of Some Tetrazole Acetamide Derivatives as Novel Non-Carboxylic PTP1B
inhibitors. Bioorg Chem. 2019. 92:103221. doi:10.1016/j.bioorg.2019.103221

27. Shekouhy M, Karimian S, Moaddeli A, Faghih Z, Delshad Y, Khalafi-Nezhad A. The Synthesis and
Biological Evaluation of Nucleobases/Tetrazole Hybrid Compounds: A New Class of Phosphodiesterase
Type 3 (PDE3) Inhibitors. Bioorg Med Chem. 2020. 28:115540. doi.10.1016/j.bmc.2020.115540.

28. Zhang L-H, Zhang Z-H, Li M-Y, Wei Z-Y, Jin X-J, Piao H-R. Synthesis and Evaluation of the HIF-
1α Inhibitory Activities of Novel Ursolic Acid Tetrazole Derivatives. Bioorg Med Chem Lett. 2019.
29:1440–5. doi:10.1016/j.bmcl.2019.04.028.

29. Bahadorikhalili S, Ma'mani L, Mahdavi H, Shafiee A. Copper Supported β-Cyclodextrin Functionalized
PEGylated Mesoporous Silica Nanoparticle-Graphene Oxide Hybrid: An Efficient and Recyclable
Nano-Catalyst for Straightforward Synthesis of 2-Arylbenzimidazoles and 1, 2, 3-Triazoles.Micropo
Mesopo Mat. 2018. 262: 207–16. doi.10.1016/j.micromeso.2017.11.046.

30. Basu P, Bhanja P, Salam N, Dey TK, Bhaumik A, Das D. et al. Silver Nanoparticles Supported Over
Al_2O_3@Fe_2O_3 Core-Shell Nanoparticles as an Efficient Catalyst for One-Pot Synthesis of 1,2,3-Triazoles
and Acylation of Benzyl Alcohol. Mol Catal. 2017. 439: 1–40. doi.10.1016/j.mcat.2017.05.005.

31. Chetia M, Gehlot PS, Kumar A, Sarma D. A Recyclable/Reusable Hydrotalcite Supported Copper
Nanocatalyst for 1,4-Disubstituted-1,2,3-Triazole Synthesis via Click Chemistry Approach. Tetrahedron
Lett. 2018. 59 397–401. doi.10.1016/j.tetlet.2017.12.051.

32. Elayadi H, Ali MA, Mehdi A, Lazrek HB. Nano Crystalline CuO: Synthesis and Application as
an Efficient Catalyst for the Preparation of 1, 2, 3-Triazole Acyclic Nucleosides via 1, 3-Dipolar
Cycloaddition. Cat Commun. 2012. 26:155–8. doi.10.1016/j.catcom.2012.05.016.

33. Haghighat M, Shirini F, Golshekan M. Efficiency of $NaHSO_4$ Modified Periodic Mesoporous
Organosilica Magnetic Nanoparticles as a New Magnetically Separable Nanocatalyst in the Synthesis of
[1, 2, 4]Triazolo Quinazolinone / Pyrimidine Derivatives. J Mol Struct. 2018. 1171: 168–78. doi.10.1016/
j.molstruc.2018.05.112.

34. Mahdavinasab M, Hamzehloueian M, Sarrafi Y. 2019. Preparation and Application of Magnetic
Chitosan/Graphene Oxide Composite Supported Copper as a Recyclable Heterogeneous Nanocatalyst in
the Synthesis of Triazoles. I J Bio Macromol. 2018. 138:764–72. Doi.10.1016/j.ijbiomac.2019.07.013.

35. Naeimi H, Shaabani R. Preparation and Characterization of Functionalized Graphene Oxide Cu (I) complex: A facile and Reusable Nanocatalyst for Microwave Assisted Heterocyclization of Alkyl Halides
with Alkynes and Sodium Azide. Cat Commun. 2016. 87:6–9.

36. Alyari M, Mehrabani MG, Allahvirdinesbat M, Safa KD, Kafil HS, Panahi PN. Ultrasound Assisted
Synthesis of Thiazolidine Thiones Containing 1, 2, 3-Triazoles using Cu/TiO_2. Arkivoc. 2017. 4:145–
57. doi.10.24820/ark.5550190.p009.761.

37. Darroudi M, Rouh H, Hasanzadeh M, Shadjou N. Cu/SiO_2-Pr-NH-Benz as a Novel Nanocatalyst for
the Efficient Synthesis of 1, 4-Disubstituted Triazoles and Propargyl Amine Derivatives in an Aqueous
Solution. Heliyon. 2021. 78:6766. doi.10.1016/j.heliyon.2021.e06766.

38. Raj JP, Gangaprasad DI, Vajjiravel M, Karthikeyan K, Elangovan J. CuO-Nanoparticles Catalyzed
Synthesis of 1,4-Disubstituted-1,2,3-Triazoles from Bromoalkenes. J Chem Sci. 2018. 130: 44.
doi.10.1007/s12039-018-1452-1.

39. Alonso F, Moglie Y, Radivoy G, Yus M. Multicomponent Click Synthesis of 1, 2, 3-Triazoles from
Epoxides in Water Catalyzed by Copper Nanoparticles on Activated Carbon. J Org Chem. 2011.
76:8394–405. doi.10.1021/jo2016339.

40. Alonso F, Moglie Y, Radivoy G, Yusa M. Multicomponent Synthesis of 1, 2, 3-Triazoles in Water
Catalyzed by Copper Nanoparticles on Activated Carbon. J Org Chem. 2011. 76:8394–405. doi.10.1021/
jo2016339.

41. Sharghi H, Khalifeh R, Doroodmanda MM. Copper Nanoparticles on Charcoal for Multicomponent Catalytic Synthesis of 1, 2, 3-Triazole Derivatives from Benzyl Halides or Alkyl Halides, Terminal Alkynes and Sodium Azide in Water as a "Green" Solvent. Adv Synth Cat. 2009. 351:207–18. doi.10.1002/adsc.200800612.

42. Iniyavan P, Balaji GL, Sarveswari S, Vijayakumar V. CuO Nanoparticles: Synthesis and Application as an Efficient Reusable Catalyst for the Preparation of Xanthene Substituted 1, 2, 3-Triazoles via Click Chemistry. Tetrahedron Lett. 2015. S0040–4039(15):01146–6. doi.10.1016/j.tetlet.2015.07.016.

43. Rajabi-Moghaddam H, Naimi-Jamal MR, Tajbakhsh M. Fabrication of Copper (II)-Coated Magnetic Core-Shell Nanoparticles $Fe_3O_4@ SiO_2$-2-Aminobenzohydrazide and Investigation of its Catalytic Application in the Synthesis of 1, 2, 3-Triazole Compounds. Sci Rep. 2021. 11:2073. doi.10.1038/s41598-021-81632-7.

44. Maleki A, Panahzadeh M, Eivazzadeh-Keihan R. Agar: A Natural and Environmentally-Friendly Support Composed of Copper Oxide Nanoparticles for the Green Synthesis of 1, 2, 3-Triazoles. Green Chem Lett Rev. 2019. 12:395–406. doi.10.1080/17518253.2019.1679263.

45. Halder M, Islam MM, Singh P, Roy AS, Islam SM, Sen K. Sustainable Generation of Ni(OH)$_2$ Nanoparticles for the Green Synthesis of 5-Substituted 1H-Tetrazoles: A Competent Turn on Fluorescence Sensing of H_2O_2. ACS Omega. 2018. 3: 8169–80. doi. 10.1021/acsomega.8b01081.

46. Boominathan M, Pugazhenthiran N, Nagaraj M, Muthusubramanian S, Murugesan S, Bhuvanesh N. Nanoporous 3Titania Supported Gold Nanoparticles Catalyzed Green Synthesis of 1, 2, 3-Triazoles in Aqueous Medium. ACS Sustain Chem. Eng. 2013. 1(11):1405–11. doi.10.1021/sc400147r.

47. Chetia M, Ali AA, Bordoloi A, Sarma D. Facile Route for the Regioselective Synthesis of 1, 4-Disubstituted 1,2,3-Triazole Using Copper Nanoparticles Supported on Nanocellulose as Recyclable Heterogeneous Catalyst. J Chem Sci. 2017. 129:1211–17. doi:10.1007/s12039-017-1318-y.

48. Saha R, Arunprasath D, Sekar G. Surface Enriched Palladium on Palladium-Copper Bimetallic Nanoparticles as Catalyst for Polycyclic Triazoles Synthesis. J Cat. 2019. 377:673–83. doi.10.1016/j.jcat.2019.07.063.

49. Khalil KD, Riyadh SM, Gomha SM, Ali I. Synthesis, Characterization and Application of Copper Oxide Chitosan Nanocomposite for Green Regioselective Synthesis of [1, 2, 3]Triazoles. *Int J Bio Macromol.* 2019. 130:928–37. doi.10.1016/j.ijbiomac.2019.03.019.

50. Sharma N, Gupta M, Chowhan B, Frontera A. Magnetically Separable Nanocatalyst (IL@CuFe$_2$O$_4$-L-Tyr-TiO$_2$/TiTCIL): Preparation, Characterization and its Applications in 1, 2, 3-Triazole Synthesis and in Photodegradation of MB. J Mol Strut. 2020. 1224:129029. doi:10.1016/j.molstruc.2020.129029.

51. Rezaei F, Amrollahi MA, Khalifeh R. Design and Synthesis of Fe$_3$O$_4$@SiO$_2$/Aza-crown Ether-Cu(II) as a Novel and Highly Efficient Magnetic Nanocomposite Catalyst for the Synthesis of 1,2,3-Triazoles, 1-Substituted 1H-Tetrazoles and 5-Substituted 1H-Tetrazoles in Green Solvents. Inorganica Chim Acta. 2019. S0020–1693:31672–4.

52. Salimi M, Abadi FEN, Sandaroos R. Fe$_3$O$_4$@Hydrotalcite-NH$_2$-CoII NPs: A Novel and Extremely Effective Heterogeneous Magnetic Nanocatalyst for Synthesis of the 1-Substituted 1H-1, 2, 3, 4-Tetrazoles. Inorg Chem Commun. 2020. 122:108287. doi.10.1016/j.inoche.2020.108287.

53. Tamoradi T, Ghorbani-Choghamarani A, Ghadermazi M. CoFe$_2$O$_4$@glycine-M (M= Pr, Tb and Yb): Three Green, Novel, Efficient and Magnetically-Recoverable Nanocatalysts for Synthesis of 5-Substituted 1H-Tetrazoles and Oxidation of Sulfides in Green Condition. Solid State Sci. 2019. 88: 81–94. doi.10.1016/j.solidstatesciences.2018.10.011.

54 Zarchi MAK, Darbandizadeh SSA, Abadi M. Dendron-Functionalized Fe$_3$O$_4$ Magnetic Nanoparticles with Palladium Catalyzed CN Insertion of Aryl Halides for the Synthesis of Tetrazoles and Benzamide. J Organomet Chem. 2019. 880, 196–212. doi.org/10.1016/j.jorganchem.2018.11.006.

55. Behrouz S. Highly Efficient Three-Component Synthesis of 5-Substituted-1H-tetrazoles From Aldehydes, Hydroxylamine, and Tetrabutylammonium Azide using Doped Nano-Sized Copper(I) Oxide (Cu$_2$O) on Melamine-Formaldehyde Resin. J Saudi Chem Soc. 2017. 21:220–8. doi.10.1016/j.jscs.2016.08.003.

56. Hosseini-Sarvari M, Najafvand-Derikvandi S. Nano TiO$_2$/SO$_4^{2-}$ as a Heterogeneous Solid Acid Catalyst for the Synthesis of 5-Substituted-1H-Tetrazoles. Comptes Rendus Chimie. 2014. 10:1007–12. doi.10.1016/j.crci.2013.11.002.

57. Kritchenkov AS, Egorov AR, Krytchankou IS, Dubashynskaya NV, Volkova OV, Shakola TV. et al. Synthesis of Novel 1H-Tetrazole Derivatives of Chitosan via Metal Catalyzed 1,3-Dipolar Cycloaddition.

Catalytic and Antibacterial Properties of [3-(1H-Tetrazole-5-Yl)Ethyl] Chitosan and its Nanoparticles. Int J BioMacromol. 2019. 132:340–50. doi:10.1016/j.ijbiomac.2019.03.153.

58. Mani P, Sharma C, Kumar S, Awasthi SK. Efficient Heterogeneous Silver Nanoparticles Catalyzed One-Pot Synthesis of 5-Substituted 1*H*-Tetrazoles. J Mol Cat A: Chem. 2014. 392:150–6. doi.10.1016/j.molcata.2014.05.008.

59. Moradi P, Hajjami M, Tahmasbi B. Fabricated Copper Catalyst on Biochar Nanoparticles for the Synthesis of Tetrazoles as Antimicrobial Agents. Polyhedron. 2019. S0277–5387: 30606-0. doi.10.1016/j.poly.2019.114169.

60. Nikoorazm M, Erfani Z. Core-shell Nanostructure (Fe$_3$O$_4$@MCM-41@Cu-P2C) as a Highly Efficient and Recoverable Nanocatalyst for the Synthesis of Polyhydroquinoline, 5-Substituted 1H-Tetrazoles and Sulfides. *Chem Phy Lett*. 2019. 737:136784. doi:10.1016/j.cplett.2019.136784.

61. Padmaja RD, Rej S, Chanda K. Environmentally Friendly, Microwave-Assisted Synthesis of 5-Substituted 1*H*-Tetrazoles by Recyclable CuO Nanoparticles via (3+2) Cycloaddition of Nitriles and NaN$_3$. Chin J Cat. 2017. 38:1918–24. doi:10.1016/S1872-2067(17)62920-6.

62. Zamani L, Mirjailli BB, Zomorodian K, Zomorodian S. Synthesis and Characterization of 5-Substituted 1H-Tetrazoles in the presence of Nano-TiCl$_4$. SiO$_2$. South Afr J Chem. 2015. 68:133–7.

63. Abdolahi-Alibeik M, Moaddeli A. Cu-MCM-41 Nanoparticles: An Efficient Catalyst for the Synthesis of 5-Substituted 1*H*-Tetrazoles via [3+2] Cycloaddition Reaction of Nitriles and Sodium Azide. J Chem Sci. 2016. 128:93–9. doi.10.1007/s12039-015-1005-9.

64. Sreedhar B, Kumar AS, Yada D. CuFe$_2$O$_4$Nanoparticles: A Magnetically Recoverable and Reusable Catalyst for the Synthesis of 5-Substituted 1*H*-Tetrazoles. Tetrahedron Lett. 2011. 52:3565–9. doi:10.1016/j.tetlet.2011.04.094.

65. Tamoradi T, Veisi H, Karmakar B, Gholami J. A Competent Green Methodology for the Synthesis of Aryl Thioethers and 1*H*-Tetrazole Over Magnetically Retrievable Novel CoFe$_2$O$_4$@L-Asparagine Anchored Cu, Ni Nanocatalyst. Mat Sci Engin C. 2018. 107: 110260. doi.10.1016/j.msec.2019.110260.

66. Jani MA, Bahrami K. Synthesis of 5-Substituted 1*H*-Tetrazoles and Oxidation of Sulfides by Using Boehmite Nanoparticles/Nickel-Curcumin as a Robust and Extremely Efficient Green Nanocatalyst. Appl Organomet Chem. 2020. 34:6014. doi:10.1002/aoc.6014.

67. Baskaya G, Esirden I, Erken E, Sen F, Kaya M. Synthesis of 5-Substituted-1H-Tetrazole Derivatives Using Monodisperse Carbon Black Decorated Pt Nanoparticles as Heterogeneous Nanocatalysts. J Nanosci Nanotech. 2017. 17:1992–9. doi.10.1166/jnn.2017.12867.

68. Ghorbani-Choghamarani A, Taherinia Z. High Catalytic Activity of Peptide Nanofibres Decorated with Ni and Cu Nanoparticles for the Synthesis of 5-Substituted 1*H*-Tetrazoles and *N*-Arylation of Amines. Austr J Chem. 2017. 70:1127–37.

69. Movaheditabar P, Javaherian M, Nobakht V. CuO/Aluminosilicate as an Efficient Heterogeneous Nanocatalyst for the Synthesis and Sequential One-Pot Functionalization of 5-Substituted-1*H*-Tetrazoles. Reaction Kin Mecha Cat. 2017. 122:217–18.

70. Abadi SS, Zarchi MA. A Novel Route for the Synthesis of 5-Substituted 1-*H*Tetrazoles in the Presence of Polymer-Supported Palladium Nanoparticles. New J Chem. 2017. 41:10397–406. doi.10.1039/C7NJ02222K.

71. Agawane SM, Nagarkar JM. Synthesis of 5-Substituted 1*H*-Tetrazoles using a Nano ZnO/Co$_3$O$_4$Catalyst. Cat Sci Tech. 2012. 2:1324–7. doi.10.1039/C2CY20094E.

72. Yapuri U, Palle S, Gudaparthi O, Narahari SR, Rawat DK, Mukkanti K. et al. Ligand-free Nano Copper Oxide Catalyzed Cyanation of Aryl Halides and Sequential One-Pot Synthesis of 5-Substituted-1H-Tetrazoles. Tetrahedron Lett 54: 4732–4.DOI:10.1016/j.tetlet.2013.06.107

73. Xu DP, Xiong M, Kazemnejadi M (2021) Efficient Reduction of Nitro Compounds and Domino Preparation of 1-Substituted-1*H*-1,2,3,4-Tetrazoles by Pd(II)-Polysalophen Coated Magnetite NPs as a Robust Versatile Nanocomposite. RSC Advances 11: 12484–99. DOI: https://doi.org/10.1039/D1RA01164B

74. Attia YA, Mohamed YMA, Awad MM, Alexeree S (2020) Ag-Doped ZnO Nanorods Catalyzed Photo-Triggered Synthesis of Some Novel (1H-Tetrazol-5-yl)-Coumarin Hybrids. J Organomet Chem 919: 121320.

75. Pawar HR, Chikate RC (2020) One Pot Three Component Solvent Free Synthesis of N-Substituted Tetrazoles using RuO$_2$/MMT Catalyst. J Mol Stru. 1225: 128985. DOI: http://dx.doi.org/10.1016/j.molstruc.2020.128985

76. Nasrollahzadeh M, Sajjadi M, Tahsili MR, Shokouhimehr M, Varma RS (2019)Synthesis of 1-Substituted 1*H*-1, 2, 3, 4-Tetrazoles using Biosynthesized Ag/Sodium Borosilicate Nanocomposite. ACS Omega. 4:8985–9000. DOI: https://doi.org/10.1021/acsomega.9b00800

77. Naeimi H, Kiani F (2015) Ultrasound-Promoted One-Pot Three Component Synthesis of Tetrazoles Catalyzed by Zinc Sulfide Nanoparticles as a Recyclable Heterogeneous Catalyst. Ultrason Sonochem 27: 408–15. https://doi.org/10.1016/j.ultsonch.2015.06.008

78. Khorramabadi V, Habibia D, Heydari S (2020)Facile Synthesis of Tetrazoles Catalyzed by the New Copper Nano-Catalyst. Green Chem Lett Rev. 13: 50–9. DOI: https://doi.org/10.1080/17518253.2020.1726505

79. Kargar PG, Bagherzade G (2021) The Anchoring of a Cu(II)-Salophen Complex on Magnetic Mesoporous Cellulose Nanofibers: Green Synthesis and an Investigation of its Catalytic Role in Tetrazole Reactions Through a Facile One-Pot Route. RSC Adv 11: 19203–20. DOI: https://doi.org/10.1039/D1RA01913A

80. Sarrafioun F, Jamehbozorgi S, Ramezani M (2019) Synthesis of Tetrazoles Catalyzed by Novel Cobalt Magnetic Nanoparticles. Russ J Org Chem 55: 1777–84. DOI: https://doi.org/10.1134/S1070428019110216

81. Naeimi H, Kiani F, Moradian M (2014) ZnS Nanoparticles as an Efficient and Reusable Heterogeneous Catalyst for Synthesis of 1-Substituted-1*H*Tetrazoles Under Solvent-Free Conditions. J Nanoparticle Res 16: 2590. DOI: https://doi.org/10.1007/s11051-014-2590-0

82. Ariannezhad M, Habibi D, Heydari S (2019) Synthesis of Tetrazoles from Amines Mediated by New Copper Nanocatalyst. Russ J Org Chem 55: 1591–7. DOI:https://doi.org/10.1134/S1070428019100208

9 Nanocatalysed Synthesis and Biological Significance of Imidazoles, Hydantoins, Oxazoles, and Thiazoles

Surbhi Dhadda,[1] *Nidhi Jangir,*[1] *Shikha Agarwal,*[2]
Arvnabh Mishra,[3] *and Dinesh Kumar Jangid*[1]

[1] Department of Chemistry (Centre of Advanced Study), University of Rajasthan, JLN Marg, Jaipur, Rajasthan, India
[2] Synthetic Organic Chemistry Laboratory, Department of Chemistry, MLSU, Udaipur, Rajasthan, India
[3] Department of Industrial Chemistry, ISTAR, C. V. M. University, Vallabh Vidyanagar Anand, India

9.1 INTRODUCTION

Imidazole, benzimidazole, hydantoin, oxazole, benzoxazole, thiazole, and benzothiazole derivatives are recognized as treasured molecules in medicinal, agricultural, and pharmaceutical chemistry. The heterocycles bearing these moieties are reported to be present in numerous biologically active molecules and natural products. In the past few years, synthetic organic chemistry has been linked to green chemical approaches through which environmentally benign routes are supposed to be designed and used. Some of the eco-friendly and sustainable protocols include the use of nanomaterial as a catalyst, the use of a green solvent or no solvent, and the use of alternative conventional thermal methods, namely ultrasonic and microwave irradiation.

Organic chemistry can be divided into several classes, of which heterocycles form by far the leading class and are of enormous prominence industrially, biologically, and certainly for the efficiency of any advanced human civilization. Almost all the biologically active agrochemicals and pharmaceuticals are heterocyclic scaffolds, as are innumerable modifiers and additives used in manufacturing units as diverse as information storage, reprography, plastics, and cosmetics. Nitrogen (N), sulphur (S), and oxygen (O) containing heterocyclic systems exist in widely held natural products that contribute to gigantic structural multiplicity, and further, they retain biological activity more generally (Figure 9.1). Therapeutic chemists have exploited this last characteristic in creating a number of tiny drug molecules in current use. This chapter considers the fundamentals of heterocyclic chemistry and its manifestation in natural products such as vitamins, antibiotics, DNA, and amino acids. The scope and variability of the subject is imitated in the composition of heterocycles and partially in a range of areas on the amalgamation of these heterocyclic compounds, and other choices are extensively emphasized.

The basic introduction, synthetic protocols and biological applications of the following heterocycles are described in this chapter:

9.2   Imidazoles
9.3   Hydantoins

DOI: 10.1201/9781003141488-9

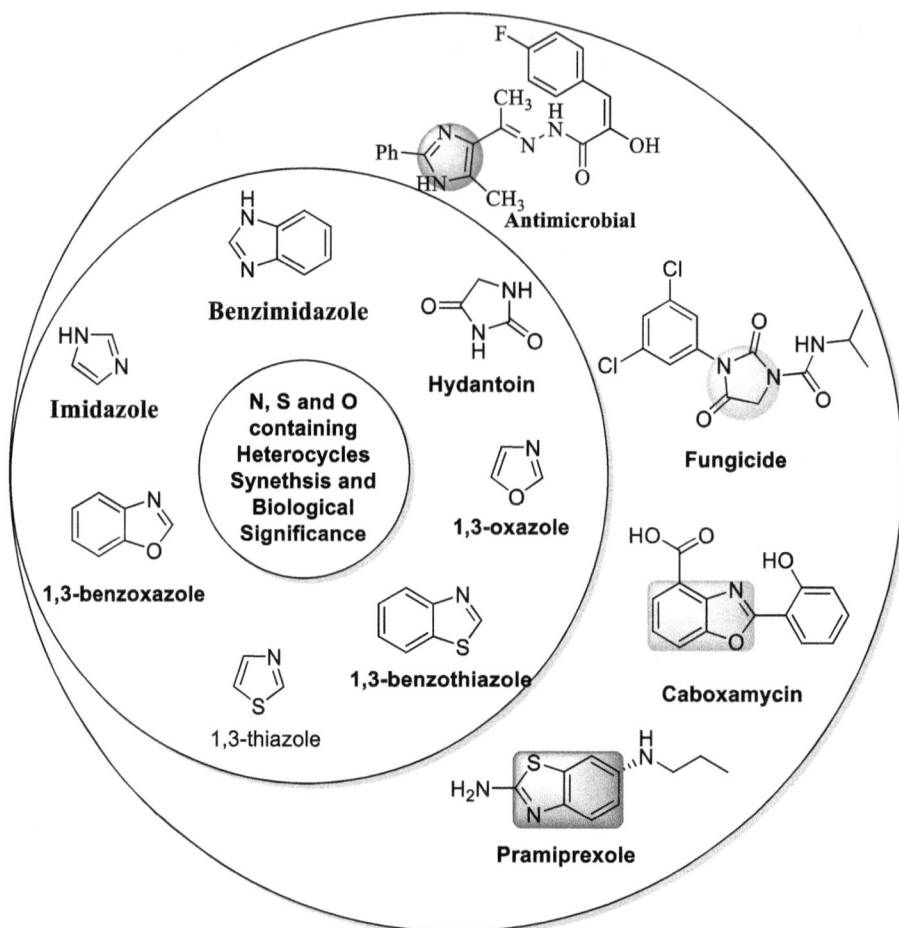

FIGURE 9.1   N, S and O containing heterocycles and their biological significance

9.4   Oxazoles
9.5   Thiazoles

9.2   IMIDAZOLE

Imidazole (Figure 9.2a) is a five-membered heterocycle containing a nitrogen atom at the 1,3-position. The imidazole ring is an integral part of various significant natural products such as nucleic acid, histamine, purine, and histidine. The imidazole ring is the key component of many biologically significant compounds and shows various pharmaceutical properties such as antibacterial, antifungal, analgesic, anti-inflammatory, antidepressant, anti-tubercular, anticancer, anti-leishmanial, and anti-viral properties.[1-3] Imidazole remedies have wide use in resolving several outlooks in medical prescriptions. Several procedures for the preparation of imidazoles and their numerous structural transformations offer massive possibilities in the area of pharmaceutical chemistry.

Benzimidazole (Figure 9.2b) is also a heterocyclic aromatic compound that is a combination of a benzene and an imidazole ring and has the molecular formula $C_7H_6N_2$. Imidazole and its benzofused derivatives have aromatic moiety and so are highly stable due to resonance (Figure 9.3). In research, benzimidazole has a huge variety of uses as a material for the preparation of many bioactive scaffolds. Many anthelmintic remedies, such as triclabendazole, mebendazole, and albendazole, belong to

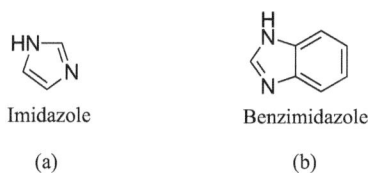

FIGURE 9.2   The structure of imidazole (a) and benzimidazole (b)

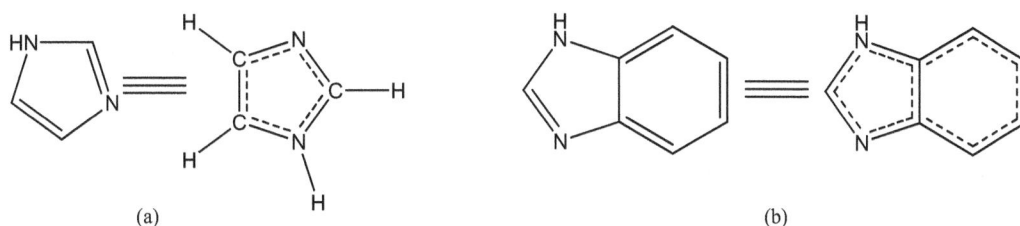

FIGURE 9.3   Resonance hybrid of (a) imidazole and (b) benzimidazole

the benzimidazole class of compounds. The proton-pump inhibitors (antacids) lansoprazole, omeprazole, rabeprazole, and pantoprazole have a benzimidazole ring. Other pharmacological drugs that feature benzimidazole are galeterone, dovitinib, and mavatrep, as well the benzimidazole opioids, such as etonitazene.

9.2.1   Synthesis of Imidazole and Benzimidazole Derivatives

Maleki et al.[4] reported the synthesis of a new catalytic system sulfonated Fe_3O_4@PVA nanostructure. This Fe_3O_4@PVA sulfonic acid-based superparamagnetic nanocatalyst was used for the preparation of 2,4,5-triarylimidazole derivatives in ethanol through a three-component one-pot reaction between benzil or benzoin, ammonium acetate, and aldehyde derivatives (Scheme 9.1). The catalyst is reusable and inexpensive and can be recycled simply by using an external magnet due to the high magnetic characteristic of the catalyst without any significant loss of its catalytic activity. The advantages of this protocol are highly efficient synthesis, high atom economy, use of environmentally benign reaction conditions, and cheap solvent.

Thwin et al.[5] synthesized bioactive polysubstituted pyrroles and 1,2,4,5-tetrasubstituted imidazole derivatives on the reaction of a wide range of aldehydes, amines, benzil, and ammonium acetate catalyzed by Cu@imine/Fe_3O_4 magnetic nanoparticles (MNPs) under solvent-free conditions (Scheme 9.2). The catalyst showed extraordinary reactivity for the desired synthesis of a spectrum of imidazoles under mild reaction conditions in short reaction times and was recycled and reused without any substantial loss in reactivity and yields. This synthetic protocol displayed a number of advantages, such as being eco-friendly, facile, and efficient, giving excellent yields, easy workup, easy purification of the products, short reaction time, low cost, easy separation, and high reusability of the catalyst.

Varzi et al.[6] prepared hybrid nanocatalyst ZnS-$ZnFe_2O_4$ and then reported the synthesis of 2,4,5-triaryl-1H-imidazole derivatives from different aromatic aldehydes, benzil, and ammonium acetate in ethanol under ultrasonication at 70°C using ZnS-$ZnFe_2O_4$ as a catalyst (Scheme 9.3). This procedure has numerous benefits, such as high yields, the use of an eco-friendly solvent, simple isolation of products, high efficacy of the heterogeneous catalyst, short reaction times, mild reaction conditions, and chromatography-free purification. ZnS-$ZnFe_2O_4$ MTMO showed high catalytic activity and could be recovered by simply using an external magnet and reused several times in organic transformations.

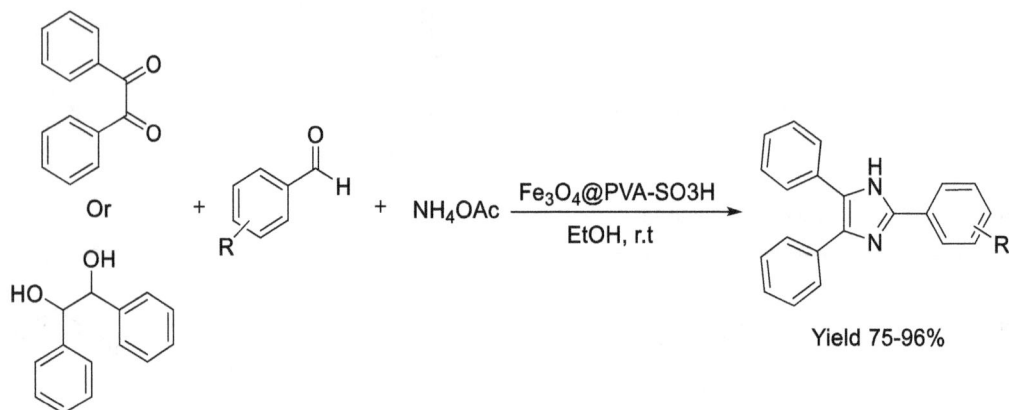

SCHEME 9.1 Synthesis of Fe3O4@PVA-SO3H and their catalytic use for the synthesis of 2,4,5-triaryl-1H-imidazoles

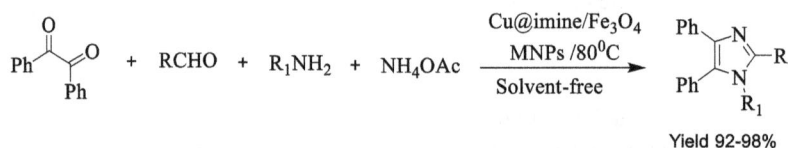

SCHEME 9.2 Synthesis of 1,2,4,5-tetrasbstituted imidazoles derivatives using Cu@imine/Fe3O4 MNPs as a catalyst

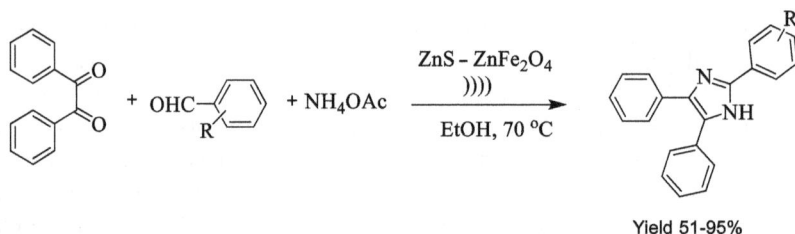

SCHEME 9.3 Synthesis of 2,4,5-triaryl-1H-imidazoles catalyzed by ZnS-ZnFe$_2$O$_4$ MTMO

The synthesis of 2,4,5-trisubstituted imidazoles was reported by Mardani et al.[7] by a three-component reaction of aromatic aldehydes, benzil, and ammonium acetate using reusable, low-cost, eco-friendly Fe$_3$O$_4$ nanoparticles (NPs) under a low-power microwave in solvent-free conditions (Scheme 9.4). The use of Fe$_3$O$_4$ MNPs was introduced as environmentally benign, heterogeneous, and reusable, and was easily separable from the reaction mixture catalyst. This procedure has many advantages, such as moderate-to-excellent yields, environmental acceptability, easy workup, short reaction time, atom economy, low-cost under solvent-free conditions, low-power microwave irradiation, and simple removal of catalyst.

Nejatianfar et al.[8] introduced an environmentally benign, effective, and simple method for the production of 2,4,5-trisubstituted and 1,2,4,5-tetrasubstituted imidazoles catalyzed by Cu(II) immobilized on a guanidinated epibromohydrin-functionalized γ-Fe$_2$O$_3$@TiO$_2$ (γ-Fe$_2$O$_3$@TiO$_2$-EG-Cu(II) nanocatalyst through a condensation reaction under solvent-free conditions. Several

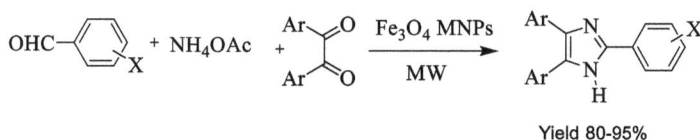

SCHEME 9.4 Synthesis of trisubstituted imidazoles using Fe_3O_4 MNPs under solvent-free and microwave irradiation conditions

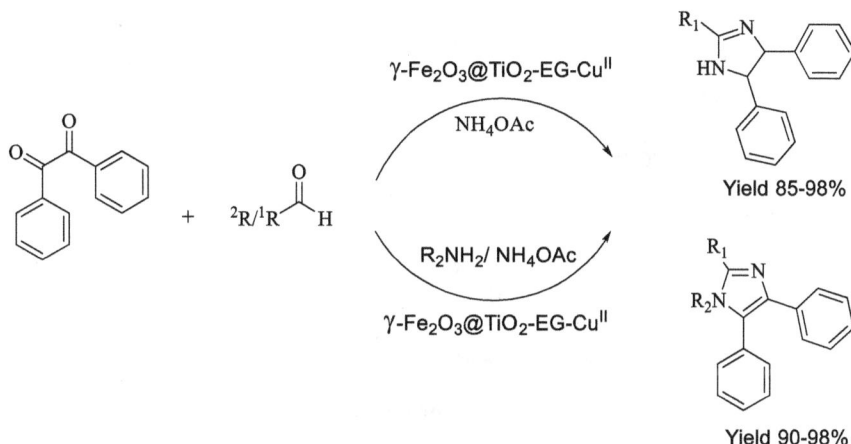

SCHEME 9.5 Synthesis of 2,4,5-trisubstituted and 1,2,4,5-tetrasubstituted imidazoles in the presence of γ-Fe2O3@TiO2-EG-Cu (II) nanocatalyst

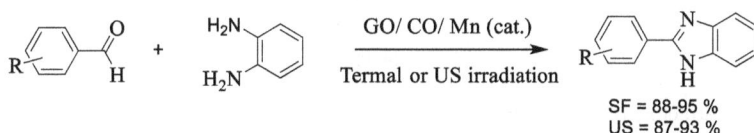

SCHEME 9.6 Synthesis of benzimidazole derivatives

aldehydes, benzil, ammonium acetate, and amines were reacted to synthesized desired imidazole derivatives using γ-Fe_2O_3@TiO_2-EG-Cu(II) as a reusable nanocatalyst (Scheme 9.5). This magnetic catalyst has many benefits, such as being non-volatile, green, thermally robust, efficient, easy to handle, non-explosive, recoverable and reusable numerous times without any noticeable loss of its catalytic activity. The current synthetic procedure has several advantages, such as short reaction time, excellent yields of products, green reaction media, high atom economy, easy procedure, and a variety of substrates.

Karami et al.[9] prepared a novel nanocatalyst, Co/Mn metal oxide supported on graphene oxide sheets for the formation of benzimidazole derivatives from 1,2-benzenediamine and corresponding aldehydes in water under ultrasound irradiation (Scheme 9.6). The reaction showed several benefits, such as simple operation and easy workup, excellent yield of desired products, mild conditions, short reaction time, non-toxic and inexpensive catalyst, an eco-friendly procedure, and reusability of catalyst. The structures of biologically active imidazole and benzimidazole derivatives are shown in (Figure 9.4).

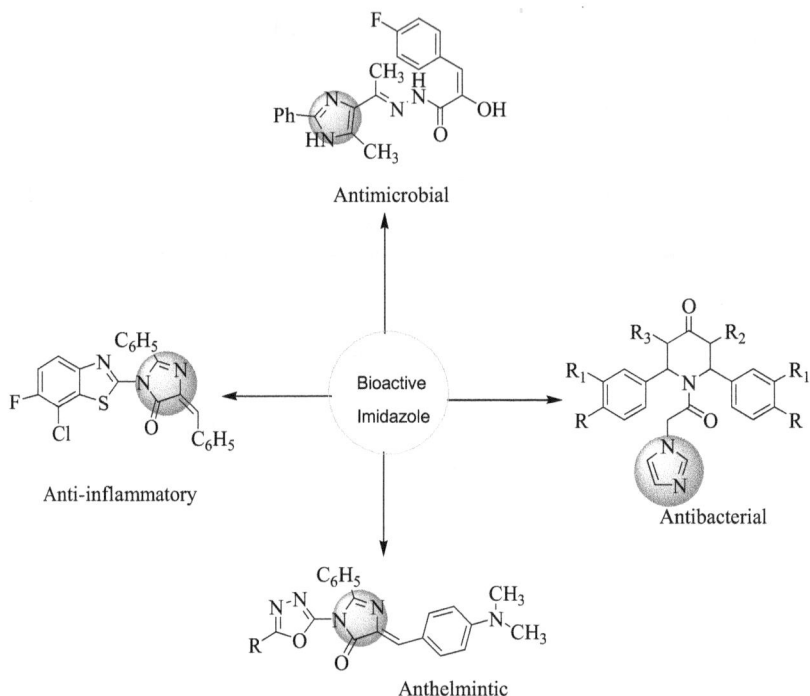

FIGURE 9.4   Some biologically active imidazole and benzimidazole derivatives

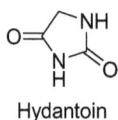

Hydantoin

FIGURE 9.5   The structure of hydantoin

9.3   HYDANTOIN

Hydantoin, or glycolylurea (Figure 9.5), is an oxidized compound of imidazolidine and was first separated by Adolf von Baeyer in 1861 when he was studying uric acid. The hydantoin moiety is a vital structural moiety that exists in a range of biologically potent compounds[10] and is used to treat many human diseases. Depending on the nature of substitution on the hydantoin ring, a wide range of pharmacological properties, for example, anti-ulcer, anti-muscarinic, anti-arrhythmic, anticonvulsant, antiviral, and anti-diabetic agents,[11] have been identified. Some hydantoin derivatives have also been used as platelet aggregation inhibitors, as well as antidepressants.[12]

9.3.1   Synthesis of Hydantoin Derivatives

Safari et al.[13] reported the synthesis of 5-substituted hydantoins by reaction of aldehydes, ammonium carbonate, and zinc cyanide in the presence of magnetic Fe_3O_4-chitosan NPs in an ethanol-acetic acid-water system (1:1:1) (Scheme 9.7). The naturally occurring biopolymer on the deacetylation-formed chitin chitosan is one of the main components of the shells of crustaceans. In many reactions, chitosan is used as a green catalyst in its native form and even as solid support for the functioning

$$RCHO + (NH_4)_2CO_3 + Zn(CN)_2 \xrightarrow[\substack{EtOH/AcOH/H_2O \\ 60^0C}]{Fe_3O_4 - Chitosan\ nps}$$

Yield 80-97%

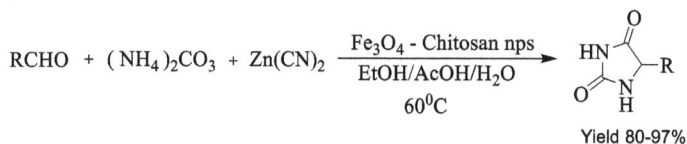

SCHEME 9.7 The synthesis of 5-substituted hydantoin derivatives

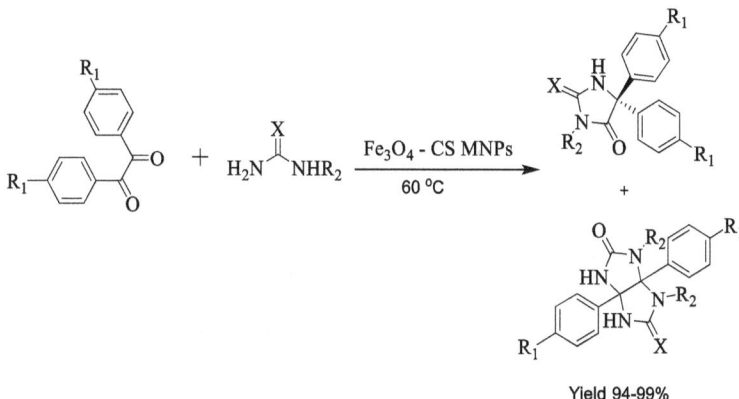

Yield 94-99%

SCHEME 9.8 Synthesis of 5,5-diphenylhydantoins and 5,5-diphenyl-2-thiohydantoins

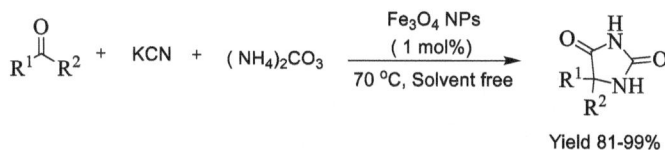

Yield 81-99%

SCHEME 9.9 Synthesis of hydantoin derivatives by using Fe_3O_4 NPs as catalyst

of many reactions. It displays many benefits, such as reusability, non-toxicity, biocompatibility, low cost, operational simplicity, biodegradability, and renewability. This reaction showed many important features, such as low cost, mild reaction conditions, use of green chemistry principles, and a renewable and reusable catalyst.

Safari et al.[14] reported the synthesis of 5,5-diphenylhydantoins and 5,5-diphenyl-2-thiohydantoins catalyzed by magnetic Fe_3O_4-chitosan NPs efficiently from substituted urea or thiourea, and benzil derivatives (Scheme 9.8). Fe_3O_4-chitosan NPs were set up to be an effortlessly prepared, recoverable and reusable organocatalyst. It was easily recovered under a magnetic field without considerable loss of its catalytic activity, even after several runs. This protocol has several advantageous features, such as environmental friendliness, operational simplicity, low catalyst loading, and reusability of the catalyst.

Safari et al.[15] reported the one-pot, facile, and rapid production of 5,5-disubstituted hydantoins catalyzed by magnetic Fe_3O_4 NPs under solvent-free conditions by a multi-component reaction of potassium cyanide, aldehydes and ketones (carbonyl compounds), and ammonium carbonate (Scheme 9.9). The use of MNPs as a catalyst makes this approach green and sustainable. This procedure has numerous advantages, such as excellent yields, very easy execution of approach, short reaction time, simplicity, use of a reusable magnetic catalyst, and simple separation of the catalyst from the reaction mixture just by using an external magnet.

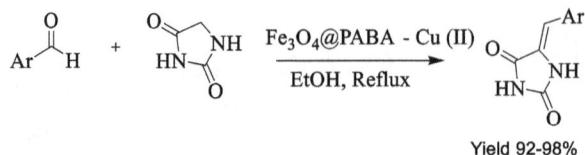

SCHEME 9.10 Synthesis of 5-arylidenthiazolidine-2,4-dione and 5-arylidene-imidazolidine-2,4-dione derivatives catalyzed by Fe3O4@PABA-Cu (II) MNPs

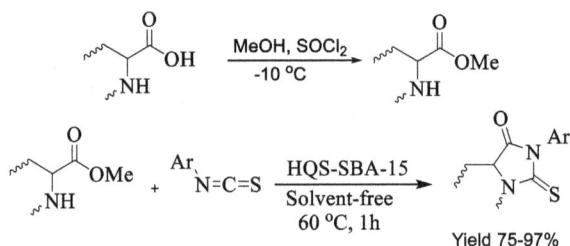

SCHEME 9.11 Synthesis of 2-thiohydantoin catalyzed by HQS-SBA-15

Esam et al.[16] suggested an efficient and novel synthetic approach to produce 5-arylidenthiazolidine-2,4-diones and 5-arylidene-2-imidazolidine-2,4-dione derivatives by aldol condensation between various heteroaromatic aldehydes and hydantoin or thiazolidine-2,4-dione scaffolds in ethanol, and catalyzed by recoverable nanocatalyst Fe$_3$O$_4$@PABA-Cu(II) MNPs (Scheme 9.10). This method presented numerous noteworthy factors, such as easy workup, simple separation of the catalyst from products, non-toxic nature and environmentally benign catalyst characteristics, catalyst reusability, lower formation of byproducts, efficiency, excellent yields, and short reaction time. The nanocatalyst Fe$_3$O$_4$@PABA-Cu(II) was easily recovered by a magnet and is a good replacement for a homogenous mineral catalyst that cannot be recovered. The surface-modified MNPs are green and are a reusable nanosized catalyst with excellent activity and PABA as a biocompatible and non-toxic compound that serves as an efficient bridge between Fe$_3$O$_4$ and Cu particles to form a stable and leak-free nanocatalyst.

Vavsari et al.[17] reported the one-pot preparation of 2-thiohydantoin derivatives on the reaction of α-aminoester, and isothiocyanate derivatives catalyzed by new renewable mesoporous silica SBA-15 functionalized with 8-hydroxyquinoline-5-sulfonic acid (HQS-SBA-15) nanocatalyst under solvent-free conditions (Scheme 9.11). The novel catalyst displayed many merits, such as easy handling, excellent recyclability with high catalytic activity, low catalyst amount used, and recovery. Thus, this approach is found to be mild, green, and economical, with a high yield of products for this reaction.

Maiti et al.[18] reported a green synthetic procedure for the preparation of oxo- and thiohydantoin counterparts fused with tetrahydro-β-carboline supported by a novel ionic liquid (IL) initiated by thermal and microwave irradiation. With various carbonyl compounds, IL-bound tryptophan underwent a Pictet-Spengler reaction to produce the IL-immobilized tetrahydro-β-carbolines in aqueous isopropanol media. With various isocyanates and isothiocyanate, the successive reaction of substituted tetrahydrocarboline derivatives provided a three-dimensional combinatorial library in a traceless manner. This reaction involves the coupling of Boc-protected L-tryptophan to hydroxyl ethylmethylimidazoliumtetrafluoroborate (Scheme 9.12). The main importance of using an IL soluble support was its straight easy monitoring capacity using standard analytical techniques and its eco-friendliness. Most hydantoin derivatives are biologically active, and their structures are shown in (Figure 9.6).

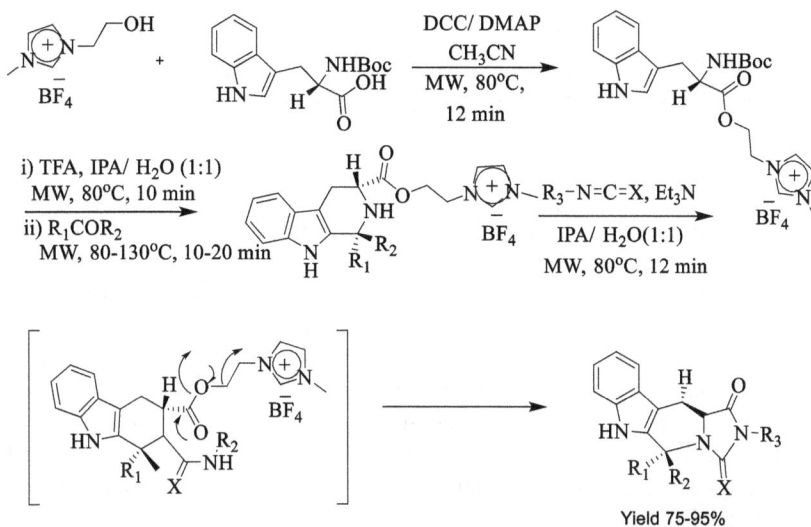

SCHEME 9.12 Synthesis of Hydantoin fused with tetrahydro-β-carboline supported by IL

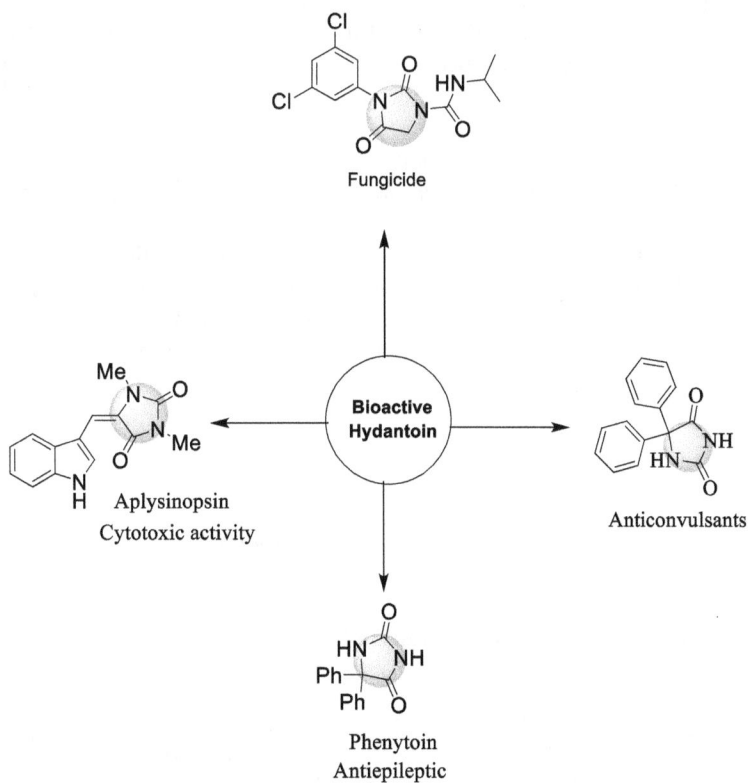

FIGURE 9.6 Some biologically active hydantoin derivatives

9.4 OXAZOLES

Oxazole (Figure 9.7a) is a five-membered heterocyclic compound containing an oxygen and a nitrogen atom at the 1,3-position. These are aromatic in nature but less aromatic than thiazoles. The derivatives of oxazole are very important because they could be used as intermediates for the construction of other new biologically active molecules. The oxazole ring is the key component of many pharmacologically important compounds that possess a wide range of biological properties, such as antimicrobial,[19] anticancer,[20] anti-tubercular,[21] anti-inflammatory,[22] anti-diabetic,[23] anti-obesity,[24] and antioxidant properties,[25] and oxazole derivatives are also useful in the formation of synthetic intermediates and could be used as chemical scaffolds in combinatorial chemistry.

Benzoxazole (Figure 9.7b) is also an aromatic heterocycle that has a benzene-fused oxazole ring and the molecular formula C_7H_5NO. Benzoxazole itself has very few practical aspects. It has a large variety of uses in research as a starting material for the synthesis of many bioactive scaffolds and has many reactive sites that allow for functionalization at the ring due to highly stability (Figure 9.8). It is found as a chemical structure in many pharmaceutical drugs such as flunoxaprofen and tafamidis. Benzoxazole belongs to the group of antifungal agents with anti-allergic, antioxidant, anti-parasitic, and anti-tumoral activity.

9.4.1 SYNTHESIS OF OXAZOLE AND BENZOXAZOLE DERIVATIVES

Ziarati et al.[26] reported the synthesis of a series of bioactive benzoxazoles from a mixture of aldehyde and o-Phenylenediamine with $NiFe_{2-x}Eu_xO_4$ MNPs as a catalyst in water as solvent under conventional method and ultrasonication (Scheme 9.13). This synthetic protocol has many benefits compared with other methods, such as simplicity, mild reaction conditions, efficiency, ultrasound-mediated, the use of safe and cheap solvents, the use of green reusable $NiFe_{2-x}Eu_xO_4$ MNPs as a catalyst, and high yields of products. The catalyst used in this procedure has several advantages, such as being magnetically separable, easily synthesized in laboratories, recoverable, and recyclable.

Fekri et al.[27] synthesized novel benzoxazole derivatives by the reaction of aryl aldehydes with 2-aminophenol catalyzed by $NiFe_2O_4@SiO_2@$amino glucose (Scheme 9.14). This approach has many advantages, such as high-to-excellent yields, cost-efficiency, environmental friendliness, waste reduction, short reaction times, ease of separation and reusability of the magnetic catalyst,

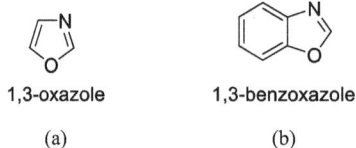

1,3-oxazole   1,3-benzoxazole

(a)   (b)

FIGURE 9.7   Structure of (a) oxazole and (b) benzoxazole

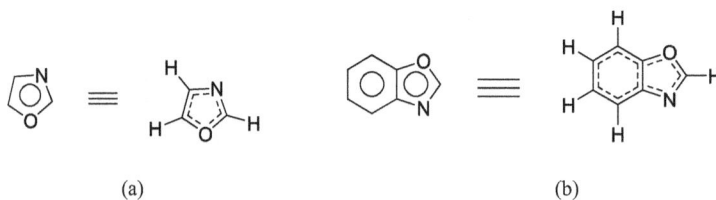

(a)   (b)

FIGURE 9.8   Resonance hybrid of (a) oxazole and (b) benzoxazole

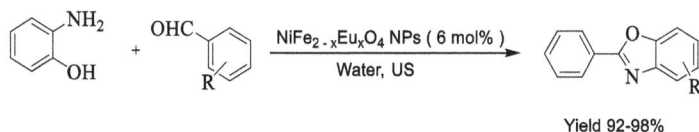

SCHEME 9.13 NiFe$_2$-xEuxO$_4$ MNPs catalyzed preparation of benzoxazoles

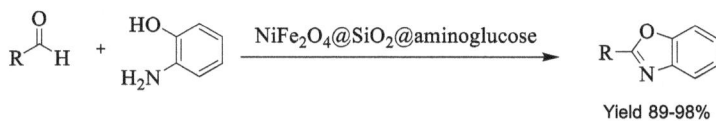

SCHEME 9.14 Synthesis of benzoxazoles using NiFe2O4@SiO2@amino glucose catalyst

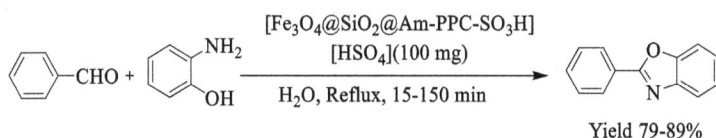

SCHEME 9.15 Synthesis of benzoxazoles using MNPs as catalyst

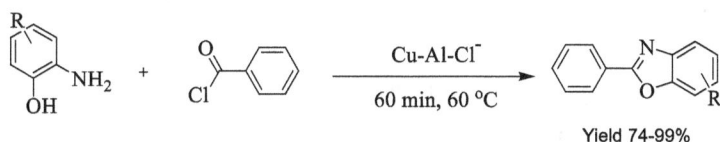

SCHEME 9.16 Synthesis of 2-phenyl benzoxazole derivatives

and simple workup. The synthesized catalyst NiFe$_2$O$_4$@SiO$_2$@amino glucose is novel and can be effortlessly recovered and reused for successive reaction cycles.

Sayyahi et al.[28] successfully prepared a novel magnetic nanoparticle-based heterogeneous acidic catalyst [Fe$_3$O$_4$@SiO$_2$@Am-PPC-SO$_3$H] [HSO$_4$] which was used in the synthesis of benzoxazoles from the reaction of aldehyde and o-aminophenol in aqueous media (Scheme 9.15). The catalyst was retrievable, sustainable, and separated magnetically, which shows excellent reusability without significant loss of its activity. Some of the advantages include products synthesized in high yields, mild reaction conditions, short reaction time, and environmental friendliness.

Benzoxazoles were synthesized by Gupta et al.[29] on the facile reaction of benzoyl chloride, 2-amino phenol, and Al-Cu-Cl hydrotalcite as heterogeneous nanocatalyst under solvent-free conditions (Scheme 9.16). This protocol was more efficient as compared to other reported synthetic procedures as it had lower catalyst loading, clean reaction profiles, mild reaction conditions, cost efficiency, atom economy, easy workup, and a recyclable and reusable catalyst that did not lose its activity even after five runs. Benzoxazoles are the key components of bioactive heterocycles, and the structures of these heterocycles are shown in (Figure 9.9).

9.5 THIAZOLES

Thiazole (Figure 9.10a) is a five-membered heterocyclic compound containing a sulphur and a nitrogen atom at the 1,3-position. They are planar and aromatic in nature, but more aromatic than oxazoles. The thiazole ring is notable as a component of the vitamin thiamine (B$_1$). Other

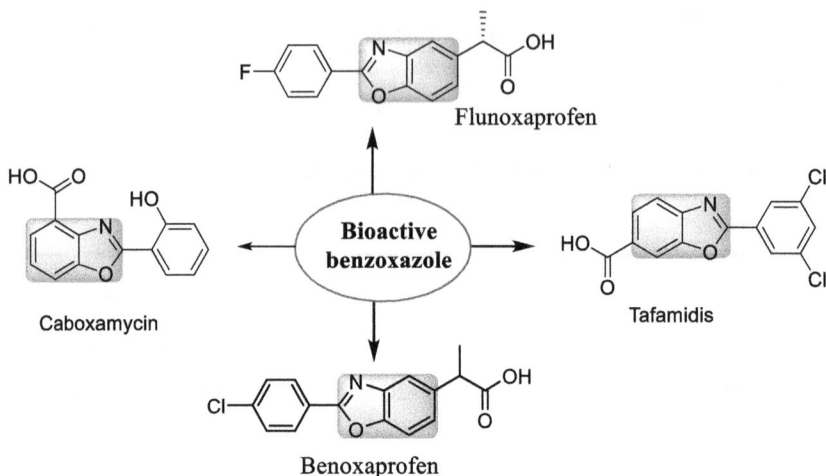

FIGURE 9.9 Structure of bioactive benzoxazoles

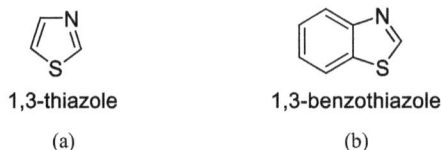

FIGURE 9.10 Structure of (a) thiazole and (b) benzothiazole

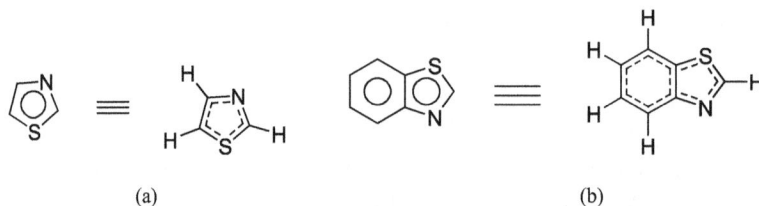

FIGURE 9.11 Resonance hybrid of (a) thiazole and (b) benzothiazole

compounds of thiazole take in rhodanine and the rhodanine red dye, and the yellow dye primuline is prepared from it. Some examples of drugs synthesized from thiazoles are thiazolsulfone (promizole), sulfasuxidine, and sulfathiazole. Thiazole-based derivative 2-mercaptobenzothiazole (mertax) is utilized to speed up the vulcanization of rubber. Furthermore, thiazoles have displayed promising antimicrobial, antifungal,[30,31] antitumor, and antiviral activities,[32–36] as well as many other biological applications.[37–39]

Benzothiazole (Figure 9.10b) is also an aromatic heterocyclic compound. It contains a benzene-fused thiazole ring with the molecular formula C_7H_5NS and is stabilized through resonance (Figure 9.11). It is present in naturally synthesized peptides and utilized in the expansion of peptidomimetics (i.e., molecules that mimic the function and structure of peptides). Benzothiazoles display a wide spectrum of pharmacological applications such as antioxidant,[40] anti-inflammatory, antimicrobial,[41] antiviral, and anticancer[42] activities. In current years, some benzothiazole derivatives have found solicitation in medicinal and bioorganic chemistry and in the advancement of proven drugs such as lubeluzole, pramipexole, ethoxzolamide, probenazole, bentaluron, and zopolrestat.[43]

9.5.1 Synthesis of Thiazole and Benzothiazole Derivatives

Hangirgekar et al.[44] reported the synthesis of pharmaceutically active hydrazinyl thiazole through a simple and efficient method with high-to-excellent yields of products from the three-component, one-pot condensation of thiosemicarbazide phenyl tosylates, and substituted aryl aldehydes in the catalytic influence of magnetic Fe_2O_3 NPs in water as solvent (Scheme 9.17). This synthetic protocol has many outstanding features, such as an eco-friendly approach, mild reaction conditions, use of green solvent, and excellent yields. The catalyst was easily recovered and reused many times in small amounts without any significant loss of its catalytic effect.

Shaterian et al.[45] prepared Fe_3O_4@vitamin B_1 as an efficient and inexpensive heterogeneous nanocatalyst for the production of novel trisubstituted 1,3-thiazole derivatives by a one-pot, three-component reaction of cyclic 1,3-dicarbonyls, thioamides, and arylglyoxal monohydrate in an aqueous medium (Scheme 9.18). Some advantages of this methodology are short reaction times, high yields, simple operation, use of green solvent, cost-effectiveness, eco-friendly nature, simple preparation of the catalyst from commercially available materials, and high catalytic activity that makes it sustainable, economic, and in convention with some green chemistry protocols. Vitamin B_1 stabilized on Fe_3O_4 MNPs is a superparamagnetic, highly efficient, retrievable nanocatalyst that is magnetically removable and retains its strength after reutilizing without detectable activity loss.

Gundala et al.[46] reported that the three-component one-pot amalgamation of different aldehydes/ketones, thiosemicarbazide, and different phenacyl bromides in the catalytic influence of copper oxide NPs dispersed on titanium dioxide in water yielded a collection of hydrazinyl-thiazoles (Scheme 9.19). The significant features of this method are a clean reaction profile, green approach,

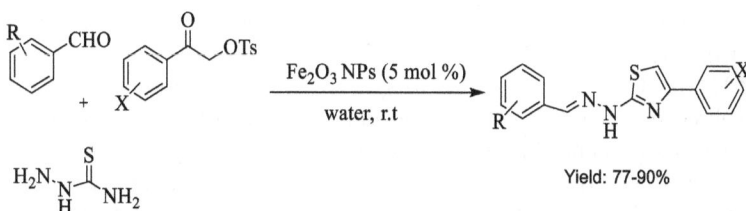

SCHEME 9.17   Magnetic Fe_2O_3 NPs catalyzed synthesis of hydrazinylthiazoles

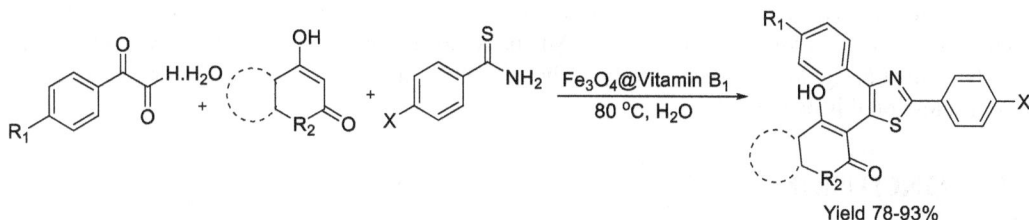

SCHEME 9.18   Synthesis of 1,3-thiazoles catalyzed by Fe3O4@vitamin B_1 MNPs

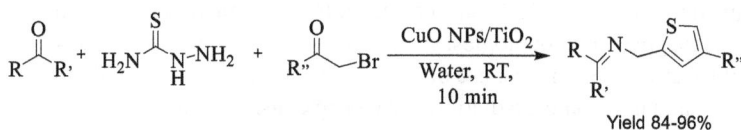

SCHEME 9.19   Multi-component synthesis of diversified hydrazinyl-thiazoles catalyzed by CuO NPs/TiO$_2$ in water

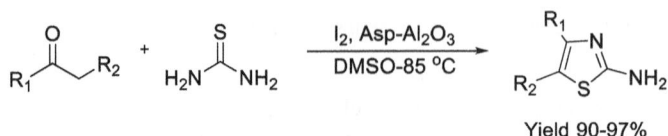

Yield 90-97%

SCHEME 9.20   Asp-Al$_2$O$_3$ NPs catalyzed thiazoles synthesis

broad substrate scope, short reaction time, ease of operation, scalability, no chromatographic puri-fication required, high yields at low catalyst loading, and potential for comprehensive applications in pharmacological industries. The catalyst used in this protocol was recoverable and reusable without any noteworthy loss of its activity. Additionally, the high catalytic performance of CuONPs/TiO$_2$ was due to the high dispersity of the catalyst in water, followed by the interaction of organic substrates with CuONPs.

Zamegar et al.[47] reported the preparation of asparagine functionalized aluminium oxide (Asp-Al$_2$O$_3$) NPs by a two-step procedure that involved the grafting of Al$_2$O$_3$ with 3-chloropropyltrimethoxysilane (CPTMS) and successive organo-functionalization using aspara-gine amino acid. Then 2-aminothiazoles were synthesized by a one-pot reaction of thiourea, methylcarbonyls, and iodine as an oxidizing reagent catalyzed by the Asp-Al$_2$O$_3$ organo-nanocatalyst at 85°C in dimethylsulfoxide (DMSO) (Scheme 9.20). The benefits of this improved procedure include a green approach, an environmentally safe route, clean conditions, short reaction time, simple workup, excellent yield of products with high purity, easy separation of products, reusability of the nanocatalyst, and suitable handling. In addition, immobilization of organocatalysts on the Al$_2$O$_3$ surface was stable under the catalytic reaction conditions, which suggests that they can be reused efficiently. Initially, Al$_2$O$_3$ NPs were produced by a precipitation method and reformed with 3-chloropropyltrimethoxysilane (CPTMS).

A modified Hantzsch method was used to synthesize novel 4-thiazolylpyrazoles by Beyzaei et al.[48] on the three-step reaction of malononitrile, triethyl orthoacetate, and phenylhydrazine through acid-catalysis (Scheme 9.21). Thionation of pyrazole was then carried out by phos-phorus pentasulfide (P$_4$S$_{10}$) to give 5-amino-3-methyl-1-phenyl-1H-pyrazole-4-carbothioamide in the presence of MgO NPs as catalyst under solvent-free conditions. Lastly, cyclocondensation of thioamide with α-bromoketones made 4-thiazolylpyrazoles. This synthetic procedure is better than other methods because of greater efficiency, excellent yields in shorter reaction times, and environmental friendliness. As a final point, the newly synthesized compounds were tested for in vitro antibacterial activities against a range of pathogenic bacteria. All derivatives displayed moderate-to-good activities (Figure 9.12). All the synthesized compounds displayed inhibitory effects against *S. agalactiae* successfully, although antibiotics such as penicillin and ceftriaxone were useless on this pathogen.

9.6   CONCLUSION

Imidazoles are highly interesting heterocyclic moieties as they represent a number of biologically and pharmacologically active molecules. These heterocyclic scaffolds are the building blocks of sev-eral natural products and drug molecules. As scientists move towards environmentally green chem-istry, a new branch of chemistry has been introduced to synthetic organic and inorganic chemistry. In the past few years, green methodologies, such as the use of catalysts that can be further reutilized, less or no use of hazardous chemicals, use of green solvents, and the use of alternate energy sources such as microwave and ultrasonic irradiation, have been considered for the production of imidazole, hydantoin, oxazole, and thiazole-containing heterocycles. Furthermore, in all the reactions, products

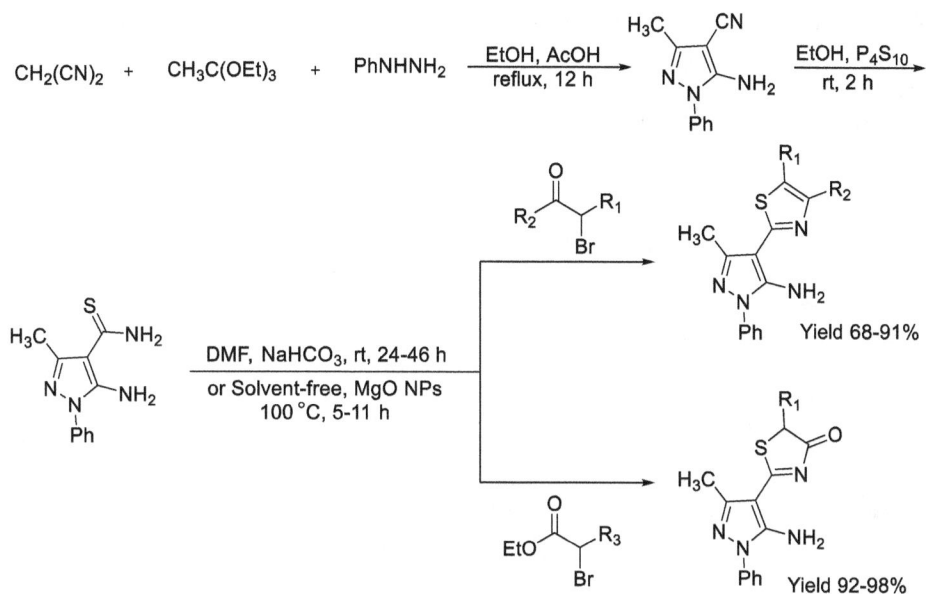

SCHEME 9.21   Synthesis of Hantzschthiazole derivatives

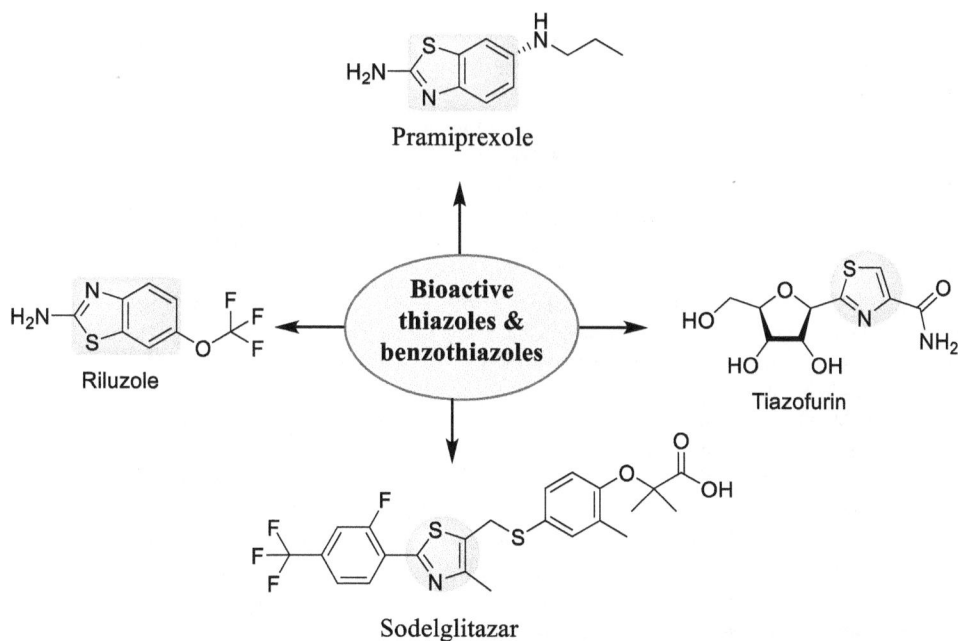

FIGURE 9.12   Structure of bioactive thiazoles and benzothiazoles

were formed in excellent yields and in short times without the use of volatile organic solvents and in the presence of reusable catalysts and green reaction media. In this chapter, we have summarized the synthesis of imidazole, hydantoin, oxazole, and thiazole derivatives using eco-friendly approaches, and with examples of heterocycles with medicinal potential.

REFERENCES

1. Congiu C, Cocco MT, Onnis V. (2008). Design, synthesis, and in vitro antitumor activity of new 1,4-diarylimidazole-2-ones and their 2-thione analogues. Bioorg Med Chem Lett. 18: 989–993. https://doi.org/10.1016/j.bmcl.2007.12.023.

2. Venkatesan AM, Agarwal A, Abe T, Ushirogochi HO, Santos D, Li Z, Francisco G, Lin YI, Peterson PJ, Yang Y, Weiss WJ, Shales DM, Mansour TS. (2008). 5,5,6-Fused tricycles bearing imidazole and pyrazole 6-methylidene penems as broad-spectrum inhibitors of β-lactamases. Bioorg Med Chem. 16:1890–1902. https://doi.org/10.1016/j.bmc.2007.11.006.

3. Roman G, Riley JG, Vlahakis JZ, Kinobe RT, Brien JF, Nakatsu K, Szarek WA. (2007). Heme oxygenase inhibition by 2-oxy-substituted 1-(1H-imidazol-1-yl)-4-phenylbutanes: Effect of halogen substitution in the phenyl ring. Bioorg Med Chem. 15:3225–3234. https://doi.org/10.1016/j.bmc.2007.02.034.

4. Maleki A, Rahimi J, Valadi K. (2019). Sulfonated Fe_3O_4@PVA superparamagnetic nanostructure: Design, in-situ preparation, characterization and application in the synthesis of imidazoles as a highly efficient organic–inorganic Bronsted acid catalyst. Nano-Structures & Nano-Objects. 18:100264. https://doi.org/10.1016/j.nanoso.2019.100264.

5. Thwin M, Mahmoudi B, Olga A, Ivaschukc, Qahtan A, Yousif. (2019). An efficient and recyclable nanocatalyst for the green and rapid synthesis of biologically active polysubstituted pyrroles and 1,2,4,5- tetrasubstituted imidazole derivatives. RSC Adv. 9:15966–15975. https://doi.org/10.1039/C9RA02325A.

6. Varzi Z, Maleki A. (2019). Design and preparation of ZnS-$ZnFe_2O_4$: A green and efficient hybrid nanocatalyst for the multicomponent synthesis of 2,4,5-triaryl-1H-imidazoles. Appl Organometal Chem. 5008. https://doi.org/10.1002/aoc.5008.

7. Mardani HR, Forouzani M, Emami R. (2019). Efficient and green synthesis of trisubstituted imidazoles by magnetically nanocatalyst and microwave assisted. Asian Journal of Green Chem. 3:525–535.

8. Nejatianfar M, Akhlaghinia B, Jahanshahi R. (2018). Cu (II) immobilized on guanidinated epibromohydrin-functionalized γ-Fe_2O_3@TiO_2 (γ-Fe_2O_3@TiO_2-EG-Cu(II)): A highly efficient magnetically separable heterogeneous nanocatalyst for one-pot synthesis of highly substituted imidazoles. Appl Organometal Chem. 32(2):4095. https://doi.org/10.1002/aoc.4095.

9. Karami AY, Manaf M, Ghodrati K, Khajavi R, Hojjati M. (2020). Nanoparticles supported graphene oxide and its application as an efficient and recyclable nano-catalyst in the synthesis of imidazole derivatives in ultrasound solvent-free condition. Int Nano Lett. 10:89–95. https://doi.org/10.1007/s40089-020-00297-8.

10. Meusel M, Gutschow M. (2004). Recent developments in hydantoin chemistry. A review. Org Pre Proced Int. 36 (5):391–443. https://doi.org/10.1080/00304940409356627.

11. (a) Thenmozhiyal JC, Wong PTH, Chui WK. (2004). Anticonvulsant activity of phenylmethylenehydantoins: A structure-activity relationship study. J Med Chem. 47(6):1527–1535. https://doi.org/10.1021/jm030450c. (b) Khanfar MA, Sayed KA El. (2010). Phenylmethylene hydantoins as prostate cancer invasion and migration inhibitors. CoMFA approach and QSAR analysis. Eur J Med Chem. 45(11):5397–5405. https://doi.org/10.1016/j.ejmech.2010.08.066.

12. (a) Wessels FL, Schwan TJ, Pong SF. (1980). Synthesis and antidepressant activity of 5- (4-dimethylaminobenzyl) imidazolidine-2,4-dione. J Pharm Sci. 69(9):1102–1104. https://doi.org/10.1002/jps.2600690933. (b) Caldwell AG, Harris CJ, Stepney R, Whittaker N. (1980). Heterocyclic prostaglandin analogues. Part 2. Hydantoins and other imidazole analogues. J Chem Soc Perkin Trans. 1:495–505. https://doi.org/10.1039/P19800000495.

13. Safari J, Javadian L. (2016). Fe_3O_4-chitosan nanoparticles as a robust magnetic catalyst for efficient synthesis of 5-substituted hydantoins using zinc cyanide. Iran J Catal. 6(1):57–64.

14. Safari J, Javadian L. (2014). Chitosan decorated Fe_3O_4 nanoparticles as a magnetic catalyst in the synthesis of phenytoin derivatives. RSC Adv. 4:48973–48979. https://doi.org/10.1039/C4RA06618A.

15. Safari J, Javadian L. (2013). A one-pot synthesis of 5,5-disubstituted hydantoin derivatives using magnetic Fe_3O_4 nanoparticles as a reusable heterogeneous catalyst. Comptes Rendus Chimie. 16(12):1165–1171. https://doi.org/10.1016/j.crci.2013.06.005.

16. Esam Z, Malihe A, Bekhradnia A, Mohammadi M, Tourani S. (2020). A Novel Magnetic Immobilized Para-Aminobenzoic Acid-Cu (II) Complex: A Green, Efficient and Reusable Catalyst for Aldol Condensation Reactions in Green Media. Catal Letters. 150:3112–3131. https://doi.org/10.1007/s10562-020-03216-w.

17. Vavsari VF, Ziarani GM, Balalaie S, Latifi A, Karimi M, Badiei A. (2016). New functionalized 8-hydroxyquinoline-5-sulfonic acid mesoporous silica (HQS-SBA-15) as an efficient catalyst for the synthesis of 2-thiohydantoin derivatives. Tetrahedron Lett. 72(35):5420–5426. https://doi.org/10.1016/j.tet.2016.07.034.

18. Maiti B, Chanda K, Sun CM. (2009). Traceless Synthesis of Hydantoin Fused Tetrahydro-carboline on Ionic Liquid Support in Green Media. Org Lett. 11(21):4826–4829. https://doi.org/10.1021/ol901857h.

19. Zhang W, Liu W, Jiang X, Jiang F, Zhuang H, Fu L. (2011). Design, synthesis and antimicrobial activity of chiral 2-(substituted-hydroxyl)-3-(benzo[d] oxazol-5-yl) propanoic acid derivatives. Eur J Med Chem. 46(9):3639–3650. https://doi.org/10.1016/j.ejmech.2011.05.028.

20. Kumar D, Kumar NM, Sundaree S, Johnson EO, Shah K. (2010). An expeditious synthesis and anticancer activity of novel 4-(3′-indolyl) oxazole. Eur J Med Chem. 45(3):1244–1249. https://doi.org/10.1016/j.ejmech.2009.12.024.

21. Moraski GC, Chang M, Villegas-Estrada A, Franzblau SG, Mollmann M, Miller MJ. (2010). Structure-activity relationship of new anti-tuberculosis agents derived from oxazoline and oxazole benzyl esters. Eur J Med Chem. 45(5):1703–1716. https://doi.org/10.1016/j.ejmech.2009.12.074.

22. Eren G, Unlu S, Nuñezv MT, Labeaga L, Ledo F, Entrena A, Ea Banoglu, Costantino G, Şahin MF (2010) Synthesis, biological evaluation, and docking studies of novel heterocyclic diaryl compounds as selective COX-2 inhibitors. Bioorg Med Chem. 18:6367–6376. https://doi.org/10.1016/j.ejmech.2009.12.074.

23. Ashton WT, Sisco RM, Dong H, Lyons KA, He H, Doss GA, Leiting B, Patel RA, Wu JK, Marsilio F, Thornberry NA, Weber AE. (2005). Dipeptidyl peptidase IV inhibitors derived from β-aminoacylpiperidines bearing a fused thiazole, oxazole, isoxazole, or pyrazole. Bioorg Med Chem Lett. 15(9):2253–2258. https://doi.org/10.1016/j.bmcl.2005.03.012.

24. Jadhav RD, Kadam KS, Kandre S, Guha T, Reddy MMK, Brahma MK, Deshmukh NJ, Dixit A, Doshi L, Potdar N, Enose AA, Vishwakarma RA, Sivaramakrishnan H, Srinivasan S, Nemmani KVS, Gupte A, Gangopadhyay AK, Sharma R. (2012). Synthesis and biological evaluation of isoxazole, oxazole, and oxadiazole containing heteroaryl analogs of biarylureas as DGAT1 inhibitors. Eur J Med Chem. 54:324–342. https://doi.org/10.1016/j.ejmech.2012.05.016.

25. Parveen M, Ali A, Ahmed S, Malla AM, Alam M, Silva PSP, Silva MR, Lee DU. (2013). Synthesis, bioassay, crystal structure and ab initio studies of Erlenmeyer azlactones. Spectrochim Acta A Mol Biomol Spectrosc. 104:538–545. https://doi.org/10.1016/j.saa.2012.11.054.

26. Ziarati A, Ali SN, Mehdi RN, Ganjali MR, Badiei A. (2017). Sonication method synergism with rare earth based nanocatalyst: Preparation of $NiFe_2–xEuxO_4$ nanostructures and its catalytic applications for the synthesis of benzimidazoles, benzoxazoles, and benzothiazoles under ultrasonic irradiation. J Rare Earths. 35(4):374–381. https://doi.org/10.1016/S1002-0721(17)60922-0.

27. Fekri LZ, Nikpassand M, Shariati S, Aghazadeh B, Zarkeshvari R, pour NN. (2018). Synthesis and characterization of amino glucose-functionalized silica-coated $NiFe_2O_4$ nanoparticles: A heterogeneous, new and magnetically separable catalyst for the solvent-free synthesis of 2,4,5–trisubstituted imidazoles, benzo[d]imidazoles, benzo[d]oxazoles and azo-linked benzo[d]oxazoles. J Organomet Chem. 871:60–73. https://doi.org/10.1016/j.jorganchem.2018.07.008.

28. Sayyahi M, Gorjizadeh M, Sayyahi S. (2018). Fe_3O_4@SiO_2@Am-PPC-SO_3H] [HSO_4]: A new magnetic solid acid nanocatalyst for the synthesis of benzoxazole derivatives. Iran J Catal. 8(3):203–211.

29. Gupta R, Sahu PK, Srivastava SK, Agarwal DD. (2017). Environmental benign synthesis of novel double layered nano catalyst and their catalytic activity in synthesis of 2-substituted benzoxazoles. Catal Commun. 92(10):119–123. https://doi.org/10.1016/j.catcom.2017.01.005.

30. Ghafil RAA, Rajaa AAG. (2019). Schiff-Chalcone derivatives (preparation, investigation, antibacterial assay). Int J Pharm Res. 11(1):657–666.

31. Jawad AM, Aljamali NM. (2020). Innovation, preparation of cephalexin drug derivatives and studying of (toxicity & resistance of infection). Int J Psychosoc Rehabilitation. 24(04):3754–3767. https://doi.org/10.37200/IJPR/V24I4/PR201489.

32. Kadhium AJ, Hussein AAA, Aljamali NM. (2020). Invention of imidazole &thiazole-sulfazane ligands (synthesis, spectral investigation, microbial behavior) for the first time. Int J Pharm Res. 12(2). https://doi.org/10.31838/ijpr/2020.12.02.0151.

33. Mohmd M, Aljamali NM, Abbas NA. (2018). Preparation, spectral investigation, thermal analysis, biochemical studying of new (oxadiazole - five membered ring)-ligands. J Glob Pharma Technol. 10(1):20–29.

34. Mohmd M, Aljamali NM, Shubber WA, Abdalrahman SA. (2018). New azomethine- azo hetero-cyclic ligands via cyclization of ester. Research J Pharm and Tech. 11(6). https://doi.org/10.5958/0974-360X.2018.00472.9.

35. Aljamali NM. (2019). The various preparation methods in synthetic chemistry, 1st edition. Evincepub Publishing.

36. Ala JK, Mhammed JH, Aljamali NM. (2020). Thiazole amide derivatives (synthesis, spectral investigation, chemical properties, antifungal assay). NeuroQuantology. 18(1):16–25.

37. Jawad AM, Aljamali NM. (2020). Innovation, preparation of cephalexin drug derivatives and studying of (toxicity & resistance of infection). Int J Psychosoc Rehabilitation. 24(04):3754–3767. https://doi.org/10.37200/IJPR/V24I4/PR201489.

38. Aljamali NM, Jawad AM, Aseel FK, Bahar NAAA, Nour AAA. (2019). Review in chemical structures of common compounds. International Journal of Chemical Synthesis and Chemical Reactions. 5(1):1–15.

39. Mhmed M, Aljamali NM, Abdalrahman SA, Shubber WA. (2018). Formation of oxadiazole derivatives ligands from condensation and imination reaction with references to spectral investigation, thermal and microbial assay. Biochem Cell Arch. 18(1): 847–853.

40. Uremis N, Uremis MM, Tolun FI. (2017). Synthesis of 2-substituted benzothiazole derivatives and their *in vitro* anticancer effects and antioxidant activities against pancreatic cancer cells. Anticancer Res. 37:6381–6389. https://doi.org/ 10.21873/anticanres.12091.

41. Jha KK, Samad A, Kumar Y. (2010). Design, synthesis and biological evaluation of 1,3,4-oxadiazole derivatives. Eur J Med Chem. 45:4963–4967. https://doi.org/10.1016/j.ejmech.2010.08.003.

42. Aboraia AS, Abdel-Rahman HM, Mahfouz NM, EI-Gendy MA. (2006). Novel 5-(2-hydroxyphenyl)-3-substituted-2,3-dihydro-1,3,4-oxadiazole-2-thione derivatives: Promising anticancer agents. Bioorg Med Chem. 14:1236–1246. https://doi.org/10.1016/j.bmc.2005.09.053.

43. Seth S. (2015). A comprehensive review on recent advances in synthesis & pharmacotherapeutic potential of benzothiazoles. Antiinflamm Antiallergy Agents Med Chem. 14(2):98–112(15). https://doi.org/10.2174/1871523014666150528110703.

44. Gurav R, Surve SK, Babar S, Choudhari P, Patil D, More V, Sankpal S, Hangirgekar S. (2020). Rust-derived Fe_2O_3 nanoparticles as a green catalyst for the one-pot synthesis of hydrazinyl thiazole derivatives. Org Biomol Chem. 18:4575–4582. https://doi.org/10.1039/D0OB00109K.

45. Shaterian HR, Molaei P. (2019). Fe_3O4@vitamin B1 as a sustainable superparamagnetic heterogeneous nanocatalyst promoting green synthesis of trisubstituted 1,3-thiazole derivatives. Appl Organometal Chem. 4964. https://doi.org/10.1002/aoc.4964.

46. Reddy GT, Kumar G, Reddy NCG. (2018). Water-mediated one-pot three-component synthesis of hydrazinyl-thiazoles catalyzed by copper oxide nanoparticles dispersed on titanium dioxide support: A green catalytic process. Adv Synth Catal. 360(5):995–1006. https://doi.org/10.1002/adsc.201701063.

47. Zarnegar Z, Shokrani Z, Safari J. (2019). Asparagine functionalized Al_2O_3 nanoparticle as a superior heterogeneous organocatalyst in the synthesis of 2-aminothiazoles. J Mol Struct. https://doi.org/10.1016/j.molstruc.2019.02.080.

48. Beyzaei H, Aryan R, Molashahi H, Zahedi MM, Kermani AS, Ghasemi BMM, Manesh. (2017). MgO nanoparticle-catalyzed, solvent-free Hantzsch synthesis and antibacterial evaluation of new substituted thiazoles. J Iran Chem Soc. 14(5):1023–1031. https://doi.org/10.1007/s13738-017-1052-x.

10 Nanocatalysed Synthesis of Pyrazoles, Indazoles, and Pyrazolines

Divyani Gandhi,[1] *Ayushi Sethiya,*[1] *Nusrat Sahiba,*[1]
Dinesh Kumar Jangid,[2] *and Shikha Agarwal*[1]
[1] Synthetic Organic Chemistry Laboratory, Department of Chemistry, MLSU, Udaipur, Rajasthan, India
[2] Department of Chemistry (Centre of Advanced Study), University of Rajasthan, JLN Marg, Jaipur, Rajasthan, India

10.1 INTRODUCTION

Green chemistry and catalysis science are important aspects of sustainability. Recently, nanoparticles have drawn a huge interest in the sciences because of their diverse applications in catalysis. Nanocatalysis is a fascinating field in organic synthesis due to its numerous advantages, such as having a highly porous nature, a large surface area, a lower quantity requirement, mild reaction conditions, and being recyclable. Scientists are continuously modifying nanocatalysts to improve their selectivity and effectiveness. These catalytic systems may lead to the large-scale production of pharmaceutically and industrially significant products with fewer by-products for the next millennium. This chapter will give an extensive overview of the emerging field of nanomaterials in synthetic applications of heterocyclic entities, including pyrazoles, indazoles, and pyrazolines.

Nanocatalysis is a promising front-line in catalysis where catalytic activity depends on particle size and shape, and the number of surface atoms. Due to a high surface area and reactive morphologies, they have several key benefits, such as high atom efficiency, simple isolation of products, and versatile recyclability.[1,2] Nanocatalysts are heterogeneous catalysts with a high surface-to-volume ratio and bear a large number of catalytic sites that interact with reaction components efficiently. The reactivity and selectivity of the nanostructures is mainly determined by the energy of surface atoms.[3–5]

Nanoparticles with catalytic activity have drawn ample attention for use in chemical reactions as they are capable of increasing the rate of chemical reactions and yields. They can be easily recovered and recycled from a reaction mixture and thus possess the benefits of both heterogeneous and homogeneous catalysis simultaneously.[6,7] Nanocatalysis is significant for societal development as it fastens the process of converting raw materials into important chemicals in an effective, economical, and sustainable way.[8–10] A new era of chemistry that blends the benefits of multicomponent reactions and nanostructured catalysts has emerged as an important field in science for the progress of sustainable and green methods of organic synthesis.[11–14] Over the past decades, a plethora of applications of heterocycles in drug discovery has led to the development of several novel methods with nanocatalyst support and is of immense interest to synthetic chemists.[15–17] This chapter includes a detailed array of the nanocatalyzed synthesis of heterocyclic moieties, namely pyrazoles, indazoles, and pyrazolines.

DOI: 10.1201/9781003141488-10

10.1.1 PYRAZOLES

Pyrazole, a five-membered heterocycle with two nitrogen atoms and a core framework in a vast library of heterocycles, has promising fluorescent, agrochemical, and biological properties.

Dickinson et al.[18] published the first report of pyrazole synthesis in 1964, where they used cyanoethylene and hydrazine to obtain aminocyanopyrazoles. Since then, the synthesis of pyrazole has been the subject of important research with a wide range of reagents and conditions. Some recent researchers have reported the synthesis of pyrazole derivatives with ionic liquids,[19] iodine,[20] metal oxide,[21] and photocatalysts[22], among others.

Pyrazoles are found in synthetic products and many natural compounds and show far-reaching biological activities. Many commercially existing drugs are derived from pyrazole core entities, including sulfaphenazole (antibacterial drug), celecoxib (anti-inflammatory drug), rimonabant (anti-obesity drug), mepiprazole (anxiolytic drug), pyrazofurin (anticancerdrug), deracoxib (anti-inflammatory drug), difenamizole (anti-inflammatory drug), lonazolac (non-steroidal anti-inflammatory drug(NSAID)) (Figure 10.1). Some pyrazole-bearing heterocyclic compounds were found to show inhibition of human immunodeficiency virus (HIV)-1 reverse transcriptase and interleukin (IL)-1 synthesis,[23] as well as antibacterial,[24] antimalarial,[25] anti-AIDS,[26] anti-hyperglycaemic,[27] anticancer,[28,29] antidepressant,[30,31] anticonvulsant,[32] anti-pyretic,[33,34] analgesic,[35] anti-leukaemia,[36] and antioxidant[37,38] properties, among others. Pyrazole derivatives also have applications in pesticidal,

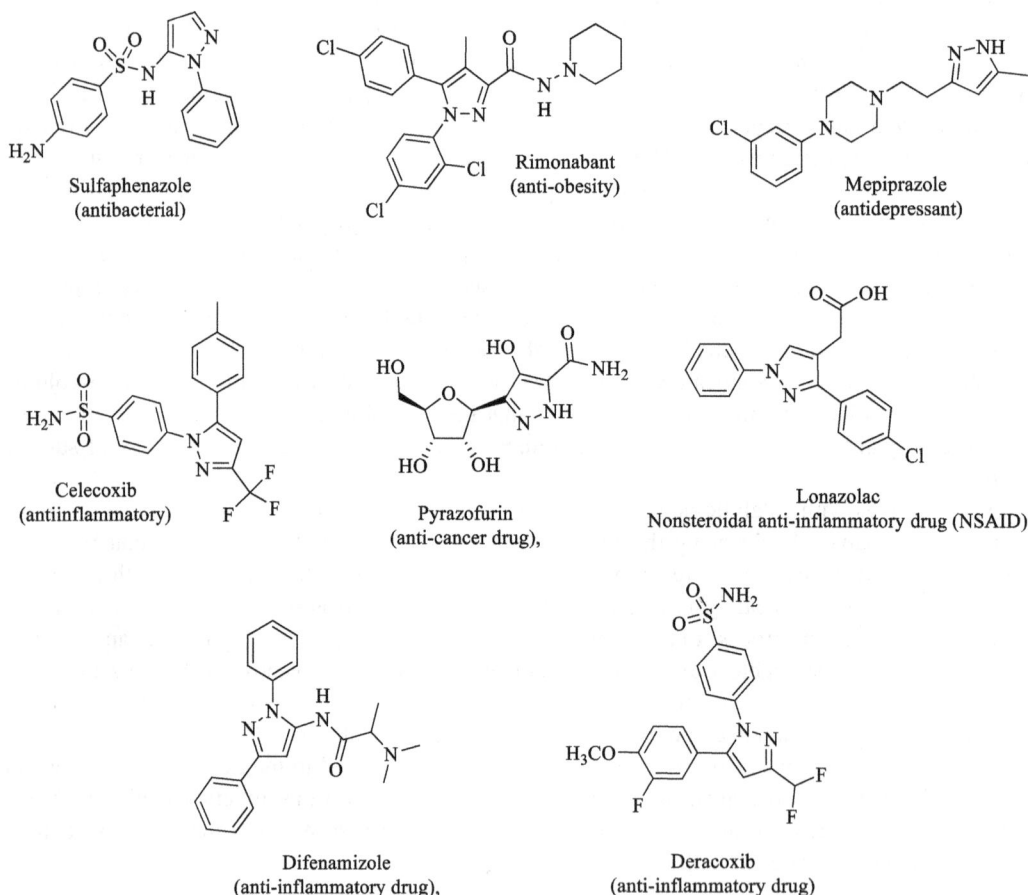

FIGURE 10.1 Marketed drugs containing pyrazole heterocycles as the core structural unit

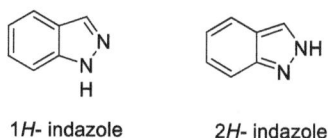

1H- indazole   2H- indazole

FIGURE 10.2 Tautomeric forms of indazoles

herbicidal,[39] and insecticidal[40] activities. Owing to their characteristic features, the use of pyrazole scaffolds is very significant for drug discovery.

10.1.2 INDAZOLES

Nitrogen bearing heterocycles, such as indazoles, are of immense significance and bear promising applications in medicinal chemistry.[41] Emil Fischer described indazole as a pyrazole ring fused with a benzene ring. They are also called isoindazolone or benzpyrazole. They generally contain two tautomeric forms, 1H- and 2H-indazole (Figure 10.2). 1H-indazole is the predominant tautomer[42] and is more thermodynamically stable than 2H-indazole.

Molecules possessing the indazole structural motif are profoundly found in nature and have gigantic biological activities in antitumour,[43] antimicrobial,[44] anti-HIV,[45] antidepressant,[46] anti-platelet,[47] anti-inflammatory,[48] anticancer,[49] and anti-spermatogenic agents,[50] and neuroprotective sodium channel modulators,[51] among others.

Some indazole derivatives have been found to possess more affinity for the imidazoline I_2 receptor and a high affinity for oestrogen receptor β and 5-HT$_{1A}$ receptors. The derivatives of indazole are also utilized as optoelectronic chromophores in the fabrication of devices such as OLEDs,[52] dye-pigments,[53] and agricultural purposes.[54] These derivatives are also found in dyes, herbicides, and sweeteners. Moreover, in addition to these biological activities, indazole scaffolds also exhibit photophysical properties for potential theranostic applications.[55]

Several approved drugs, namely lonidamine, bendacort, niraparib, bendazac, granisetron, pazopanib, benzydamine, axitinib, APINACA, and gamendazole, have the indazole nucleus in their molecular structural framework (Figure 10.3). Owing to the discovered potent bioactivity of indazole moieties, several research groups have developed a number of synthetic strategies.

10.1.3 PYRAZOLINE

Pyrazoline, sometimes referred to as dihydropyrazole, is a five-membered heterocycle with two adjacent nitrogenatoms and only one endocyclic double bond. Depending on the position of the double bond, three types of pyrazolines exist:1-pyrazoline, 2-pyrazoline, and 3-pyrazoline (Figure 10.4). 2-pyrazoline is the most attractive and important among all types of pyrazolines for frequent studies.[56]

In the nineteenth century, Fischer and Knoevenagel prepared 2-pyrazolines, employing α,β-unsaturated aldehydes/ketones with phenylhydrazine in glacial AcOH under reflux, which became one of the most popular methods. In 1996, Appendino et al.[57] explored the synthesis of a taxol-pyrazoline conjugate leading to the first appearance of cytotoxic pyrazoline in the literature, followed by a steady growth of pyrazoline in this field.

Pyrazoline compounds are electron-rich nitrogen-bearing heterocycles and perform a number of biological activities, such as antimicrobial,[58] anti-inflammatory,[59] anticancer,[60] anti-amoebic,[61] anti-nociceptive,[62] antidepressant,[63] anti-tubercular,[64] amine oxidase inhibitory,[65] cholesterol acyltransferase inhibitory,[66] COX-2 inhibitory,[67] and MAO-inhibitory activities,[68] among others. They have been proven to be highly versatile performers in various applications such as in fluorescent probes in chemosensors, organic electronics, hole-transport materials, brightening agents

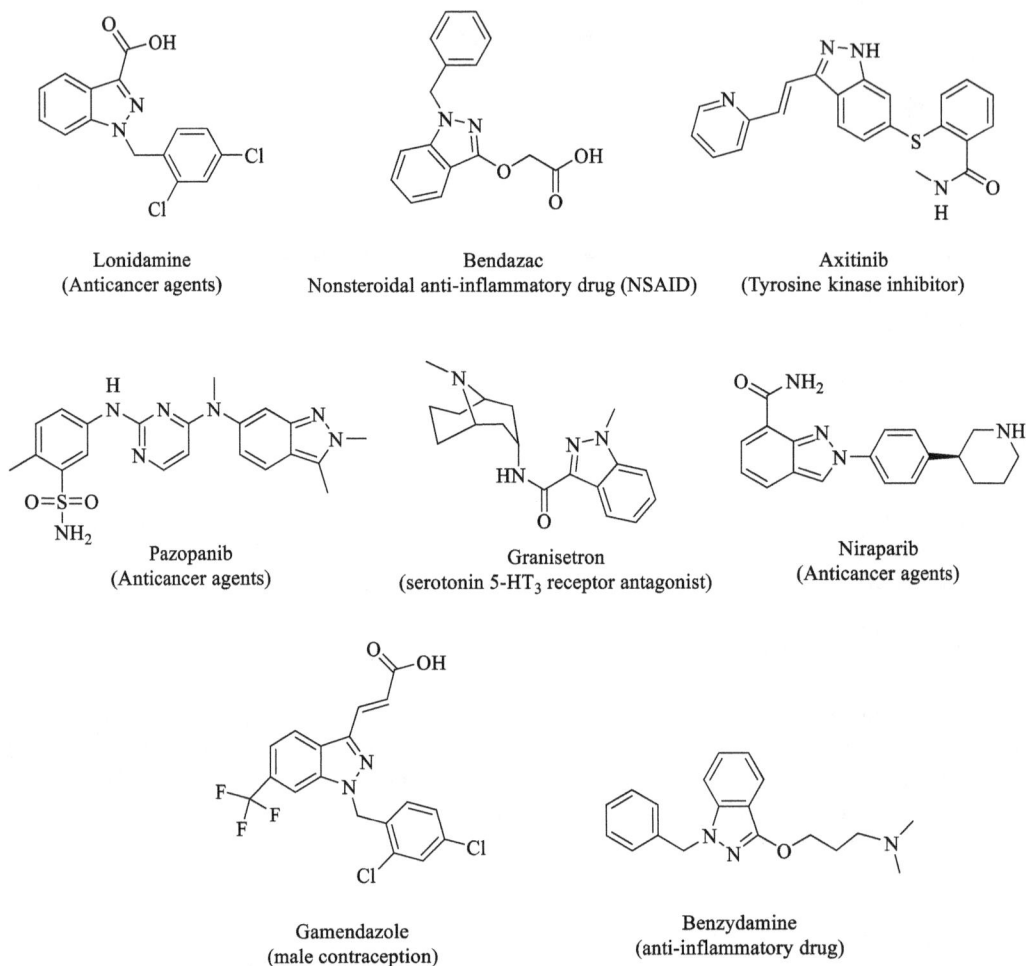

Lonidamine
(Anticancer agents)

Bendazac
Nonsteroidal anti-inflammatory drug (NSAID)

Axitinib
(Tyrosine kinase inhibitor)

Pazopanib
(Anticancer agents)

Granisetron
(serotonin 5-HT$_3$ receptor antagonist)

Niraparib
(Anticancer agents)

Gamendazole
(male contraception)

Benzydamine
(anti-inflammatory drug)

FIGURE 10.3 Approved drugs with an indazole core and pharmaceutical properties

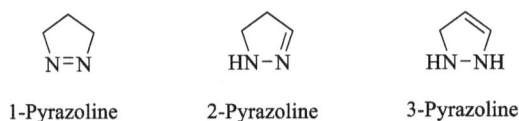

1-Pyrazoline   2-Pyrazoline   3-Pyrazoline

FIGURE 10.4 Types of pyrazoline

in synthetic fibres, papers, textiles, recognition of transition metal ions, electrophotography, and electroluminescence.[69–74]

Modern drugs that contain the pyrazoline nucleus include aminophenazone (also known as aminopyrine, amidopyrine, or pyramidon), which has analgesic, anti-inflammatory, and anti-pyretic properties; metamizole, which is a painkiller, spasm and fever reliever with anti-inflammatory properties; phenazone (also known as phenazon) as an anti-pyrine or analgesic; phenylbutazone as an NSAID; sulfinpyrazone as auricosuric medication for the treatment of gout; and oxyphenbutazone as an NSAID, among others (Figure 10.5).

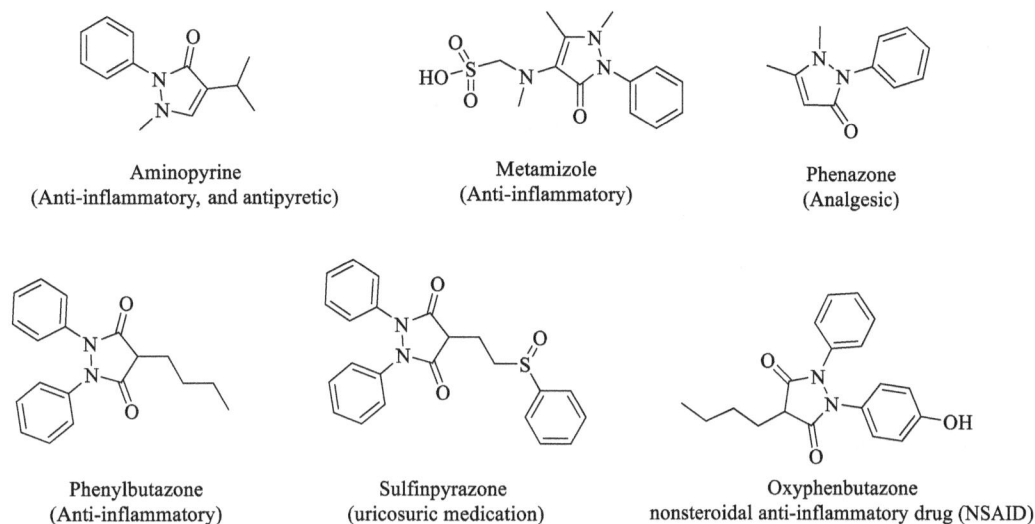

FIGURE 10.5 Some pharmacologically active drug molecules containing a pyrazoline nucleus

10.2 SYNTHETIC ASPECTS ASSOCIATED WITH NANOMATERIALS

A diverse range of synthetic methods have been developed for pyrazoles, indazoles, and pyrazolines in recent years, owing to their wide-ranging bioactivities. However, to date, most of the attention has been directed towards their synthesis by employing nanocatalysts to overcome the problem of selectivity and reactivity.

10.2.1 Synthesis of Pyrazole Derivatives by Nanocatalysis

Nanocrystalline $ZnZr_4(PO_4)_6$ ceramics[75] as a robust catalyst was applied for the preparation of methyl-6-amino-5-cyano-4-aryl-2,4-dihydropyrano[2,3-c]pyrazole-3-carboxylate derivatives via a one-pot reaction of aldehydes, hydrazine hydrate, malononitrile, dimethyl acetylenedicarboxylate in an aqueous medium (Scheme 10.1). The successful results were also attributed to a CeO_2 nanoparticles (NPs) catalyst,[76] prepared by the co-precipitation method with post-annealing in air.

Chen et al.[77] explored nanocatalysts with the magnetic RuIII@CMC/Fe_3O_4 organic–inorganic hybrid using a self-assembly strategy. Ru(III) integrated with magnetic nanosized CMC/Fe_3O_4 was developed and fabricated by a simple process of $RuCl_3$ and Na–CMC/Fe_3O_4 organic–inorganic hybrid. The high catalytic activity can be attributed to the distinctive innate Lewis-acid property of Ru(III), chelated with both carboxyl groups (COOH) and free OH groups of CMC.

Magnetic Fe_3O_4 NPs acted as heterogeneous catalysts for a multi-component one-pot reaction of hydrazine hydrate, malononitrile, benzaldehyde, and ethyl acetoacetate for the design of dihydropyrano[2,3-c]pyrazoles and was optimized under different reaction conditions.[78] The scope of the nanocatalyst in the model reaction was further extended with ZnO@PEGNPs,[79] core–shell structured magnetic silica-supported propylamine/molybdate complex (Fe_3O_4@SiO_2/Pr-NQMo[Mo_5O_{18}]),[80] magnetized dextrin nanocomposite,[81] poly(ethylene imine)-modified magnetic halloysite nanotubes (Fe_3O_4@HNTs-PEI),[82] amino-functionalized silica-coated cobalt oxide nanostructures(Co_3O_4@SiO_2-NH_2),[83] yttrium iron garnets ($Y_3Fe_5O_{12}$),[84] magnetic nano-[$CoFe_2O_4$],[85] $CoCuFe_2O_4$ magnetic nanocrystals,[86] $H_3PW_{12}O_{40}$ immobilized on aminated epibromohydrin-functionalized Fe_3O_4@SiO_2NPs(Fe_3O_4@SiO_2-EP-NH-HPA),[87] among others (Scheme 10.2).

Nanomagnetic complex lanthanum strontium magnesium oxide $La_{0.7}Sr_{0.3}MnO_3$ (LSMO) was employed for the synthesis of 1,4-dihydropyrano[2,3-c]pyrazol-5-yl cyanides by a one-pot condensation reaction of malononitrile, aromatic aldehydes, and 3-methyl-1-phenyl-2-pyrazolin-5-one

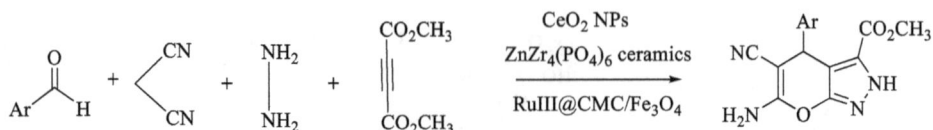

SCHEME 10.1 Nanoparticles as catalyst in the synthesis of pyrazole derivatives

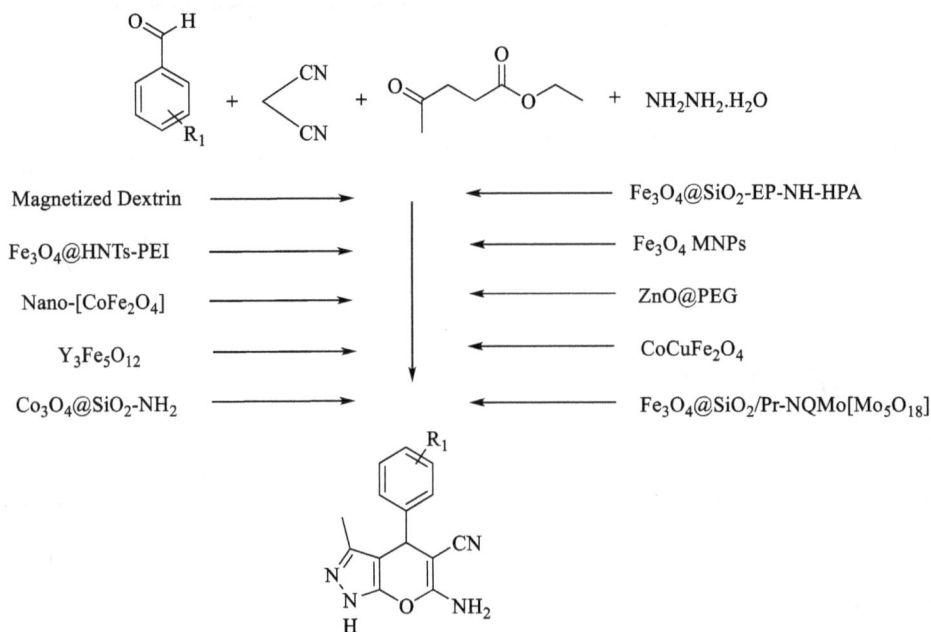

SCHEME 10.2 Nanoparticles as catalyst in the synthesis of pyrano[2,3-c]pyrazoles

in ethanol using ultrasound irradiation.[88] This protocol was extended with various nanocatalyst supports, such as novel Fe_3O_4-supported propane-1-sulfonic acid-grafted graphene oxide quantum dots (Fe_3O_4@GOQD-O-(propane-1-sulfonic acid),[89] nano-titania sulfuric acid (15-nm TSA),[90] sulfonic acid-functionalized titanomagnetite ($Fe_{3-x}Ti_xO_4$@SO_3H) NPs,[91] amino acid ionic liquid tetrabutylammonium asparaginate (TBAAsp) immobilized on titanomagnetite ($Fe_{3-x}Ti_xO_4$) NPs in an organosilane compound (TMSP) [$Fe_{3-x}Ti_xO_4$@TMSP@TBAAsp],[92] Fe_3O_4-magnetized N-pyridin-4-amine-functionalized graphene oxide [Fe_3O_4@GO-N-(pyridin-4-amine)],[93] tungstic acid immobilized 3-chloropropyl-grafted TiO_2-coated Fe_3O_4NPs (Fe_3O_4@TiO_2@$(CH_2)_3OWO_3H$)[94] and magnetic NPsNiFe$_2O_4$@SiO_2-$H_3PW_{12}O_{40}$, synthesized by the chemical support of Keggin ($H_3PW_{12}O_{40}$) heteropolyacid (HPA) on silica-coated NiFe$_2O_4$ magnetic NPs[95], among others (Scheme 10.3).

Rakhtshah et al.[96] composed a strategy for 5-aminopyrazole-4-carbonitrile derivatives by the condensation of phenylhydrazine, malononitrile, and substituted benzaldehydes in an equimolar ratio. The effect of catalyst and temperature was studied in the presence of dioxomolybdenum complex supported on silica-coated magnetite NPs (Fe_3O_4@Si@MoO_2) in the temperature range 25°C–100°C. The best results were attained in the presence of 0.02 g catalyst at room temperature. Further examination on the model reaction was done using NPs as catalysts with heterogeneous, glucose-coated super paramagnetic NPs (Glu@Fe_3O_4).[97] After accomplishing the reaction, the superparamagnetic nanocatalyst was separated from the medium with the help of an external

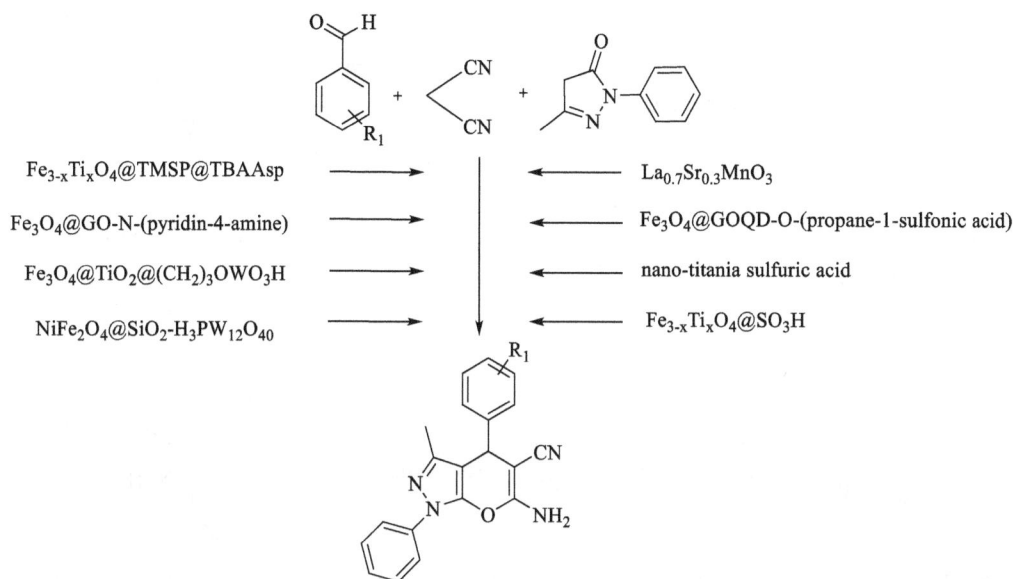

SCHEME 10.3 Nanoparticles as catalyst in the synthesis of 1,4-dihydropyrano[2,3-c]pyrazol-5-yl cyanides.

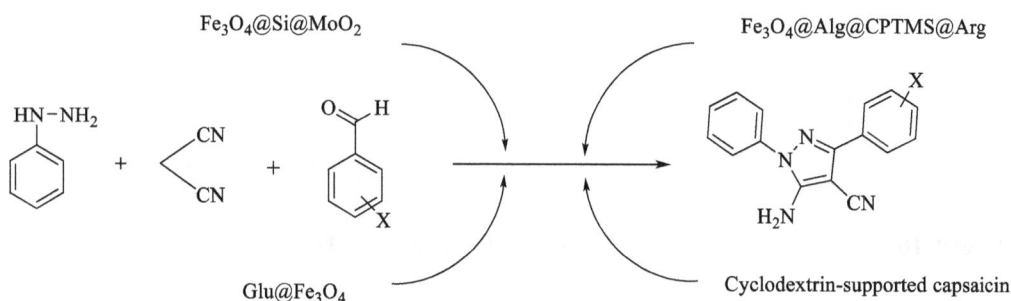

SCHEME 10.4 Nanoparticles as catalyst in the synthesis of 5-aminopyrazole-4-carbonitrile derivatives

magnet, then washed, dried and used for another reaction run. The catalyst showed excellent results for four repeated cycles with slight deterioration in its catalytic activity. Cyclodextrin-supported capsaicin NPs were also used by Arora et al.[98]

The Fe_3O_4@Alg@CPTMS@Arg[99] hybrid inorganic–organic material catalyst was used as support for the synthesis of pyrazoles. These NPs were developed using layer-by-layer techniques by grafting L-arginine (L-arg) to Fe_3O_4@Alg using 3-chloropropyltrimethoxysilane (CPTMS) as a linker. Fe_3O_4@Alg was prepared by in situ co-precipitation of iron(III) and iron(II) chloride in the presence of alginate (Alg) (Scheme 10.4).

Spiro[indoline-3,4'-pyrano[2,3-c]pyrazole] derivatives were explored using β-CD/EP as a basic heterogeneous catalyst and stationary micro-vessel, and a mixture of phenylhydrazine, ethyl acetoacetate, isatin, and malononitrile or ethyl cyanoacetate under a solvent-free environment. The β-cyclodextrin-epichlorohydrin nanosponge polymer (β-CD/EP) was synthesized from the step-wise polymerization reaction of β-cyclodextrin with epichlorohydrin under basic conditions.[100] To broaden the scope of this protocol, nano-silica supported 1,4-diazabicyclo[2.2.2]octane was used as a novel catalyst. Nano-SiO_2/DABCO,[101] a new heterogeneous basic catalyst, was synthesized using SiO_2, DABCO, and $SOCl_2$. Firstly, nano silica gel and thionyl chloride produced nano silica

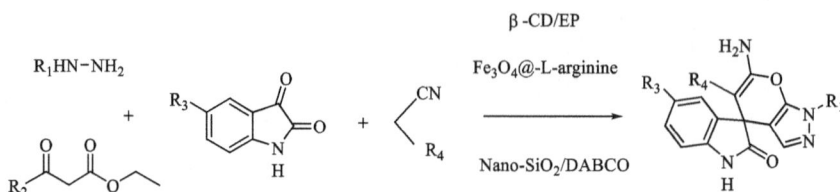

SCHEME 10.5 Nanoparticles as catalyst in the synthesis of methyl-6-amino-5-cyano-4-aryl-2,4-dihydropyrano[2,3-*c*]pyrazole-3-carboxylates

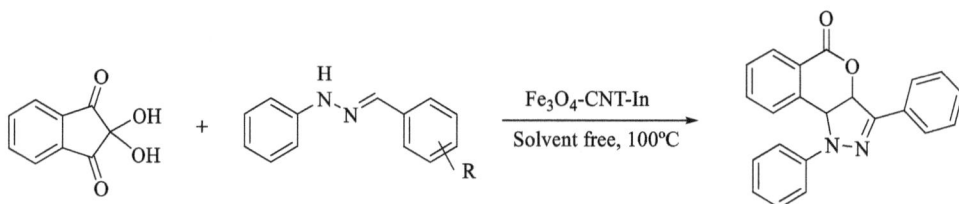

SCHEME 10.6 The use of Fe$_3$O$_4$-CNT-In nanoparticles for preparation of isochromeno[4,3-c]pyrazole-5(1*H*)-one derivatives

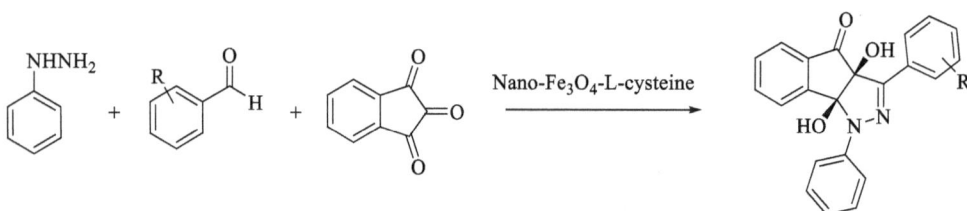

SCHEME 10.7 Synthesis of indeno[1,2-c]pyrazol-4(1H)-ones by Nano-Fe$_3$O$_4$–L-cysteine

chloride, which was then dried. The silica-chloride produced was treated with DABCO in EtOH at reflux to obtain nano-SiO$_2$/DABCO. Afterwards, the model reaction was performed using various amounts of heterogeneous solid Brønsted basic catalysts. Fe$_3$O$_4$@-L-arginine nanocomposite and 8 mol% was found to be the best experimental condition for the reaction[102] (Scheme 10.5).

A novel magnetically retrievable catalytic system involving indium NPs on a magnetic carbon nanotube (Fe$_3$O$_4$-CNT-In) was prepared by Akbarzadeh et al.,[103] who innovated a highly stable support for the green synthesis of isochromeno[4,3-c]pyrazole-5(1*H*)-one derivatives from the reaction of ninhydrin and arylhydrazones under a solvent-free environment. The catalyst was separated from the reaction mixture with the help of an external magnet and retrieved for five cycles while maintaining its efficiency (Scheme 10.6).

Ghomi et al.[104] demonstrated nano-Fe$_3$O$_4$–L-cysteine catalyst for the synthesis of indeno[1,2-c]pyrazol-4(1H)-ones using phenylhydrazine, aromatic aldehydes, and indan-1,2,3-trione at room temperaturein acetonitrile. Magnetic NPs were developed via co-precipitation of Fe(II) and Fe(III) ions in the presence of NaOH (Scheme 10.7).

An efficient heterogeneous hybrid catalyst (HPA-F-HNTs) was prepared by the functionalization of halloysite clay nanotubes by γ-aminopropyltriethoxysilane followed by immobilization of a Keggin-type heteropolyacid, phosphotungstic acid. The developed catalyst was employed for the preparation of pyrazolopyranopyrimidine derivatives via a multi-component reaction of benzaldehyde,

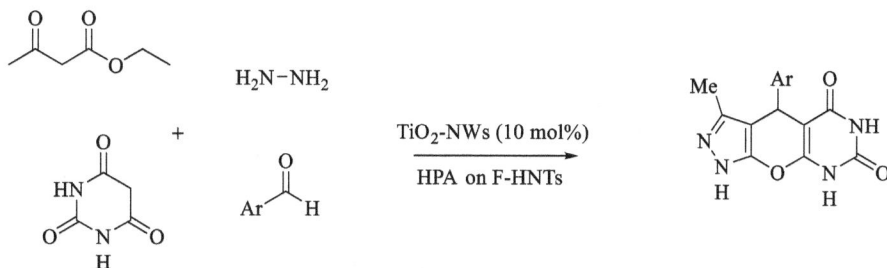

SCHEME 10.8   Preparation of pyrazolopyranopyrimidine using HPA-F-HNTs and TiO$_2$ nanowires

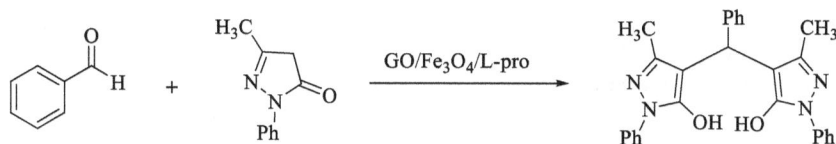

SCHEME 10.9   Synthesis of bis-pyrazole derivatives catalyzed by GO/Fe$_3$O$_4$/L-proline nano hybrid

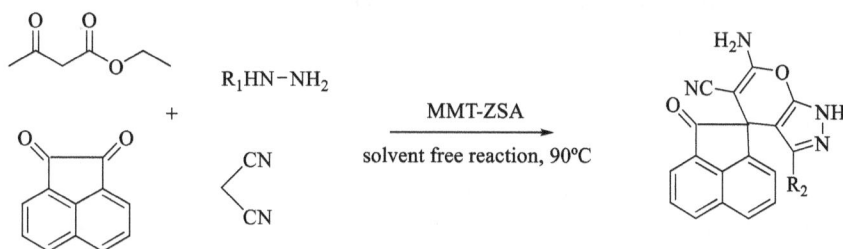

SCHEME 10.10   Synthesis of pyranopyrazoles using MMT-ZSA

hydrazine hydrate, ethyl acetoacetate, and barbituric acid.[105] Further, a catalytic amount of TiO$_2$ nanowires was also investigated by Dastkhoon et al.[106] TiO$_2$ nanowires were prepared from commercial Degussa P25 powder. The optimum catalyst amount was found to be 10 mol% among the different employed amounts of TiO$_2$ nanowires (Scheme 10.8).

A highly preferred greener process for a one-pot pseudo three-component reaction of benzaldehyde (1 eq.) and 3-methyl-1-phenyl-2-pyrazolin-5-one (2 eq.) was developed to examine the effects of superparamagnetic GO/Fe$_3$O$_4$/L-proline.[107] GO/Fe$_3$O$_4$/L-proline was obtained from the non-covalent immobilization of L-proline on graphene oxide/Fe$_3$O$_4$ nanocomposite, and the optimization studies showed that the best results were achieved by carrying out the reaction with 0.05 g of GO/Fe$_3$O$_4$/L-proline. The reusability of the catalyst was efficiently maintained during eight consecutive cycles (Scheme 10.9).

Zwitterionic sulfamic acid[108] functionalized nanoclay (MMT-ZSA) was developed and synthesized using montmorillonite K10 as a template, 3-aminopropyltriethoxysilane as a linker, and ClSO$_3$H as an SO$_3$H source. The catalytic MMT-ZSA was applied for the synthesis of dihydropyrano[2,3-c] pyrazoles via a multi-component one-pot reaction of hydrazine hydrate, β-keto ester, malononitrile, and carbonyl compounds (1,2-diketones and substituted benzaldehydes) under a solvent-free environment (Scheme 10.10).

10.2.2 NANOCATALYZED SYNTHESIS OF INDAZOLE DERIVATIVES

Triazolo[1,2-a]indazole-triones (TAITs) was developed using a three-component condensation reaction of 4-phenylurazole, dimedone, aryl aldehydes, and SiO_2-coated ZnO (ZnO@SiO_2) NPs[109] as heterogeneous catalysts in deionized water under ultrasound conditions. The catalyst was efficiently recyclable for six runs without significant loss in activity. Meanwhile, several reaction protocols were developed for their preparation using silica NPs (nano SiO_2-OSO_3H) prepared from rice husk ash[110] as acatalyst, "free"KCC-1 NPs[111] as a catalyst, silica-supported $La_{0.5}Ca_{0.5}CrO_3$ NPs (S-LCCO)[112] as new perovskite-type oxide, mesoporous aluminosilicate (AlKIT-5),[113] and silica-supported perchloric acid ($HClO_4$–SiO_2),[114] among others (Scheme 10.11).

Quinuclidin-3-thiol supported on propylsilane-functionalized silica-coated $FeNi_3$NPs ($FeNi_3$/quinuclidine), a magnetically separable catalyst, was developed by Sadeghzadeh et al.[115] This protocol was also catalyzed by a nanomagnetic organic–inorganic hybrid catalyst (Fe@Si-Gu-Prs)[116] and was synthesized by the chemical anchoring of Preyssler heteropolyacid ($H_{14}[NaP_5W_{30}O_{110}]$) onto the surface of modified Fe_3O_4 magnetic NPs with a guanidine-propyl-trimethoxysilane linker (Scheme 10.11).

SnO_2NPs[117] as a heterogeneous catalyst was used for 2H-indazolo[2,1-b]phthalazine-triones using a solvent-free one-pot reaction of phthalhydrazide, aryl aldehydes, and dimedone/1,3-cyclohexanedione. Furthermore, N-propylsulfamic acid supported onto magnetic Fe_3O_4NPs (MNPs-PSA)[118] combines the advantages of heterogeneous and homogeneous SA-based systems and make it promising for use in industrial applications. Phenyl sulfonic acid functionalized mesoporous SBA-15 silica, a hydrophobic solid acid catalyst, was also used by Veisi et al.[119] The catalyst was synthesized through silanization of activated mesoporous SBA-15 with diphenyldichlorosilane (DPCS). Then, silylation and sulfonation took place.

MNPs-guanidine(i.e.,guanidine supported on magnetic NPs Fe_3O_4), a novel base nanocatalyst, was also described by Atashkar et al.[120] The supported catalyst could be easily separated from the reaction mixture using an external magnet and reused 18 times with little loss of activity. With the promising results in the protocol, nano-alumina sulfuric acid (nano-ASA),[121] a solid acid catalyst, was also depicted by Kiasat et al. (Scheme 10.12).

γ-Al_2O_3/BF_n/Fe_3O_4 NPs[122] were used as a robust heterogeneous catalyst for the preparation of 2H-indazolo[2,1-b]phthalazine-triones using phthalic anhydride, dimedone, hydrazine monohydrate,

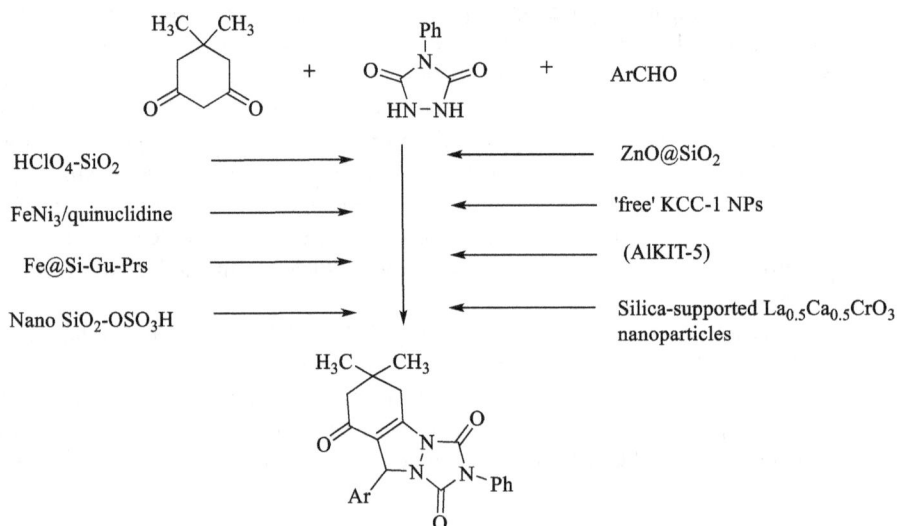

SCHEME 10.11 Preparation of triazolo[1,2-a]indazole-triones using nanocatalyst

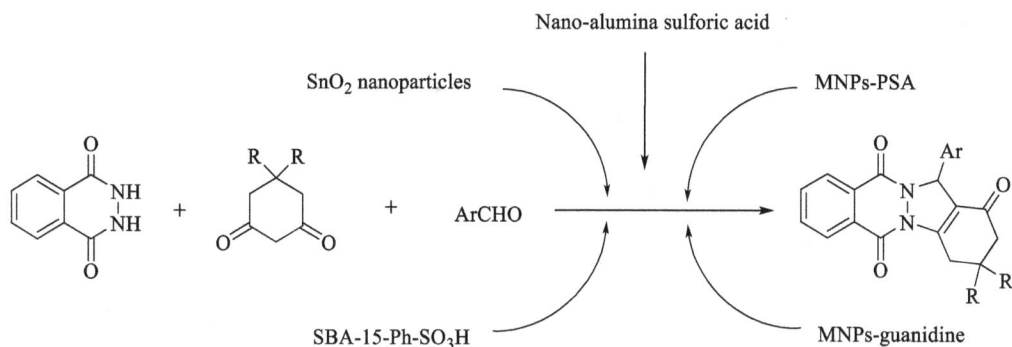

SCHEME 10.12   Synthesis of 2*H*-indazolo[2,1-b]phthalazine-triones in the presence of nanocatalysts

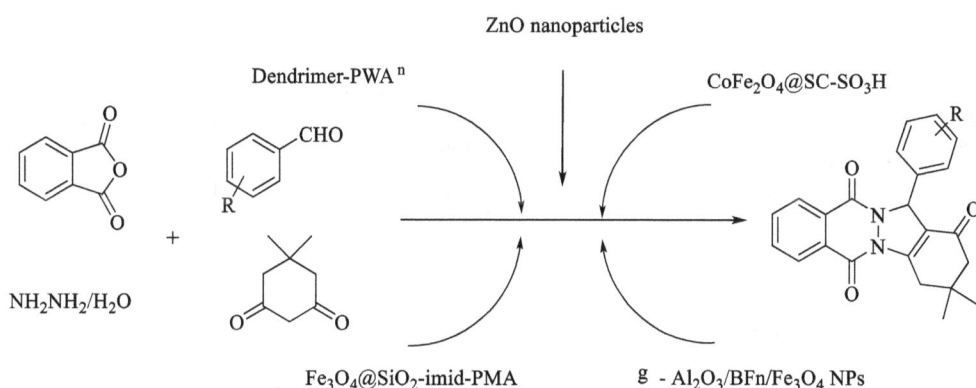

SCHEME 10.13   Synthesis of 2*H*-indazolo[2,1-b]phthalazine-triones using nanocatalyst

and substituted aromatic aldehydes. The best results were obtained at 80°C using 8mg of nano-γ-$Al_2O_3/BF_n/Fe_3O_4$ under a solvent-free environment. Considering the above protocol, and in continuation of nanocatalysts and sustainable synthesis, Zhao et al.[123] evaluated the catalytic reactivity of magnetic $CoFe_2O_4$ chitosan sulfonic acid nanoparticle, and Shaterian et al.[124]employed ZnO NPs in a range of organic transformations (Scheme 10.13).

Dendrimer-encapsulated phosphotungstic acid NPs immobilized on nanosilica (Dendrimer-PWA^n) with surface NH_2 groups were synthesized, and their structural and surface studies were evaluated by Esmaeilpour et al.[125] for this protocol.

The reaction was also carried out using $Fe_3O_4@SiO_2$-imid-PMA, and the products were produced in high yields in a short reaction time under both a solvent-free environment at 80°C and ultrasonic irradiation. The catalyst can be easily separated using an external magnetic field in a few minutes without the need fortedious filtration or a centrifugation process[126] (Scheme 10.13).

A CuO nanocatalysed[127] synthesis of 2*H*-indazoles was developed from sodium azide, 2-bromobenzaldehyde, and 1^0 amines without using any ligand. The CuO nanocatalyst worked effectively during the formation of the intermolecular C–N bond followed by the intramolecular N–N bond. Concerning the advantages of the nanocatalytic system, the literature studies also demonstrated several other catalysts, namely novel metal acetylacetonates covalently anchored onto amine-functionalized silica/starch composite[128] ASS-Cu(acac)$_2$, decorated peptide nanofibers with Cu NPs (CuNP-PNF)[129] through simple technology of self-assembly in aqueous solution, nanocomposite CuO@CB[6][130] by immobilizing CuO NPs on cucurbit[6]uril support, heterogeneous copper NPs on charcoal (Cu/C) catalyst[131], and Cu(II) complex obtained

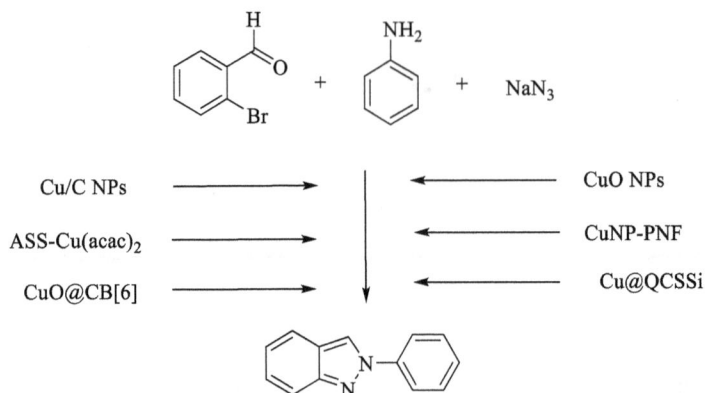

SCHEME 10.14 Multi-component synthesis of 2*H*-indazoles in the presence of nanocatalyst

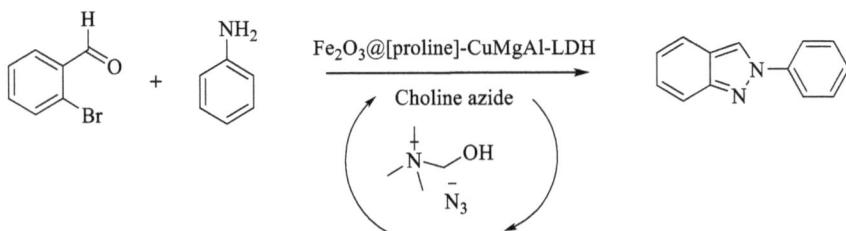

SCHEME 10.15 One-pot synthesis of 2*H*-indazole using Fe2O3@[proline]–CuMgAl–LDH

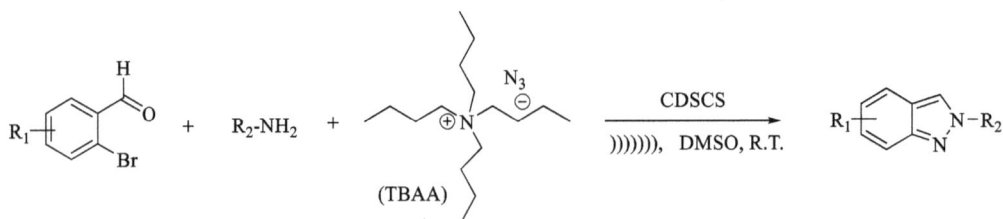

SCHEME 10.16 Synthesis of 2*H*-indazoles using CDSCS

from 2-oxoquinoline-3-carbaldehyde Schiff base supported on amino-functionalized silica (Cu@ QCSSi)[132], among others (Scheme 10.14).

A simple method was used through consecutive condensation in choline azide media that played the dual role of reagent and solvent in the presence of a novel magnetic core–shell Fe_2O_3@[pro-line]–CuMgAl–L(ayered)D(ouble)H(ydroxide) and acted as a highly efficient bifunctional catalytic system. To this end, Cu(II) was combined with Mg and Al in the LDH structure and L-proline was intercalated between the LDH layer to carry out the synthesis of 2*H*-indazoles[133] (Scheme 10.15).

To broaden the scope of this protocol, ultrasonic irradiation and copper-doped silica cuprous sulphate nanocatalyst (CDSCS) influenced the progression of the synthesis of 2*H*-indazoles. However, tetrabutylammonium azide (TBAA) not only behaved as an azide source but extensively promoted the reaction due to its phase transfer catalytic nature[134] (Scheme 10.16).

In this connection, 2-bromobenzaldehydes, substituted amines, and [bmim]N_3 as an azide source using Cu/aminoclay/reduced graphene oxide nanohybrid (Cu/AC/r-GO nanohybrid), was used as a highly efficient heterogeneous catalyst to afford 2*H*-indazoles in excellent yields[135] (Scheme 10.17).

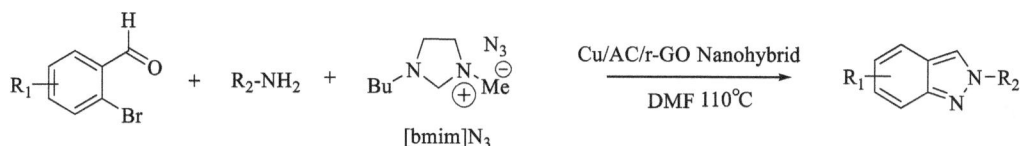

SCHEME 10.17 Three-component synthesis of 2H-Indazoles by Cu/Aminoclay/reduced graphene oxide nanohybrid

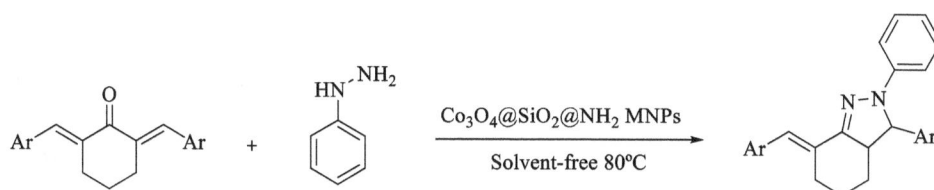

SCHEME 10.18 Synthesis of 7-benzylidene-2,3-diphenyl-3,3a,4,5,6,7-hexahydro-2H-indazole in the presence of $Co_3O_4@SiO_2@NH_2$ nanocomposite

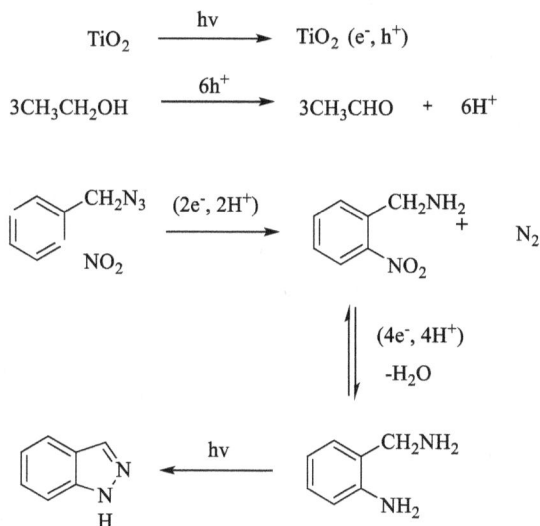

SCHEME 10.19 Nano-titania mediated green synthesis of indazole from 2-nitrobenzyl azides

Ghasemzadeh et al.[136] developed a facile and environmentally benign synthesis of 7-benzylidene-2,3-diphenyl-3,3a,4,5,6,7-hexahydro-2H-indazole derivatives using $Co_3O_4@SiO_2@$ NH_2 nanocomposites. The Co_3O_4NPs were coated with amino-functionalized SiO_2 ($SiO_2@$(3-aminopropyl)triethoxysilane) as an organic shell via a three-step method (Scheme 10.18).

Selvam et al.[137] demonstrated the high efficiency of semiconductor catalysts, nanotitania TiO_2-P25, and Ag/Pt doped TiO_2 NPs in UV and solar light that made the reaction facile for the synthesis of indazoles. The catalyst provided a microheterogeneous centre for oxidation and reduction. The oxidation of alcohol to aldehyde and the reduction of azide to amine occurred simultaneously. Initially, the solvent ethanol was oxidized to aldehyde and 2-nitrophenyl azide was reduced to 2-nitroaniline and then to diamine, which underwent photocyclization to provide indazole (Scheme 10.19).

The efficiency of N-TiO_2NPs as a green heterogeneous photocatalyst was evaluated by Selvam et al.[138] 2-phenylindazoles were obtained by reductive cleavage of azoxybenzene in methanol at

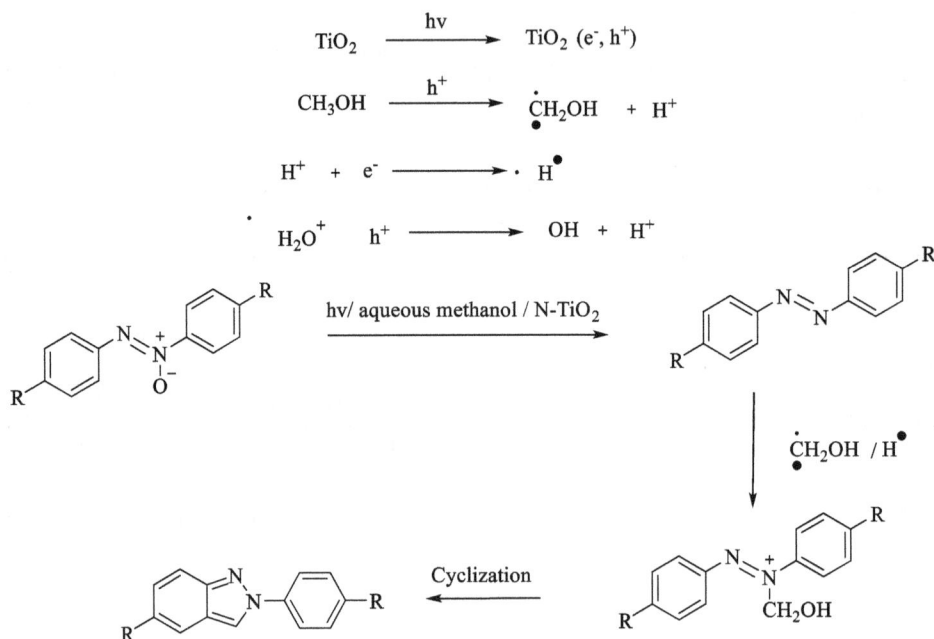

SCHEME 10.20 Reductive cleavage of azoxybenzenes to 2-phenyl indazoles in methanol in the presence of mesoporous nitrogen-doped nano titania

room temperatureunder N_2 atmosphere using N-TiO$_2$NPs. N-doped TiO$_2$ photocatalyst was prepared using nanotitania from titanyl nitrate and the nitrogen precursor hydrazine hydrate by a simple wet impregnation method. In reductive cleavage, nano N-TiO$_2$ was found more effective as compared to the prepared TiO$_2$, which showed that the nitrogen-doped TiO$_2$ improved the photoactivity of TiO$_2$ (Scheme 10.20).

10.2.3 Synthesis of Pyrazolines with the Support of a Nanocatalyst

Esfahani et al.[139] developed nanorod vanadatesulfuric acid (VSA) as a green catalyst for the preparation of 1,3,5-triaryl-2-pyrazolines (TAPs). Initially, chalcones were synthesized via substituted acetophenones and aromatic aldehydes. Subsequently, the synthesized chalcones were reacted with phenylhydrazine for the synthesis of TAPs in refluxing ethanol. The catalyst VSA nanorods were easily prepared by the reaction between sodium metavanadate and chlorosulfonic acid (1:1 mole ratio) in dry chloroform. Gharib et al.[140] further reported the fabrication of 1,3,5-triaryl pyrazoline derivatives using Preyssler heteropolyacid supported on nano-SiO$_2$, $H_{14}[NaP_5W_{30}O_{110}]$/SiO$_2$NPs (Scheme 10.21).

Aliyan et al.[141] reported the magnetically recoverable catalyst γ-Fe$_2$O$_3$@SiO$_2$-PW$_{12}$, which was synthesized by the immobilization of $H_3PW_{12}O_{40}$ on the surface of silica-encapsulated γ-Fe$_2$O$_3$ NPs using the wet impregnation method and assessed its catalytic activity for the synthesis of 1,3,5-triaryl-2-pyrazolines. The heterogeneous catalyst possessed a high separation efficiency and high surface area. As part of continuing efforts for further improvement towards green chemistry, the catalytic performance of caesium salt of phosphotungstic acid nanocast CsHPW ($Cs_{2.5}H_{0.5}PW_{12}O_{40}$) materials for the model reaction was demonstrated by Fazaeli et al.[142] (Scheme 10.22).

Cobalt-doped ZnS NPs[143] were used to synthesize pyrazolones using phenylhydrazine and ethyl acetoacetate in solvent-free conditions with excellent regioselectivity using infrared irradiation. Co-doped ZnS NPs were found to be about 40-fold more active under infrared radiation than the conventional method. The activity and selectivity of ZnS NPs were increased by the doping of Co, as

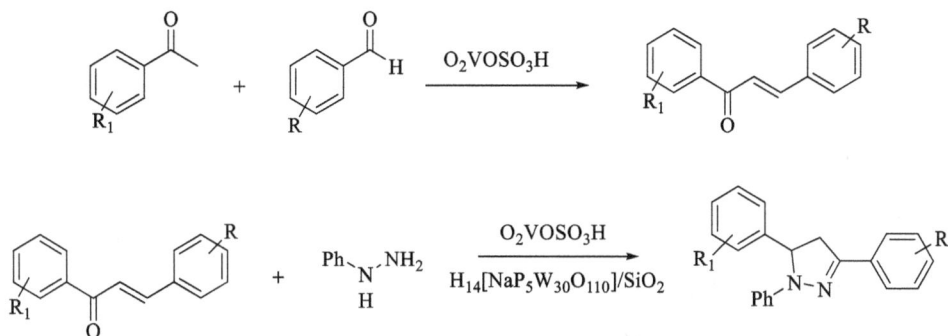

SCHEME 10.21   Nanoparticles-assisted synthesis of 1,3,5-triaryl-2-pyrazoline (TAP) derivatives

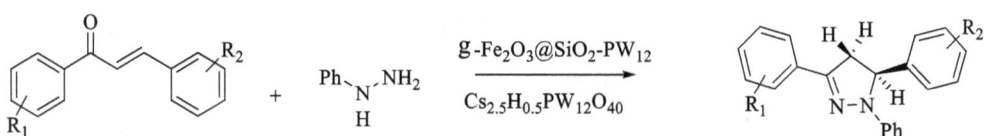

SCHEME 10.22   Synthesis of pyrazoline derivatives using nanocatalyst

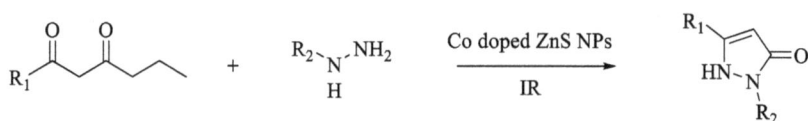

SCHEME 10.23   Synthesis of cobalt-doped ZnS nanoparticlesassisted pyrazolone derivatives

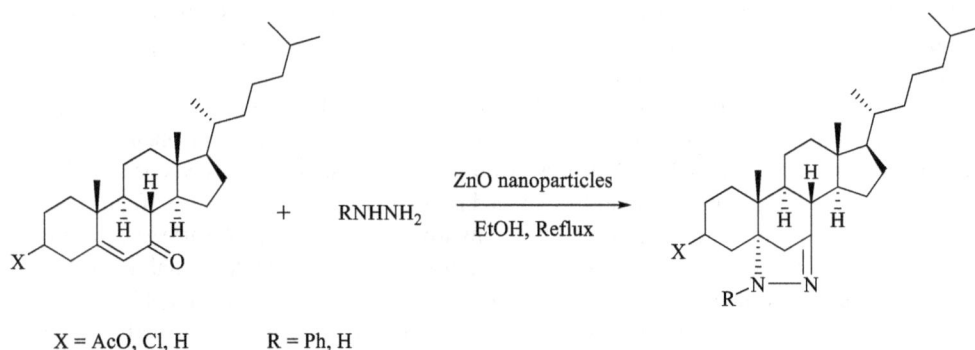

X = AcO, Cl, H   R = Ph, H

SCHEME 10.24   Synthesis of 5α-cholestano[5,7-cd] pyrazoline derivative over ZnO nanoparticles

exemplified by their high TOF value. The developed catalyst played the role of both catalyst and susceptor and increased the overall capacity of the reaction mixture to absorb infrared radiation (Scheme 10.23).

Shamsuzzaman[144] reported the biological synthesis of ZnO NPs using *Candida albicans* as an eco-friendly reducing and capping agent and applied them in the synthesis of steroidal pyrazolines from α,β-unsaturated steroidal ketones and hydrazine hydrate/phenylhydrazine hydrate in ethanol under reflux conditions (Scheme 10.24).

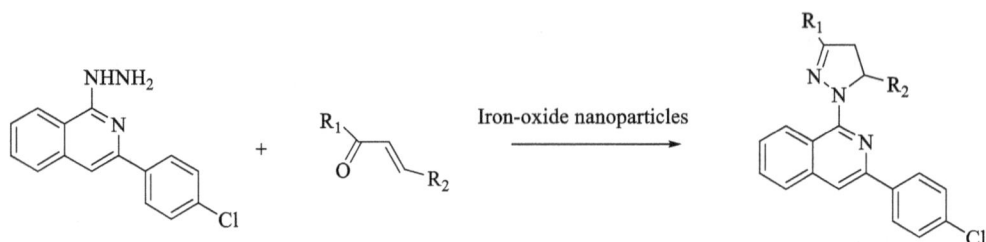

SCHEME 10.25 Cyclization of hydrazine and chalcones in the presence of iron-oxide nanoparticles

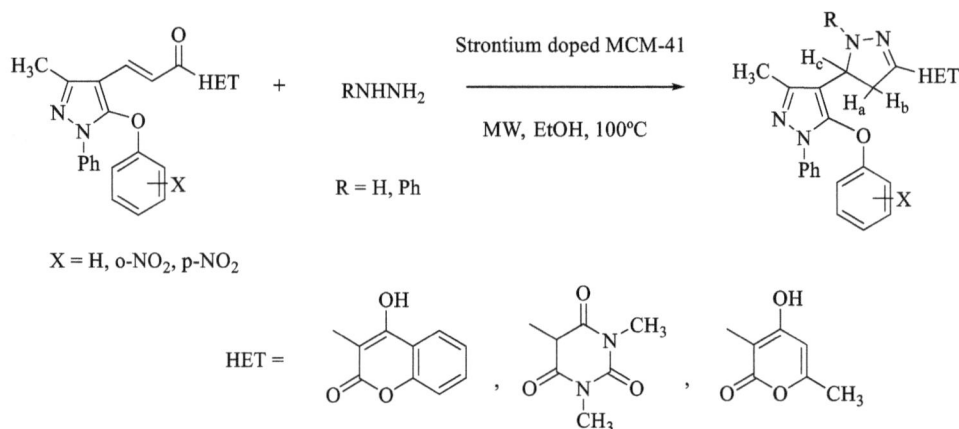

SCHEME 10.26 Synthesis of phenoxy pyrazolyl pyrazoline derivatives using strontium-doped MCM-41 (Sr-MCM-41)

Chitosan templates were employed for the synthesis of iron-oxide NPs by controlled heat treatment when diversified chalcones were reacted with 1-hydrazino-3-(4-chlororpheny)isoquinoline to convert into 1-(4,5-dihydropyrazol-1-yl)isoquinolines[145] (Scheme 10.25).

Siddiqui et al.[146] reported strontium-doped MCM-41 (Sr-MCM-41) as a heterogeneous catalyst using a simple impregnation method. Their catalytic activity was explored for phenoxy pyrazolyl pyrazoline derivatives under MWI (3–5 min) using EtOH as a solvent, and excellent yields (96–98%) were obtained. The catalyst could be recycled for up to five cycles (Scheme 10.26).

A series of 7-amino-1,3-dioxo-1,2,3,5-tetrahydropyrazolo[1,2-a][1,2,4]triazole derivatives were developed from a cyclocondensation reaction of arylaldehydes, malononitrile, and 4-phenylurazole using magnetic Fe_3O_4 NPs coated by (3-aminopropyl)-triethoxysilane (APTES–MNPs)[147] as a catalyst under a thermal solvent-free environment. The results showed that the catalyst APTES–MNPs (7 mol%) afforded products in 6 minutes with 90% yield under solvent-free conditions. Further, the reaction was performed using nanocrystalline (NC) magnesium oxide catalyst by Naeimi et al.[148] and the reusability of the NC MgO was examined several times with no loss in the catalytic activity.

Further, Cu-doped ZnO hollow sphere nanostructures were used by Maleki et al.[149] The reaction worked best at 80°C under a solvent-free environment using 0.020 g Cu-ZnO hollow spheres as a catalyst (Scheme 10.27).

The combination of IL and a heterogeneous catalyst results in an enhanced reaction rate by immobilizing IL on the surface of the support material. [MSPP]HSO$_4$@nSiO$_2$ as the heterogeneous acidic ionic liquid[150] was prepared by the impregnation of AIL, 4-methyl-1-(3-sulfopropyl)pyridinium

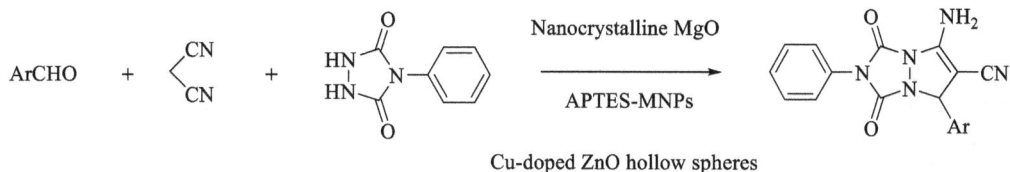

SCHEME 10.27 One-pot synthesis of pyrazolo[1,2-a][1,2,4]triazole derivatives catalyzed by nanostructures

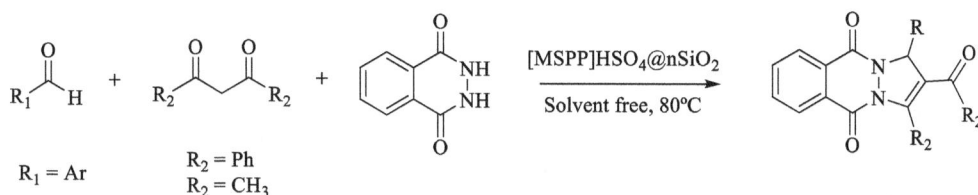

SCHEME 10.28 Synthesis of 1*H*-pyrazolo[1,2-b]phthalazinedione derivatives supported by [MSPP]HSO4@nSiO2 catalyst

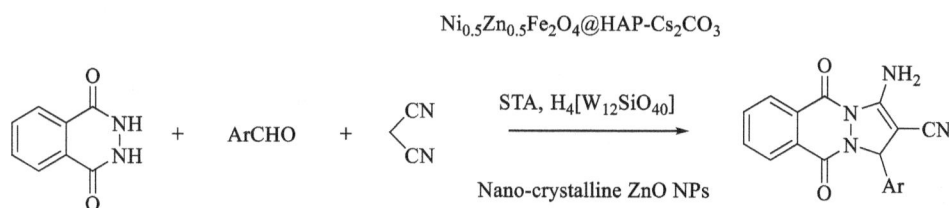

SCHEME 10.29 Synthesis of 1*H*-pyrazolo[1,2-b]phthalazinedione derivatives catalysed by nanoparticles

hydrogen sulfate [MSPP][HSO$_4$], and immobilized on silica NPs in ethanol at 25°C. Further, the catalyst was obtained by evaporating solvent and drying under vacuum at 100°C. The catalytic activity of the developed catalyst was investigated for the synthesis of substituted pyrazolo[1,2-*b*] phthalazine-5,10- diones. Finally, 6 mol% of catalyst [MSPP]HSO$_4$@nSiO$_2$ worked well at 80°C in solvent-free media (Scheme 10.28).

ZnO NPs possess an amphoteric structure bearing both Lewis acid and base properties. Azarifar et al.[151] explored a three-component cyclocondensation reaction between malononitrile, aromatic aldehydes, and phthalhydrazide for the synthesis of 1*H*-pyrazolo[1,2-b]phthalazine-5,10-diones in the presence of nanocrystalline ZnO NPs (Scheme 10.29).

Maleki et al.[152] employed a nanomagnetic basic catalyst of caesium carbonate (Cs$_2$CO$_3$) supported on hydroxyapatite-coated Ni$_{0.5}$Zn$_{0.5}$Fe$_2$O$_4$ magnetic NPs (Ni$_{0.5}$Zn$_{0.5}$Fe$_2$O$_4$@HAP-Cs$_2$CO$_3$) (NZF@HAP-Cs) for the synthesis of 1*H*-pyrazolo[1,2-b]phthalazine-5,10-diones. The special properties of Cs$_2$CO$_3$ provided adequate basic sites for the excellent catalytic activity of NZF@HAP-Cs. Furthermore, the magnetically separable catalyst could be reused at least five times without any loss in its catalytic activity and could be recovered from the reaction mixture easily using an external magnet (Scheme 10.29).

In continuation, silicotungstic acid (STA, H$_4$[W$_{12}$SiO$_{40}$])[153] coated on amino-functionalized Si–magnetite NPs was used for the synthesis of 1*H*-pyrazolo[1,2-b]phthalazinediones. The magnetite NPs were prepared using modified co-precipitation aided by the sonication method, and the silica coating was done using the Stöber method (Scheme 10.29).

10.3 CONCLUSIONS

This chapter explored the emerging potential of nanomaterials for the synthetic strategies of heterocyclic scaffolds such as pyrazoles, indazoles, and pyrazolines, as well as an overview of their applications. There has been a huge upsurge in recent trends for recoverable nanomaterials to develop highly efficient chemical processes. The nanomaterials covered also exhibit high selectivity, activity, stability, recoverability, and recyclability. We believe that this work will arouse more research interest in the nanocatalytic synthesis of biologically active heterocycles.

REFERENCES

1. Polshettiwar V, Luque R, Fihri A, Zhu H, Bouhrara M, Basset JM. (2011). Magnetically recoverable nanocatalysts.Chem. Rev.111:3036–3075.
2. Astruc D. (2020). Introduction: Nanoparticles in catalysis. Chem. Rev. 120:461–463.
3. Min Y, Akbulut M, Kristiansen K, Golan Y, Israelachvili J. (2008). The role of interparticle and external forces in nanoparticle assembly. Nat. Mater. 7:527–538.
4. Astruc D, Lu F, Aranzaes JR. (2005). Nanoparticles as recyclable catalysts: The frontier between homogeneous and heterogeneous catalysis. Angew. Chem. Int. Ed.44:7852–7872.
5. Hu H, Xin JH, Hu H, Wang X, Miao D, Liu Y. (2015). Synthesis and stabilization of metal nanocatalysts for reduction reactions - A review. J. Mater. Chem. A. 3:11157–11182.
6. Chaturvedi S, Dave PN, Shah NK. (2012). Applications of nano-catalyst in new era. J. Saudi Chem. Soc.16(3): 307–325.
7. Rossi LM, Costa NJS, Silva FP, Gonçalves RV. (2013). Magnetic nanocatalysts: Supported metal nanoparticles for catalytic applications. Nanotechnol. Rev. 2(5): 597–614.
8. Dahl JA, Maddux BLS, Hutchison JE. (2007). Toward greener nanosynthesis. Chem. Rev. 107:2228–2269.
9. Karimi B, Mansouri F, Mirzaei HM. (2015). Recent applications of magnetically recoverable nanocatalysts in c-c and c-x coupling reactions. Chem. Cat. Chem. 7: 1736–1789.
10. Sheldon RA,Arends IWCE, Hanefeld U. (2007). Green Chem. Catal. Wiley-VCH:Weinheim.
11. Chen MN, Mo LP, Cui ZS, Zhang ZH. (2019). Magnetic nanocatalysts: Synthesis and application in multicomponent reactions. Curr. Opin. Green Sustain. Chem.15:27–37.
12. Nikoorazm M,Ghobadi M. (2019). Cu-SBTU@MCM-41: As an efficient and reusable nanocatalyst for selective oxidation of sulfides an oxidative coupling of thiols. Silicon.11:983–993.
13. Shirini F, Abedini M. (2013). Application of nanocatalysts in multi-component reactions. J Nanosci. Nanotechnol.7:4838–4860.
14. Singh SB. (2018). Copper nanocatalysis in multi-component reactions: A green to greener approach. Curr. Catal.7:80–88.
15. Dhameliya TM, Donga HA, Vaghela PV, Panchal BG, Sureja DK, Bodiwala KB, Chhabria MT. (2020). A decennary update on applications of metal nanoparticles (MNPs) in the synthesis of nitrogenand oxygen-containing heterocyclic scaffolds.RSCAdv.10:32740–32820.
16. Maleki A, Azizi M, Emdadi Z. (2018). A novel poly(ethyleneoxide)-based magnetic nanocomposite catalyst for highly efficient multicomponent synthesis of pyran derivatives. Green Chem. Lett. Rev. 11:573–582.
17. Khan MU, Siddiqui ZN. (2018). Ce@STANPs/ZrO$_2$ as nanocatalyst for multicomponent synthesis of isatin-derived imidazoles under green reaction conditions. ACS Omega. 3:10357–10364.
18. Dickinson CL, Williams JK, McKusick BC. (1964). Aminocyanopyrazoles. J. Org. Chem. 29:1915–1919.
19. Srivastava M, Rai P, Singh J, Singh J. (2013). An environmentally friendlier approach-ionic liquid catalysed, water promoted and grinding induced synthesis of highly functionalised pyrazole derivatives. RSC Adv.3:16994–16998.
20. Srivastava M, Rai P, Singh J, Singh J. (2014). Efficient iodine-catalyzed one pot synthesis of highly functionalised pyrazoles in water. New J. Chem. 38:302–307.
21. Maddila S, Rana S, Pagadala R, Kankala, S, Maddila S, Jonnalagadda SB. (2015). Synthesis of pyrazole-4-carbonitrile derivatives in aqueous media with CuO/ZrO$_2$ as recyclable catalyst. Catal. Commun. 61:26–30.

22. Ding Y, Zhang T, Chen QY, Zhu C. (2016). Visible-light photocatalytic aerobic annulation for the green synthesis of pyrazoles. Org. Lett. 18:4206–4209.

23. Genin MJ, Biles C, Keiser BJ, *et al*. (2000). Novel 1,5-diphenylpyrazole nonnucleoside HIV-1 reverse transcriptase inhibitors with enhanced activity versus the delavirdine-resistant p236l mutant: Lead identification and SAR of 3- and 4-substituted derivatives. J. Med. Chem. 43(5):1034–1040.

24. Kumar SR, Arif IA, Ahamed A, Idhayadhulla A. (2016)Antiinflammatory and antimicrobial activities of novel pyrazole analogues.Saudi J. Biol. Sci. 23:614–620.

25. Bekhit AA, Hassan AM, AbdEl Razik HA, El-Miligy MM, El-Agroudy EJ,Bekhit Ael-D. (2015). New heterocyclic hybrids of pyrazole and its bioisosteres: Design, synthesis and biological evaluation as dual acting antimalarial-antileishmanial agents. Eur. J. Med. Chem. 94:30–44.

26. Sony JK, Ganguly S. (2016). A battle against AIDS: New pyrazole key to an older lock-reverse transcriptase. Int. J. Pham Pharm. Sci. 8:75–79.

27. Kees KL, Fitzgerald JJ, Steiner KE, *et al*. (1996). New potent antihyperglycemic agents in db/db mice: synthesis and structure-activity relationship studies of (4-substituted benzyl) (trifluoromethyl) pyrazoles and –pyrazolones. J. Med. Chem. 39:3920–3928.

28. AlamR,Wahi D, SinghR, SinhaD,TandonV, GroverA, Rahisuddin. (2016). Design, synthesis, cytotoxicity, Hu Topollα inhibitory activity and molecular docking studies of pyrazole derivatives as anticancer agents. Bioorg. Chem. 69:77–90.

29. Shamsuzzaman S, Siddiqui T, Alam MG, Dar AM. (2015). Synthesis, characterization and anticancer studies of new steroidal oxadiazole, pyrrole and pyrazole derivatives. J. Saudi Chem. Soc. 19:387–391.

30. Bailey DM, Hansen PE, Hlavac AG,*et al*. (1985). 3,4-Diphenyl-1H-pyrazole-1-propanamine antidepressants. J. Med. Chem. 28:256–260.

31. AzizM A, Abuo-Rahma GEDA, Hassan AA. (2009). Synthesis of novel pyrazole derivatives and evaluation of their antidepressant and anticonvulsant activities. Eur. J. Med. Chem. 44:3480–3487.

32. Michon V, Penhoat CHD, Tombret F, Gillardin JM, Lepage F, Berthon L. (1995). Preparation, structural analysis and anticonvulsant activity of 3- and 5-aminopyrazole *N*-benzoyl derivatives. Eur. J. Med. Chem. 30:147–155.

33. Malvar DDC, Ferreira RT, Castro RAD, *et al*. (2014). Antinociceptive, anti-inflammatory and antipyretic effects of 1,5-diphenyl-1*H*-pyrazole-3-carbohydrazide, a new heterocyclic pyrazole derivative. Life Sci. 95(2):81–88.

34. Pasin JSM, Ferreira APO, Saraiva ALL, *et al*. (2010). Antipyretic and antioxidant activities of 5-trifluoromethyl-4,5-dihydro-1H-pyrazoles in rats. Braz J Med Biol Res. 43:1193–1202.

35. Gursoy SA, Demirayak G, Capan K. (2000). Synthesis and preliminary evaluation of new 5-pyrazolinone derivatives as analgesic agents. Eur. J. Med. Chem. 35:359–364.

36. Baraldi PG, Beria I, Cozzi P, *et al*. (2004). Cinnamoyl nitrogen mustard derivatives of pyrazole analogues of tallimustine modified at the amidino moiety: Design, synthesis, molecular modeling and antitumor activity studies. Bioorg. Med. Chem. 12:3911–3921.

37. Nagamallu R, Kariyappa AK. (2013). Synthesis and biological evaluation of novel formyl-pyrazoles bearing coumarin moiety as potent antimicrobial and antioxidant agents. Bioorg. Med. Chem. Lett. 23:6406–6409.

38. Piyush NK, Shailesh PS, Dipak KR. (2014). Synthesis, identification and *in vitro* biological evaluation of some novel 5-imidazopyrazole incorporated pyrazoline and isoxazoline derivatives. New J. Chem. 38:2902–2910.

39. Parlow JJ. (1998). Synthesis of pyrazolecarbonylaminopyridinecarboxamides as herbicides. J. Heterocycl. Chem. 35:1493–1499.

40. Huang D, Huang M, Liu W *et al*. (2017). Design, synthesis and biological evaluation of 1H-pyrazole-5-carboxamide derivatives as potential fungicidal and insecticidal agents. Chem. Pap. 71:2053–2061.

41. Gao MC,Xu B. (2016). Transition metal-involving synthesis and utilization of N-containing heterocycles: Exploration of nitrogen sources. Chem. Rec. 16:1701–1714.

42. Teixeira FC, Ramos H, Antunes IF, Curto MJM, Teresa Duarte M, Bento I. (2006). Synthesis and structural characterization of 1-and 2-substituted indazoles: Ester and carboxylic acid derivatives. Molecules 11:867–889.

43. Qian S, Cao J,Yan Y *et al*. (2010). SMT-A07, a 3-(Indol-2-yl) indazole derivative, induces apoptosis of leukemia cells in vitro. Mol. Cell. Biochem. 345:13–21.

44. Li X, Chu S, Feher V A *et al.* (2003). Structure-based design, synthesis, and antimicrobial activity of indazole-derived SAH/MTA nucleosidase inhibitors. J. Med. Chem.46:5663–5673.
45. Han W, Pelletier JC, Hodge CN. (1998). Tricyclic ureas: A new class of HIV-1 protease inhibitors.Bioorg. Med. Chem. Lett.8:3615–3620.
46. Ikeda Y, Takano N, Matsushita H *et al.* (1979). Pharmacological studies on a new thymoleptic anti-depressant, 1-[3-(dimethylamino)propyl]-5-methyl-3-phenyl-1H-indazole (FS-32). Arzneim. Forsch.29:511–520.
47. Lee FY, Lien JC, Huang LJ *et al.* (2001). Synthesis of 1-benzyl-3-(50-hydroxymethyl-20-furyl)indazole analogues as novel antiplatelet agents. J. Med. Chem. 44:3747–3749.
48. Picciòla G, Ravenna F, Carenini G, Gentili P, Riva M. (1981). Heterocyclic compounds containing the residue of a 4-aminophenylalkanoic acid with potential anti-inflammatory activity. IV. Derivatives of 2-phenyl-2H-indazole.Farmaco Sci.36(12):1037–1056.
49. De Lena M, Lorusso V, Latorre A, Fanizza G, Gargano G, Caporusso L, Mazzei A. (2001). Paclitaxel, cisplatin and lonidamine in advanced ovarian cancer. A phase II study. *Eur. J. Cancer.* 37(3):364–368.
50. Corsi G, Palazzo G, Germani C, Barcellona PS, Silvestrini B. (1976). 1-Halobenzyl-1H-indazole-3-carboxylic acids. A new class of antispermatogenic agents. J. Med. Chem.19:778–783.
51. Clutterbuck LA, Posada CG, Visintin C *et al.* (2009). Oxadiazolylindazole sodium channel modulators are neuroprotective toward hippocampal neurons. J. Med. Chem. 52:2694–2707.
52. Zhang Y, Ma X, Chen Y*et al.* (2013). Synthesis and characterization of oxadisilole-fused 1-benzo[f]indazoles and 1-naphtho[2,3-f]indazoles. Eur. J. Org. Chem.2013:3005–3012.
53. Ullmann's Encyclopedia of Industrial Chemistry, seventh Ed. (2005). Wiley-VCH Verlag GmbH & Co. KGaA, Weinheim.
54. Mills AD, Maloney P, Hassanein E, Haddadin MJ, Kurth MJ. (2007). Synthesis of a library of 2-alkyl-3-alkyloxy-2H-indazole-6-carboxamides.J. Comb. Chem.9:171–177.
55. Catalan J, del Valle JC, Claramunt RM *et al.* (1994). Acidity and basicity of indazole and its N-methyl derivatives in the ground and in the excited state. J. Phys. Chem.98:10606–10610.
56. Matiadis D,Sagnou M. (2020). Pyrazoline hybrids as promising anticancer agents: An up-to- date over-view. Int. J. Mol. Sci.21:5507–5545
57. Appendino G, Jakupovic J, Varese M, Belloro E, Danieli B, Bombardelli E. (1996). Synthesis of 7,9-nitrogen-substituted paclitaxel derivatives. Tetrahedron Lett. 37:7837–7840.
58. Manna K, Agrawal YK. (2009). Microwave assisted synthesis of new indophenazine 1,3,5-trisubstruted pyrazoline derivatives of benzofuran and their antimicrobial activity. Bioorg. Med. Chem. Lett.19: 2688–2692.
59. Barsoum FF, Hosni HM,Girgis AS. (2006). Novel bis(1-acyl-2-pyrazolines) of potential anti-inflammatory and molluscicidal properties.Bioorg. Med. Chem. 14:3929–3937.
60. Havrylyuk D, Zimenkovsky B, Vasylenko O, Zaprutko L, Lesyk R. (2009). Synthesis of novel thiazolone-based compounds containing pyrazoline moiety and evaluation of their anticancer activity. Eur. J. Med. Chem. 44:1396–1404.
61. Abid M,Bhat AR, Athar V, Azam A. (2009). Synthesis, spectral studies and antiamoebic activity of new 1-*N*-substituted thiocarbamoyl-3-phenyl-2-pyrazolines.Eur. J. Med. Chem. 44:417–425.
62. Kaplancikli ZA, Turan-Zitouni G, Özdemir A, Can ÖD, Chevallet P. (2009). Synthesis and antinociceptive activities of some pyrazoline derivatives. Eur. J. Med. Chem. 44:2606–2610.
63. Gokhan-Kelekci N, Koyunoğlu S,Yabanoğlu S*et al.* (2009). New pyrazoline bearing 4(3*H*)-quinazolinone inhibitors of monoamine oxidase: Synthesis, biological evaluation, and structural determinants of MAO-A and MAO-B selectivity. Bioorg. Med. Chem. 17:675–689.
64. Babu VH, Manna SK, Surendran S, Srinivasan KK, Bhatt GV. (2004). Synthesis and biological evalu-ation of 1,3,5-trisubstituted pyrazolines bearing benzofuran. Ind. J. Het. Chem. 13:253–256.
65. Manna F, Chimenti F, Bolasco A *et al.* (2002). Inhibition of amine oxidases activity by 1-acetyl-3,5-diphenyl-4,5-dihydro-(1H)-pyrazole derivatives. Bioorg. Med. Chem. Lett. 12:3629–3633.
66. Jeong TS, KimK S, An SJ, Cho KH, Lee S, Lee WS. (2004). Novel 3,5-diaryl pyrazolines as human acyl-CoA: Cholesterol acyltransferase inhibitors. Bioorg. Med. Chem. Lett. 14:2715–2717.
67. Mallireddigari MR, Boominathan R, Gabriel JL, Reddy EP. (2008). Design, synthesis, and biological evaluation of 1-(4-sulfamylphenyl)-3-trifluoromethyl-5-indolyl pyrazolines as cyclooxygenase-2 (COX-2) and lipoxygenase (LOX) inhibitors. Bioorg. Med. Chem. 16:3907–3916.

68. Chimenti F, Fioravanti R, Bolasco A *et al*. (2008). Synthesis, molecular modeling studies and selective inhibitory activity against MAO of *N*1-propanoyl-3,5-diphenyl-4,5-dihydro-(1*H*)-pyrazole derivatives. Eur. J. Med. Chem. 43:2262–2267.

69. Hua S, Zhang S, Hua Y, Tao Q, Wu A. (2013). A new selective pyrazoline-based fluorescent chemosensor for Cu^{2+} in aqueous solution. Dyes Pigm. 96:509–515.

70. Kumar CK, Trivedi R, Giribabu L, Niveditha S, Bhanuprakash K, Sridhar B. (2015). Ferrocenyl pyrazoline based multichannel receptors for a simple and highly selective recognition of Hg^{2+} and Cu^{2+} ions. J. Organomet. Chem. 780:20–29.

71. Wang P, Onozawa-Komatsuzaki N, Himeda Y, Sugihara H, Arakawa H, Kasuga K. (2001). 3-(2-Pyridyl)-2-pyrazoline derivatives: novel fluorescent probes for Zn^{2+} ion. Tetrahedron Lett. 42:9199–9201.

72. Cherpak V, Stakhira P, Khomyak S *et al*. (2011). Properties of 2,6-di-tert.-butyl-4-(2,5-diphenyl-3,4-dihydro-2H-pyrazol-3-yl)-phenol as hole-transport material for life extension of organic light emitting diodes. Opt. Mater. 33:1727–1731.

73. Vandana T, Ramkumar V, Kannan P. (2016). Synthesis and fluorescent properties of poly(arylpyrazoline)'s for organic-electronics. Opt. Mater. 58:514–523.

74. Arbaciauskiene E, Kazlauskas K, Miasojedovas A *et al*. (2010). Multifunctional polyconjugated molecules with carbazolyl and pyrazolyl moieties for optoelectronic applications. Synth. Met. 160:490–498.

75. Ghomia JS, Kheirabadia MA, Alavia HS, Ziaratib A. (2016). Synthesis of methyl 6-amino-5-cyano-4-aryl-2,4-dihydropyrano[2,3-*c*]pyrazole-3-carboxylates using nano-$ZnZr_4(PO_4)_6$ as an efficient catalyst. Iranian J. Catalysis. 6(4):319–324.

76. Ghomi JS, Kheirabadi MA, Alavi HS. (2016). Environmentally benign synthesis of methyl-6-amino-5-cyano-4-aryl-2,4-dihydropyrano[2,3-*c*]pyrazole-3-carboxylates using CeO_2 nanoparticles as a reusable and robust catalyst. Z. Naturforsch. 71(11)b: 1135–1140.

77. Chen Y, Zhang Z, Jiang W, Zhang M, Li Y. (2019). RuIII@CMC/Fe_3O_4 hybrid: An efficient, magnetic, retrievable, self-organized nanocatalyst for green synthesis of pyranopyrazole and polyhydroquinoline derivatives. Mol. Divers. 23:421–442.

78. Aleem MAE, El-Remaily AA. (2014). Synthesis of pyranopyrazoles using magnetic Fe_3O_4 nanoparticles as efficient and reusable catalyst. Tetrahedron. 70:2971–2975.

79. Tabassum S, Devi KRS, Govindaraju S. (2020). An insight into the superior performance of ZnO@PEG nanocatalyst for the synthesis of 1,4-dihydropyrano[2,3-c]pyrazoles under ultrasound. Mater. Today: Proceedings. https://doi.org/10.1016/j.matpr.2020.06.283

80. Neysi M, Zarnegaryan A, Elhamifar D. (2019). Core–shell structured magnetic silica supported propylamine/molybdate complexes: an efficient and magnetically recoverable nanocatalyst. New J. Chem. 43:12283–12291.

81. Khamakani ZA, Afruzi FH, Maleki A. (2020). Magnetized dextrin: Eco-friendly effective nanocatalyst for the synthesis of dihydropyrano[2,3-c]pyrazole derivatives. Chem. Proc.

82. Hajizadeh Z, Maleki A. (2018). Poly(ethylene imine)-modified magnetic halloysite nanotubes: A novel, efficient and recyclable catalyst for the synthesis of dihydropyrano[2,3-c]pyrazole derivatives. Mol. Catal. 460:87–93.

83. Shahbazi S, Ghasemzadeh MA, Shakib P, Zolfaghari MR, Bahmani M. (2019). Synthesis and anti microbial study of 1,4-dihydropyrano[2,3-c]pyrazole derivatives in the presence of amino-functionalised silica coated cobalt oxide nanostructure as catalyst. Polyhedron. 170:172–179.

84. Sedighinia E, Badri R, Kiasat AR. (2019). Application of yttrium iron garnet as a powerful and recyclable nanocatalyst for one-pot synthesis of pyrano[2,3-c]pyrazole derivatives under solvent-free conditions. Russian J. Org. Chem. 55:1755–1763.

85. Mishra M, Nizam A, Jomon KJ, Tadaparthi K. (2019). New facile ultrasound-assisted magnetic nano-[$CoFe_2O_4$]-catalyzed one-pot synthesis of pyrano[2,3-*c*]pyrazoles. Russian J. Org. Chem. 55:1925–1928.

86. Dadaei M, Naeimi H. (2020). An environment-friendly method for green synthesis of pyranopyrazole derivatives catalyzed by $CoCuFe_2O_4$ magnetic nanocrystals under solvent-free conditions. Polycycl. Aromat. Compd. https://doi.org/10.1080/10406638.2020.1725897

87. Mohtasham NH, Gholizadeh M. (2020). Nano silica extracted from horsetail plant as a natural silica support for the synthesis of $H_3PW_{12}O_{40}$ immobilized on aminated magnetic nanoparticles (Fe_3O_4@SiO_2-EP-NH-HPA): A novel and efficient heterogeneous nanocatalyst for the green one-pot synthesis of pyrano[2,3-c]pyrazole derivatives. Res. Chem. Intermed. 46:3037–3066.

88. Azarifar A, Yami RN, Kobaisi MA, Azarifar D. (2013). Magnetic La$_{0.7}$Sr$_{0.3}$MnO$_3$ nanoparticles: Recyclable and efficient catalyst for ultrasound-accelarated synthesis of 4H-chromenes, and 4H-pyrano[2,3-c] pyrazoles. J. Iran Chem. Soc. 10:439–446.

89. Abbasabadi MK, Azarifar D, Zand HRE. (2020). Sulfonic acid-functionalized Fe$_3$O$_4$-supported magnetized graphene oxide quantum dots: A novel organic-inorganic nanocomposite as an efficient and recyclable nanocatalyst for the synthesis of dihydropyrano[2,3-*c*]pyrazole and 4*H*-chromene derivatives. *Appl. Organomet. Chem.* 34:6004–6005.

90. Azarifar D, Khatami SM, Zolfigol MA, Yami RN. (2014). Nano-titania sulfuric acid-promoted synthesis of tetrahydrobenzo[b]pyran and 1,4-dihydropyrano[2,3-c]pyrazole derivatives under ultrasound irradiation. J. Iran Chem. Soc. 11:1223–1230.

91. Azarifar D, Abbasi Y. (2016). Sulfonic acid-functionalized magnetic Fe$_{3-x}$Ti$_x$O$_4$ nanoparticles: New recyclable heterogeneous catalyst for one-pot synthesis of tetrahydrobenzo[b]pyrans and dihydropyrano[2,3-c]pyrazole derivatives. *Synth.* Commun. 46:745–758.

92. Azarifar D, Badalkhani O, Abbasi Y. (2018). Amino acid ionic liquid-based titanomagnetite nanoparticles: An efficient and green nanocatalyst for the synthesis of 1,4-dihydropyrano[2,3-c] pyrazoles. Appl. Organometal. Chem. 32:3949–3950.

93. Azarifar D, Abbasabadi MK. (2019). Fe$_3$O$_4$-supported *N*-pyridin-4-amine-grafted grapheme oxide as efficient and magnetically separable novel nanocatalyst for green synthesis of 4*H*-chromenes and dihydropyrano[2,3-*c*]pyrazole derivatives in water. Res. Chem. Intermed. 45:199–222.

94. Gholtash JE, Farahi M. (2018). Tungstic acid-functionalized Fe$_3$O$_4$@TiO$_2$:preparation, characterization and its application for the synthesis of pyrano[2,3-c]pyrazole derivatives as a reusable magnetic nanocatalyst. *RSC Adv.* 8:40962–40967.

95. Maleki B, Eshghi H, Barghamadi M, Nasiri N, Khojastehnezhad A, Ashrafi SS, Pourshiani O. (2016). Silica-coated magnetic NiFe$_2$O$_4$ nanoparticles supported H$_3$PW$_{12}$O$_{40}$; synthesis, preparation, and application as an efficient, magnetic, green catalyst for one-pot synthesis of tetrahydrobenzo[b]pyran and pyrano[2,3-c]pyrazole derivatives. Res. Chem. Intermed. 42:3071–3093.

96. Rakhtshah J, Salehzadeh S, Gowdini E, Maleki F, Baghery S, Zolfigol MA. (2016). Synthesis of pyrazole derivatives in the presence of dioxomolybdenum complex supported on silica-coated magnetite nanoparticles as an efficient and easily recyclable catalyst. RSC Adv.6:104875–104885.

97. Arora P, Rajput JK. (2017). One-pot multicomponent click synthesis of pyrazole derivatives using cyclodextrin-supported capsaicin nanoparticles as catalyst. *J.* Mater. Sci. 52:11413–11427.

98. Esfandiary N, Nakisa A, Azizi K, Azarnia J, Radfar I, Heydari A. (2017). Glucose-coated superparamagnetic nanoparticle-catalysed pyrazole synthesis in water. Appl. Organomet. Chem. 31:3641–3642.

99. Amirnejat S, Nosrati A, Javanshir S. (2020). Superparamagnetic Fe$_3$O$_4$@Alginate supported L-arginine as a powerful hybrid inorganic–organic nanocatalyst for the one-pot synthesis of pyrazole derivatives. Appl. Organomet. Chem.34:5888–5889.

100. Nasab MJ, Kiasat AR, Zarasvandi R. (2018). β-Cyclodextrin nanosponge polymer: A basic and eco-friendly heterogeneous catalyst for the one-pot four-component synthesis of pyranopyrazole derivatives under solvent-free conditions. React. Kinet. Mech.124:767–778.

101. Salehi N, Mirjalili BBF. (2018). Green synthesis of pyrano[2,3-*c*]pyrazoles and spiro[indoline-3,4'-pyrano[2,3-*c*]pyrazoles] using nano-silica supported 1,4-diazabicyclo[2.2.2]octane as a novel catalyst.Org. Prep. Proced. Int. 50:578–587.

102. Ghasemzadeh MA, Eshkevari BM, Basir MHA. (2019). Green synthesis of spiro[indoline-3,4'-pyrano[2,3-c]pyrazoles] using Fe$_3$O$_4$@-L-arginine as a robust and reusable catalyst. BMC Chem. 13:119.

103. Akbarzadeh P, Koukabi N. (2020). Magnetic carbon nanotube as a highly stable support for the heterogenization of InCl$_3$ and its application in the synthesis of isochromeno[4,3-*c*]pyrazole-5(1*H*)-one derivatives. Appl. Organomet. Chem. 34:5746–5747.

104. Ghomi JS, Ebrahimi SM. (2020). Nano-Fe$_3$O$_4$-cysteine as a superior catalyst for the synthesis of indeno[1,2-c]pyrazol-4(1H)-ones. Polycycl. Aromat. Compd.https://doi.org/10.1080/10406638.2020.1852276

105. Sadjadi S, Heravi MM, Daraie M. (2017). Heteropolyacid supported on amine-functionalized halloysite nano clay as an efficient catalyst for the synthesis of pyrazolopyranopyrimidines via four-component domino reaction. Res. Chem. Intermed. 43:2201–2214.

106. Dastkhoon S, Tavakoli Z, Khodabakhshi S, Baghernehad M, Abbasabadi MK. (2015). Nanocatalytic one-pot, four-component synthesis of some new triheterocyclic compounds consisting of pyrazole, pyran, and pyrimidinone rings. New J. Chem. 39:7268–7271.

107. Keshavarz M, Ahmady AZ, Vaccaro L, Kardani M. (2018). Non-covalent supported of l-proline on graphene oxide/Fe_3O_4 nanocomposite: A novel, highly efficient and superparamagnetically separable catalyst for the synthesis of bis-pyrazole derivatives. Molecules. 23:330–346.

108. Safari J, Ahmadzadeh M. (2017). Zwitterionic sulfamic acid functionalized nanoclay: A novel nanocatalyst for the synthesis of dihydropyrano[2,3-c]pyrazoles and spiro[indoline-3,4´-pyrano[2,3-c]pyrazole] derivatives. J. Taiwan Inst. Chem. Eng.74:14–24.

109. Verma D, Sharma V, Okram GS, Jain S. (2017). High-yield multicomponent synthesis of triazolo[1,2-a] indazoletriones using silica-coated ZnO nanoparticles as heterogeneous catalyst in the presence of ultrasound. Green Chem.19:5885–5899.

110. Hamidian H, Fozooni S, Hassankhani A, Mohammadi SZ. (2011). One-pot and efficient synthesis of triazolo[1,2-a]indazoletriones via reaction of arylaldehydes with urazole and dimedone catalyzed by silica nanoparticles prepared from rice husk. Molecules. 16:9042–9048.

111. Sadeghzadeh SM. (2016). A multicomponent reaction on a 'free' KCC-1 catalyst at room temperature under solvent free conditions by visible light. RSC Adv.6:54236–54240.

112. Zahedi N, Javid A, Mohammadi MK, Tavakkoli H. (2018). Microwave-promoted solvent free one-pot synthesis of triazolo[1,2-a] indazole-triones catalyzed by silica-supported $La_{0.5}Ca_{0.5}CrO_3$ nanoparticles as a new and reusable perovskitetype oxide. Bull. Chem. Soc. Ethiop. 32(2):239–248.

113. Chari MA, Karthikeyan G, Pandurangan A, Naidu TS, Sathyaseelan B, Javaid Zaidi SM, Vinu A. (2010). Synthesis of triazolo indazolones using 3D mesoporous aluminosilicate catalyst with nanocage structure. Tetrahedron Lett. 51:2629–2632.

114. Ardakani HA, Rakati TH. (2015). $HClO_4$-SiO_2 Nanoparticles as an efficient catalyst for three-component synthesis of triazolo[1,2-a]indazole-triones. Int. J. Chem. Nuclear Mater. Metallurgical Eng. 9:1–4.

115. Sadeghzadeh SM. (2014). Quinuclidine stabilized on $FENI_3$ nanoparticles as catalysts for efficient, green, and one-pot synthesis of triazolo[1,2-a]indazole-triones. Chem. Plus. Chem. 79:278–283.

116. Akbari M, Javid A, Moeinpour F. (2017). One-pot synthesis of triazolo[1,2-a]indazole-triones catalyzed by a novel magnetically and reusable green catalyst of Preyssler. Int. J. Heterocycl. Chem. 7(2):1–6.

117. Maheswari CS, Shanmugapriya C, Revathy K, Lalitha A. (2017). SnO_2 nanoparticles as an efficient heterogeneous catalyst for the synthesis of 2H-indazolo[2,1-b]phthalazine-triones. J. Nanostruct. Chem.7:283–291.

118. Rostami A, Tahmasbi B, Yari A. (2013). Magnetic nanoparticle immobilized n-propylsulfamic acid as a recyclable and efficient nanocatalyst for the synthesis of 2*H*-indazolo[2,1-b]phthalazine-triones in solvent-free conditions: comparison with sulfamic acid. Bull. Korean Chem. Soc. 34(5):1521–1524.

119. Veisi H, Sedrpoushan A, Faraji AR, Heydari M, Hemmatia S, Fatahia B. (2015). A mesoporous SBA-15 silica catalyst functionalized with phenylsulfonic acid groups (SBA-15-Ph-SO_3H) as a novel hydrophobic nanoreactor solid acid catalyst for a one-pot three-component synthesis of 2H-indazolo[2,1-b] phthalazine-triones and triazolo[1,2-a]indazole-triones. RSC Adv. 5:68523–68530.

120. Atashkar B,Rostami A, Gholami H, Tahmasbi B. (2015). Magnetic nanoparticles Fe_3O_4-supported guanidine as an efficient nanocatalyst for the synthesis of 2H-indazolo[2,1-b]phthalazine-triones under solvent-free conditions. Res. Chem. Intermed. 41:3675–3681.

121. Kiasat AR, Noorizadeh S, Ghahremani M, Saghanejad SJ. (2013). Experimental and theoretical study on one-pot, three-component route to 2H-indazolo[2,1-b]phthalazine-triones catalyzed by nano-alumina sulfuric acid. J. Mol. Struct. 1036:216–225.

122. Chegeni MMF, Bamoniri A, Mirjalili BBF. (2020). A versatile protocol for synthesis of 2*h*-indazolo[2,1-*b*]phthalazine triones using γ-Al_2O_3/BF_n/Fe_3O_4 as an efficient magnetic nano-catalyst. Polycycl. Aromat. Compd.https://doi.org/10.1080/10406638.2020.1735457

123. Zhao X, Hu G, Tang M, Shi T, Guo X, Li T, Zhang Z. (2014). A highly efficient and recyclable cobalt ferrite chitosan sulfonic acid magnetic nanoparticle for one-pot, four-component synthesis of 2H-indazolo[2,1-b]phthalazine-triones. RSC Adv. 4:51089–51097.

124. Shaterian HR, Mollashahi E, Biabangard A. (2013). ZnO-nanoparticles: Efficient and reusable heterogeneous catalyst for one-pot, four-component synthesis of 2h-indazolo(2,1-b) phthalazine-triones. J. Chem. Soc. Pak. 35(2):330–333.

125. Esmaeilpour M, Javidi J, Dehghani F. (2016). Preparation, characterization and catalytic activity of dendrimer-encapsulated phosphotungstic acid nanoparticles immobilized on nanosilica for the synthesis of 2*H*-indazolo[2,1-*b*] phthalazine-triones under solvent-free or sonochemical conditions. J. Iran Chem. Soc. 13:695–714.

126. Esmaeilpour M, Javidi J, Dodeji FN, Zahmatkesh S. (2016). Solvent-free, sonochemical, one-pot, four-component synthesis of 2H-indazolo[2,1-b]phthalazine-triones and 1H-pyrazolo[1,2-b]phthalazine-diones catalyzed by Fe_3O_4@SiO_2-imid-PMA^n magnetic nanoparticles. Res. Chem. Intermed. https://doi.org/10.1007/s11164-016-2462-6

127. Khatun N, Gogoi A, Basu P, Das P, Patel BK. (2014). CuO nanoparticle catalysed synthesis of 2H-indazoles under ligand free conditions. RSC Adv. 4:4080–4084.

128. Sodhi RK, Changotra A, Paul S. (2014). Metal acetylacetonates covalently anchored onto amine functionalized silica/starch composite for the one-pot thioetherification and synthesis of 2H-indazoles. Catal. Lett. 144:1819–1831.

129. Taherinia Z, Choghamarani AG, Hajjami M. (2019). Decorated peptide nanofibers with cu nanoparticles: An efficient catalyst for the multicomponent synthesis of chromeno [2,3-*d*] pyrimidin-8-amines, quinazolines and 2H-indazoles. ChemistrySelect. 4:2753–2760.

130. Verma S, Kujur S, Agrahari B, Layek S, Pathak DD. (2019). Synthesis and characterization of cucurbit[6]uril supported copper oxide nanoparticles, Cuo@cb[6]: application as nanocatalyst for the synthesis of 2*H*-indazoles. ChemistrySelect. 4:10408–10416.

131. Khalifeh R, Karimzadeh F. (2019). Copper nanoparticles supported on charcoal mediated one-pot three-component synthesis of N-substituted-2*H*-indazoles via consecutive condensation C-N and N-N bond formation. Canadian J. Chem. 97:1–23.

132. Sharghi H, Aberi M, Shiri P. (2019). Silica-supported Cu(II)–quinoline complex: Efficient and recyclable nanocatalyst for one-pot synthesis of benzimidazolquinoline derivatives and 2*H*-indazoles. Appl. Organometal. Chem. 33:4974–4975.

133. Esfandiary N, Heydari A. (2020). Fe_2O_3@[proline]–CuMgAl–LDH: A magnetic bifunctional copper and organocatalyst system for one-pot synthesis of quinolines and 2*H*-indazoles in green media. Appl. Organometal. Chem. 34:5760–5761.

134. Rad MNS. (2017). Ultrasound promoted mild and facile one-pot, three component synthesis of 2H-indazoles by consecutive condensation, CAN and NAN bond formations catalysed by copper-doped silica cuprous sulphate (CDSCS) as an efficient heterogeneous nano-catalyst. Ultrason. Sonochem. 34:865–872.

135. Behrouz S. (2017). Highly efficient one-pot three component synthesis of 2H-indazoles by consecutive condensation, C–N and N–N bond formations using cu/aminoclay/reduced graphene oxide nanohybrid. J. Heterocycl. Chem. 54:1863–1871.

136. Ghasemzadeh MA, Molaei B, Abdollahi-Basir MH, Zamani F. (2017). Preparation and catalytic study on a novel amino-functionalized silica-coated cobalt oxide nanocomposite for the synthesis of some indazoles. Acta Chim. Slov. 64:73–82.

137. Selvam K, Krishnakumar B, Velmurugan R, Swaminathan M. (2009). A simple one pot nano titania mediated green synthesis of 2-alkylbenzimidazoles and indazole from aromatic azides under UV and solar light. Catal. Commun. 11:280–284.

138. Selvam K, Balachandran S, Velmurugan R, Swaminathan M. (2012). Mesoporous nitrogen doped nano titania-A green photocatalyst for the effective reductive cleavage of azoxybenzenes to amines or 2-phenyl indazoles in methanol. Appl. Catal. A Gen. 413:213–222.

139. Esfahani MN, Daghaghale M, Taei M. (2017). Catalytic synthesis of chalcones and pyrazolines using nanorod vanadatesulfuric acid: An efficient and reusable catalyst. J. Chin. Chem. Soc. 64:17–24.

140. Gharib A, Pesyan NN, Fard LV, Roshani M. (2015). Catalytical synthesis of pyrazolines using nanoparticles of preyssler heteropolyacid supported on nano-SiO_2, $H_{14}[NaP_5W_{30}O_{110}]$/$SiO_2$: A green and reusable catalyst. American J. Heterocycl. Chem. 1(1):6–12.

141. Aliyan H, Fazaelia R, Tajsaeeda N. (2013). γ-Fe_2O_3@SiO_2-PW_{12} nanoparticles: Highly efficient catalysts for the synthesis of pyrazoline derivatives. Iranian J. Catal. 3(2):99–105.

142. Fazaeli R, Aliyan H, Tangestaninejad S, Mohammadi E, Bordbar M. (2012). Nanocasting, template synthesis, and structural studies on cesium salt of phosphotungstic acid for the synthesis of novel 1,3,5-triaryl-pyrazoline derivatives. Chinese J. Catal. 33:237–246

143. Dandia A, Parewa V, Gupta SL, Rathore KS. (2013). Cobalt doped ZnS nanoparticles as a recyclable catalyst for solvent-free synthesis of heterocyclic privileged medicinal scaffolds under infrared irradiation. J. Mol. Catal. A Chem. 373:61–71.

144. Shamsuzzaman, Mashrai A, Khanam H, Aljawfi RN. (2017). Biological synthesis of ZnO nanoparticles using C. albicans and studying their catalytic performance in the synthesis of steroidal pyrazolines. Arabian J. Chem. 10:S1530–S1536.

145. Khan FN, Manivel P, Prabakaran K, Sung Jin J, Jeong ED, Kim HG, Maiyalagan T. (2012). Iron-oxide nanoparticles mediated cyclization of 3-(4-chlorophenyl)-1-hydrazinylisoquinoline to 1-(4,5-dihydropyrazol-1-yl)isoquinolines. Res. Chem. Intermed. 38:571–582.

146. Siddiqui S, Siddiqui ZN. (2018). Strontium doped MCM-41: A highly efficient, recyclable and heterogeneous catalyst for the synthesis of phenoxy pyrazolyl pyrazolines. Catal. Lett. 148:3628–3645.

147. Shaterian HR, Moradi F. (2015). Preparation of 7-amino-1,3-dioxo-1,2,3,5-tetrahydropyrazolo [1,2-a] [1,2,4]triazole using magnetic Fe_3O_4 nanoparticles coated by (3-aminopropyl)-triethoxysilane as catalyst. Res. Chem. Intermed. 41:223–229.

148. Naeimi H, Rashid Z, Zarnani AH, Ghahremanzadeh R. (2014). Nanocrystalline magnesium oxide: an efficient promoter and heterogeneous nano catalyst for the one-pot synthesis of pyrazolotriazoles in green medium. J. Nanopart. Res. 16:2416.

149. Maleki B, Nejat R, Alinezhad H, Mousavi SM, Mahdavi B, Delavari M. (2020). Nanostructural Cu-doped ZnO hollow spheres as an economical and recyclable catalyst in the synthesis of 1*H*-pyrazolo[1,2-*b*]phthalazine-5,10-diones and pyrazolo[1,2-*a*][1,2,4]triazole-1,3-diones. Org. Prep. Proced. Int. 52(4):328–339.

150. Khalili A, Esfahani MN, Baltork IM, Tangestaninejad S, Mirkhani V, Moghadam M. (2018). Synthesis and characterization of 4-methyl-1-(3-sulfopropyl)pyridinium hydrogen sulfate as a new ionic liquid immobilized on silica nanoparticles: A recyclable nanocomposite ionic liquid for the production of various substituted phthalazine-ones. J. Mol Liq. 253:1–10.

151. Azarifar A, Yami RN, Azarifar D. (2013). Nano-ZnO: An efficient and reusable catalyst for one-pot synthesis of 1H-pyrazolo[1,2-b]phthalazine-5,10-diones and pyrazolo[1,2-a][1,2,4]triazole-1,3-diones. J. Iran Chem. Soc. 10:297–306.

152. Maleki B, Chalaki SBN, Ashrafi SS, Seresht ER, Moeinpour F, Khojastehnezhad A, Tayebee R. (2015). Caesium carbonate supported on hydroxyapatite-encapsulated $Ni_{0.5}Zn_{0.5}Fe_2O_4$ nanocrystallites as a novel magnetically basic catalyst for the one-pot synthesis of pyrazolo[1,2-b]phthalazine-5,10-diones. Appl. Organometal. Chem. 29:290–295.

153. Arora P, Rajput JK. (2018). Amelioration of $H_4[W_{12}SiO_{40}]$ by nanomagnetic heterogenization: For the synthesis of 1H–pyrazolo[1,2-b] phthalazinedione derivatives. Appl. Organometal. Chem. 32:4001–4002.

Index

Note: Page numbers in *italic* denote figures and in **bold** denote tables.

For Product Safety Concerns and Information please contact our EU
representative GPSR@taylorandfrancis.com
Taylor & Francis Verlag GmbH, Kaufingerstraße 24, 80331 München, Germany